OPIOID DEPENDENCE

Mechanisms and Treatment

OPIOID DEPENDENCE

Mechanisms and Treatment

Abraham ⸜Wikler, M. D.

Emeritus Professor of Psychiatry and Pharmacology
Department of Psychiatry
University of Kentucky Medical Center
Lexington, Kentucky

Plenum Press · New York and London

Library of Congress Cataloging in Publication Data

Wikler, Abraham, 1910-
  Opioid dependence.

  Includes index.
  1. Opioid habit. I. Title.
RC568.O58W54   616.86'3   80-21678
ISBN-13: 978-1-4684-3868-0   e-ISBN-13: 978-1-4684-3866-6
DOI: 10.1007/978-1-4684-3866-6

To my wife

Preface

A major problem in the treatment of opioid dependence has been the persistence of relapse despite detoxification and enforced prolonged abstention from drug use, with or without conventional psychotherapy and other efforts at rehabilitation. Both initial addiction and subsequent relapses are usually ascribed to the quest for opioid-produced *euphoria* in persons with character disorders. This formulation is in accord with one-half of the common sense "pleasure–pain" principle, but it ignores the other half, namely, the long-lasting *dysphoric* consequences of repeated opioid use (distressing abstinence phenomena, sexual disturbances, disruption of marital status, unemployment, enmeshment in criminal activities, arrests, and imprisonment). In any case, the pleasure–pain principle is an empty tautology since it is incapable of refutation by any conceivable objective data that might seem contradictory, inasmuch as it can be "saved" by invocation of untestable unconscious intervening variables.

Less tied to the pleasure–pain principle is the view that relapse is due to long-lasting sequelae of previous opioid addiction, resulting from complex conditioning processes, both operant and classical, involving pharmacological, environmental, social and personal variables. In this view, relapse is not simply a re-enactment of initial opioid use, but is a "disease, *sui generis*" a disease of its own kind. The factors contributing to this disease, *sui generis* are reviewed in this book. Among them are the far-reaching alterations of homeostasis produced by single doses of opioids ("antiprotective" actions, of which relief of pain is one facet), the counteradaptive responses of the central nervous system to such effects (which have been shown by use of narcotic antagonists to begin after one or a few repeated doses of morphine), the consequent development of tolerance and physical dependence (characterized not only by the easily recognized "early" abstinence syndrome but also by the more subtle, long-lasting "protracted" abstinence syndrome), the possible role of endogenous opioid peptides in all of these processes, and the operant conditioning of opioid-acquisitive behavior as well as the classical conditioning of the opioid agonist-abstinence cycle. While the persistence of such classically conditioned responses in detoxified "street addicts" can be detected by sophisticated techniques under experimental conditions (O'Brien, Greenstein, Ternes, McLellan, & Grabowski, 1979), extinction of the conditioned autonomic responses that are part of the disease, *sui generis* is more difficult to carry out. In the opinion of the author of this book, the elimination of the disease, *sui generis* is essential for the optimal prevention of relapse, in addition to therapies directed at the presumed causes of initial opioid use. How far this central theme applies to non-opioid drug dependencies (which are described very briefly in the opening chapter) is unknown at present; new techniques will have to be developed for detection of long-lasting consequences of such drug use and the conditioning processes that inevitably accompany them in man (Wikler, 1971; Ludwig, Wikler, & Stark, 1974).

The author is solely responsible for the interpretations of the data reviewed in this book. The names of the persons who have contributed importantly to elucidation of the long-term sequelae of drug dependence are too numerous to list here, but because of close association with them for many years in Lexington, Kentucky, the author's former colleagues at the NIDA Addiction Research Center (including Drs. Harris Isbell, Havelock F. Fraser, Harris E. Hill, Donald R. Jasinski and Charles W. Gorodetzky) and his present colleagues at the University of · Kentucky Medical Center (Drs. William R. Martin, Arnold M. Ludwig, John A. Dougherty and Dianne B. Miller) should be mentioned. To them the author expresses his indebtedness, not only for important research findings but also for stimulating discussions. Thanks are also due to the National Institute on Drug Abuse for its highly informative Research Monographs and to the editors of Plenum Publishing Corporation for their helpful cooperation.

A. WIKLER, M.D.
Emeritus Professor of
Psychiatry and Pharmacology

Albert B. Chandler
Medical Center
University of Kentucky
Lexington, Kentucky

REFERENCES

Ludwig, A. M., Wikler, A. and Stark, L. H., 1974, The first drink. Psychobiological aspects of craving, *Arch. Gen. Psychiat. 30:* 539–547.

O'Brien, C. P., Greenstein, R., Ternes, J., McLellan, A. T. and Grabowski, J., 1979, Unreinforced self-injections: Effects on rituals and outcome in heroin addicts in *Problems of drug dependence, 1979* (L. S. Harris, ed.), Proceedings of the 41st Annual Scientific Meeting of the Committee on Problems of Drug Dependence, Inc., Philadelphia, June 4–6, 1979, NIDA Research Monogr. 27, pp. 275–281. Superintendent of Documents, U.S. Government Printing Office, Washington, D.C.

Wikler, A., 1971, Some implications of conditioning theory for problems of drug abuse, *Behav. Sci. 16:* 92–97.

Contents

1   The Problems of Opioid and Other Drug Dependencies   1

Prevalence and Complications   1
Nonopioid Drug-Dependence Syndromes   5
    Barbiturate, Nonbarbiturate Sedative, and "Minor Tranquilizer"
        Dependence   5
    Alcohol Dependence   9
    Amphetamine Dependence   11
    Cocaine Dependence   12
    Hallucinogen Dependence   14
    Cannabis (Marijuana, Hashish) Dependence   16
    Tobacco Dependence   18
References   20

2   The Etiology of Opioid Dependence   25

Definitions and Dynamics   25
Personality Studies   30
Socioenvironmental Studies   31
Mode of Spread of Opioid Dependence   32
Prognosis   33
References   34

3   Opioid Analgesics and Opioid Antagonists   37

Opioid Analgesics   37
   Morphine   38
      Effects of Single Doses in the Nontolerant State   38
      Tolerance and Physical Dependence   45
   Heroin   48
   Methadone   48
   Meperidine   49
   Codeine   50
   d-Propoxyphene   50
   Pentazocine   51
Opioid Antagonists   51
   Nalorphine   53
      Effects of Single Doses in the Drug-Free State   53
      Tolerance and Physical Dependence   54
      Opioid-Antagonistic and Opioid-Blocking Actions in the
         Nontolerant State   55
      Opioid-Antagonistic and Opioid-Blocking Actions in the Tolerant
         State   55
   Cyclazocine   57
   Naloxone and Naltrexone   59
References   61

4   Opioid Receptors and Endogenous Opioid Peptides   69

Opioid Receptors   69
Endogenous Opioid Peptides (Enkephalins and Endorphins)   76
Possible Functions of Enkephalins and Endorphins   79
   Analgesia   79
   Physical Dependence   84
   Mental Disorders   86
References   90

5   Mechanisms of Opioid Analgesia   95

The Nature of Pain and Its Relief by Morphine   95
Sites of Morphine's Antinociceptive Actions in the Central Nervous Sys-
      tem   107
   Spinal Cord   107

Brain Stem   114
Cerebral Cortex   131
References   132

6   **Theories of Tolerance to and Physical Dependence on**
      Opioids   141

General Theories of Tolerance to and Physical Dependence on
      Morphine   142
   Homeostatic Counteradaptation   142
   Cellular Counteradaptation   143
   Dual Action   143
Theories of the Mechanisms of Counteradaptation to the Agonistic Ef-
      fects of Drugs   145
   Disuse Supersensitivity   145
   Pharmacological Redundancy   147
   New Receptors   150
   Enzyme Expansion   157
   Immune Mechanisms   158
   Learning Factors   159
References   162

7   **Conditioning Processes in Opioid Dependence and in**
      Relapse   167

Operant Conditioning of Opioid-Acquisitive Behavior   171
Classical Conditioning of the Opioid Agonist-Abstinence Cycle and In-
      teroceptive Conditioning of Opioid-Seeking Behavior   178
Classical Conditioning of the Opioid-Antagonist–Precipitated Opioid-
      Abstinence Syndrome   207
Occurrence of Classically Conditioned Responses in Street Addicts   211
Implications of Conditioning Factors for Relapse and Treatment   213
References   215

8   **Diagnosis and Treatment of Opioid Dependence   219**

Diagnosis   219
   Physical Dependence   219
   Opioid Use   221

Treatment   222
  Opioid Poisoning   222
  Opioid Dependence   224
    Detoxification   224
    Detoxification Followed by Narcotic-Antagonist Maintenance   227
    Methadone Maintenance (with or without Eventual Detoxifica-
        tion)   234
    Levomethadyl Maintenance   241
References   244

Index   249

The Problems of Opioid and Other Drug Dependencies

Abuse of and dependencies on drugs of all sorts (notably alcohol, cannabis, sedatives, stimulants, and tobacco), though varying in kind and in degree, are worldwide. For a sampling of drug problems through the world, the reader is referred to Peterson (1978) and to Austin *et al.* (1978). This chapter is concerned with problems of opioid and other drug dependencies in the United States.

PREVALENCE AND COMPLICATIONS

Estimates of the prevalence of opioid dependence in the United States have been based on various sources, changing considerably over the years. These include police and prison records and the registers maintained by treatment clinics, hospitals, and some municipal health departments. Terry and Pellens (1928) estimated very roughly that the total number of opioid addicts in the period 1915–1920 was 200,000. Ball and Chambers (1970) calculated that in 1967 the number was 108,424. In 1927, the number had risen to approximately 300,000 (Center for New York City Affairs of the New School for Social Research, City Almanac, 1972). Current estimates are about 500,000 (DuPont, 1978). In estimating prevalence *rates*, the growth of the total population of the United States should be borne in mind. In 1920, the total population (all ages, both sexes) was 105,710,620; in 1970, it was 203,211,926; and in the beginning of 1978, it was estimated at 217,700,000 (World Almanac and Book of

1

Facts, 1979). Therefore, the prevalence rate in 1920 was 0.19%; if the 1970 population is used for both years, the prevalence rate in 1967 was 0.05%, and in 1972, it was 0.15%; in 1978, it was estimated at 0.23%. Apparently the prevalence rate increased three-fold between 1967 and 1972 and four-fold between 1967 and 1978. The sudden upsurge in the prevalence rate of opioid dependence between 1967 and 1972 coincided with the emergence of a youthful "counterculture" oriented toward the use of so-called soft drugs (marijuana, barbiturates, certain nonbarbiturate sedative–hypnotics, and more recently, phencyclidine). Whether or not there is any causal relationship between opioid dependence and abuse of "soft" drugs is problematic. In particular, the hypothesized relationship between previous marijuana and subsequent heroin use has been much debated (Wikler, 1974). Grinspoon (1971) ridiculed this hypothesis, pointing out that all cannabis or heroin users had previously drunk milk, eaten food, read comic books, etc., yet no one would maintain that these activities led to the use of cannabis or heroin. Such criticism is invalid, since an activity that is universal (e.g., drinking milk or eating food) cannot be tested for a statistically significant relationship with other variables that are not universal (e.g., using cannabis or heroin). What is needed is a chi-square analysis of the relationship between marijuana and heroin use, such as was applied by Pillard (1971) to marijuana and LSD ($p < 0.001$) and to marijuana and alcohol, an almost universally distributed variable (NS). In England, Paton (1968) reported a parallel increase in the number of cannabis offenses and the number of heroin addicts, and in Egypt, Soueif (1971) found a positive relationship between years of hashish consumption and the percentage of opium taken among hashish users.

   Pillard (1970) stated that no one has failed to find a statistical relationship between marijuana and the use of other drugs, legal and illegal. The widespread abuse of marijuana and other drugs, both "soft" and "hard," among contemporary youth is well illustrated by the results of national surveys made by O'Donnell et al. (1976) and Abelson et al. (1977), analyzed by Parry (1979). The data presented by Parry are from the 1977 National Survey of Drug Abuse (Abelson et al., 1977). For each drug class, the *percentage* of the random sample of young adults (18–25 years of age) who stated they "ever used" is given and, in parentheses, the *percentage* who stated they "used past month." After each percentage ("ever used" and "used past month"), an estimate is made of the total number of users, based on a projected population of 18- to 24-year-olds in the United States for 1975 of 27,535,000 or roughly 28,000,000 (Kurtz, 1969): *marijuana and/or hashish*, 60%, 16,800,000 (28%, 7,840,000); *hallucinogens*, 20%, 5,600,000 (2%, 560,000): *cocaine*, 19%,

5,320,000 (4%, 1,120,000); *heroin,* 4%, 1,120,000 (less than 0.5%, less than 140,000); *other opioids,* 13%, 3,640,000 (1%, 280,000); *stimulants,* 21%, 5,880,000 (2%, 560,000); *sedatives,* 18%, 5,040,000 (3%, 840,000); *tranquilizers,* 13%, 3,640,000 (2%, 560,000); *alcohol,* 84%, 23,520,000 (70%, 19,600,000); *cigarettes,* 68%, 19,040,000 (47%, 13,160,000). Figures for all drugs were lower but still substantial in the youth group 12–17 years of age. In older adults, aged 26 or older, the figures for all drugs except alcohol and cigarettes dropped sharply; for example, for marijuana, the percentage of the sample that stated they had "ever used" was 15% and the "used past month" category was 3%. On the other hand, Parry (1979) noted that the 14% of the youth group (aged 12–17 years) who in 1972 had tried marijuana had doubled by 1977, and that the 7% of the same group who were "current" users in 1972 had also doubled in 1977; he concluded that marijuana experience seems to "take off" after age 13, peaks at ages 22–25, drops sharply among the 26- to 34-year-olds, and almost disappears among those aged 35 and older. In a nationwide survey of the use of drugs by men aged 20–30, O'Donnell *et al.* (1976) found prevalences for drug classes that were similar to those of the 1977 National Survey of Drug Abuse (Abelson *et al.,* 1977), discussed above. For each drug class, the percentage of random sample stating "lifetime use" is followed (in parentheses) by the percentage stating "current use": *marijuana,* 55% (26%); *hallucinogens,* 22% (2%); *cocaine,* 14% (2%); *heroin,* 6% (1%); *other opioids,* 31% (2%); *stimulants,* 27% (5%); *sedatives,* 20% (3%); *alcohol,* 97% (85%); *cigarettes,* 88% (55%). These finds were quite similar to the percentages in 1975 high school male seniors, except that the 20- to 30-year-olds reported significantly higher lifetime prevalence rates for cocaine, heroin, and other opioid drugs.

An indication of current attempts to deal with this huge drug problem is afforded by DuPont's (1978) statement that there are about 250,000 people receiving drug treatment in over 3000 clinics and drug abuse programs in the United States. Nearly 40% of this large drug-abuse treatment capacity is funded by the federal government, and approximately 65% of the patients admitted to such federally funded programs are treated for heroin dependence; after heroin, the most often reported drug problems on admission are marijuana, barbiturates, and amphetamines, while cocaine, LSD, phencyclidine, and volatile solvents are reported less often. Though in comparison with the use of other drugs (marijuana, hallucinogens, cocaine and other stimulants, sedatives and tranquilizers, alcohol, and cigarettes) the prevalence of "used past month" or "current use" of heroin and other opioids is relatively low (see above), it is striking that heroin abusers preponderate in federally funded treatment programs and that the cost to the nation of heroin abuse is estimated at $6 billion a year by DuPont (1978). No estimates are available of the costs to the nation of the abuse of nonopioid drugs.

The complications of the nonmedical use of marijuana, hallucinogens, cocaine and other stimulants, sedatives and "minor tranquilizers," alcohol, and cigarettes can be very serious, but as this book is devoted mainly to opioid dependence, they will be mentioned, when appropriate, only in connection with nonopioid drug-dependence syndromes (see below). With regard to heroin and other opioids, chronic use is associated with increased death rates from suicides (Miles, 1977), violence (Sells et al., 1972), or drug overdoses (Cherubin et al., 1972). In a study by Sapira (1968), 75% of autopsies made on opioid addicts at the U.S. Public Health Service Hospital in Lexington, Kentucky, showed generalized hyperplasia of the entire lymphatic system, especially at the hilus of the liver, around the head of the pancreas, and under the pylorus; hepatomegaly was found in 30% of opioid addicts applying for admission. As a result of self-administration of opioids with contaminated needles and syringes, occasional cases of bacterial or myotic endocarditis (Wikler et al., 1942) or generalized septicemia (Wikler et al., 1943) have occurred among opioid addicts. On the other hand, maintenance on methadone for long periods of time does not produce serious medical problems (Kreek, 1973). However, even in a "protected" environment in which opioids are chronically administered experimentally to volunteers under legal conditions, the mood of the subject changes from one of initial euphoria to persistent dysphoria with hypochrondriasis and anxiety (Wikler, 1952; Haertzen & Hooks, 1969; Martin, Jasinski, Haertzen, Kay, Jones, Mansky, & Carpenter, 1973). Depression and anxiety have also been noted by Robbins and Nugent (1975) and by Robins (1979) as consequences of addiction to heroin in "nonprotected" users. Marital instability is very common among opioid addicts, and Capel et al. (1972) has reported that most older addicts are separated or divorced or have not married. That heroin addiction is associated with crime (generally nonviolent) is well known, but how much this crime is due to the criminal proclivities of heroin addicts before they began to use heroin is unclear. The weight of the evidence indicates that criminal activity increases after the first use of narcotics (Nurco & DuPont, 1977). This question is discussed in some detail by McGlothlin (1979) and Robins (1979). Because of the demands of their "habit" and the uncertainty of the supply of heroin, it is understandable that opioid addicts have a higher rate of unemployment than their non-drug-using peers (Robbins and Nugent, 1975) or than when they are abstinent from opioids (McGlothlin et al., 1977).

NONOPIOID DRUG-DEPENDENCE SYNDROMES

The features of opioid dependence, the conditioning processes involved therein, and the diagnosis and treatment of these problems are discussed in later chapters of this book. For purposes of comparison and contrast, brief descriptions are presented here of the clinical features of acute and chronic intoxication with nonopioid drugs, of tolerance to them, and of the abstinence syndromes that may ensue after they have been withdrawn abruptly. Methods of detoxification are also mentioned briefly, but discussion of treatment directed toward the prevention of relapse to use of nonopioid drugs is beyond the scope of this book.

Barbiturate, Nonbarbiturate Sedative, and "Minor Tranquilizer" Dependence

In low therapeutic doses, all of these drugs allay feelings of anxiety in man. In a social situation, such reduction of anxiety may be perceived by the subject as a "sedative" effect, though to an observer, the subject may appear to be socially disinhibited. In a solitary situation, the same dose of the drug may produce drowsiness and promote sleep. The borderline between therapeutic and intoxicating dose-schedules of these drugs is difficult to define. Experimentally, Belleville and Fraser (1957) showed that chronic administration of 100 mg of secobarbital or pentobarbital four times daily by mouth over a period of 90 days produced initial intoxicating effects (slowing of visual–manual reaction time, impairment of vertical tracing and pursuit rotor performance, increase in the hours of sleep, and increased clinical intoxication scores) to which tolerance developed at varying rates; no changes were observed in respiratory rate, blood pressure, pulse rate, rectal temperature, caloric intake, or body weight. Daily doses of secobarbital, pentobarbital, or amobarbital higher than 0.4 g/day produced grossly evident signs of intoxication that were roughly proportional to the daily dosage: ataxia, dyssynergia, nystagmus, slurring of speech, depression of the superficial abdominal reflexes, and impairment of judgment and of the sensorium. In most barbiturate-intoxicated individuals, the electroencephalogram is characterized by a mixture of rhythmic fast and slowed alpha activity. Tolerance to the intoxicating effects of barbiturates, if it develops at all, is only partial. On abrupt withdrawal of secobarbital, amobarbital, or pentobarbital, an abstinence syndrome emerges, the severity of which is again roughly proportion to the daily dosage that was obtained during chronic intoxication (Isbell et al., 1950; Fraser et al., 1958; Essig & Fraser, 1958). Thus, abrupt withdrawal of so-called short-acting barbiturates at high daily dose levels is followed first by disappearance of signs of chronic intoxication and then, within 12–24 hr, by "minor" withdrawal phenomena, including anxiety, restlessness, tremulousness, diaphoresis, increase in cardiac and respiratory rates, postural hypotension, muscle twitches, fever insomnia, anorexia, nausea, vomiting, and loss of body weight. In milder cases, these may be the only withdrawal phenomena, and they may subside within 2–5 days. However, in more severe cases, the onset of "minor" withdrawal phenomena is followed by "major" withdrawal phenomena, consisting of generalized grand mal seizures (without auras) commencing on the second or third day of "short-acting" barbiturate abstinence and continuing up to the eighth day, and/or psychoses (generally resembling alchoholic delirium tremens), beginning between the third and eighth day after abrupt drug withdrawal and lasting up to two weeks. The electroencephalogram is characterized by repetitive paroxysmal, 4-Hz high-voltage spike and slow-wave discharges during the barbiturate abstinence syndrome, even in patients who do not have clinically observable seizures. Generally, barbiturate withdrawal seizures are nonfatal, but deaths from uncontolled hyperpyrexia and delirium are not uncommon; seven fatal terminations associated with hyperpyrexia have been described (Wulff, 1959). The intensity of the "short-acting" barbiturate abstinence syndrome is directly related to the daily dose level of chronic intoxication (Fraser et al., 1958). Thus, after abrupt withdrawal from 0.9–2.2 g/day of secobarbital or pentobarbital, all 18 patients had "minor" withdrawal phenomena, 14 had generalized seizures, and 12 had delirium; of 23 patients abruptly withdrawn from 0.6–0.8 g/day of secobarbital, 14 had "minor" withdrawal phenomena, 3 had generalized seizures, and 1 had hallucinations; in 18 patients abruptly withdrawn from 0.4 g/day of secobarbital or pentobarbital, only very mild "minor" withdrawal phenomena were observed; neither of 2 patients withdrawn from 0.2 g/day of secobarbital or pentobarbital showed any withdrawal phenomena.

Though the relationship between the intensities of the abstinence syndrome following abrupt withdrawal of nonbarbiturate sedatives (glutethimide, ethinamate, ethchlorvynol, and methyprylon) and the daily dose levels of chronic intoxication with these drugs has not been documented experimentally, the clinical features of chronic intoxication and "minor" and "major" withdrawal phenomena are similar to those for the "short-acting" barbituates (Essig, 1964).

The "minor tranquilizers" (meprobamate, chlordiazepoxide, and diazepam) can likewise produce signs resembling those of barbiturate intoxication and "minor" and "major" abstinence phenomena, though in the cases of chlordiazepoxide and diazepam, the clinical incidence of "major" abstinence phenomena seems to be less than after abrupt withdrawal from high daily dose levels of "short-acting" barbiturates. In an experimental study on patients, Haizlip and Ewing (1958) found that during chronic oral administration of meprobamate, 3.2 g/day to one group and 6.4 g/day to another group for 40 days, both groups were initially sedated and ataxic but eventually became tolerant to these effects; when placebos were substituted for meprobamate, both groups showed "minor" and "major" abstinence phenomena of the barbiturate type, the latter (convulsions and hallucinatory delirioid states) being more common after withdrawal from 6.4 g/day. Haizlip and Ewing (1958) estimated that the "threshold" for appearance of significant "minor" meprobamate abstinence phenomena was between 1.2 and 3.2 g/day ("therapeutic" range, 1.2–2.4 g/day). Delayed "minor" and "major" abstinence phenomena can occur after chronic administration of high daily doses of chlordiazepoxide. Hollister *et al.* (1961) substituted placebos for chlordiazepoxide after treating five patients in daily oral doses up to 300 mg/day and six patients up to 600 mg/day for 1–7 months. During chronic administration of chlordiazepoxide, the patients complained of dizziness and showed weakness, unsteadiness, and sleepiness. After abrupt withdrawal of chlordiazepoxide, various "minor" abstinence phenomena of the barbiturate type were observed in 10 of the 11 patients; 1 patient had two generalized seizures on the 12th day after withdrawal from 300 mg/day, and 2 patients had generalized seizures on the seventh and eighth days after withdrawal from 600 mg/day of chlordiazepoxide. The onset of withdrawal convulsions appeared to coincide in time with the nearly complete disappearance of chlordiazepoxide from blood plasma, indicating that the delayed onset of withdrawal seizures was due to the slow metabolism and/or excretion of the drug. As with chlordiazepoxide, withdrawal phenomena of the barbiturate type (including seizures that may be delayed up to eight days after drug withdrawal) have been reported following abrupt discontinuation of high doses (100–150 mg/day) of diazepam (Aivazian, 1964; Hollister *et al.*, 1963). One patient developed status epilepticus (successfully treated with intravenous pentobarbital) when her supply of diazepam was temporarily exhausted; she had been treated for the "stiff-man" syndrome with diazepam, 15 mg four times daily (60 mg/day) over a long period (Cohen, 1966). Definite diazepam abstinence phenomena have been reported after abrupt withdrawal of the drug from daily doses in the "therapeutic" range. Thus, Pevnick *et al.* (1978) described a patient who had been treated for "anxiety" with 30–45 mg/day of diazepam orally for 20 months. Between the fifth and ninth days after the abrupt withdrawal of diazepam, the patient lost weight precipitately; exhibited orthostatic pulse-rate increases, increased tremors, muscle twitches, retching, and insomnia; and complained of nervousness, anorexia, nausea, abdominal pain or cramping, muscle cramps, and facial numbness. This abstinence syndrome subsided between the ninth and tenth days of diazepam abstinence (except that the patient's body weight did not return to the prewithdrawal value until the fourteenth day). Diazepam-seeking behavior was especially marked between the fifth and seventh days of abstinence but subsided thereafter. Another patient, described by Winokur et al. (1980), had been treated for nausea, abdominal distress, and mild anxiety with 5 mg of diazepam three times daily for six years; during the last two weeks of this period, he had increased the dose from 15 mg/day to 25 mg/day because of emotional upset due to a sudden death in the family. On admission to the hospital, he was first maintained on diazepam orally, 5 mg four times daily for four days; then, placebo capsules were substituted for four days, and the diazepam–placebo cycle was repeated once more. Abstinence phenonema began to develop on the second day of each abrupt withdrawal period and intensified during subsequent abstinence days. The abstinence phenomena (which were spectacularly relieved by the resumption of diazepam administration) consisted of extreme anxiety and irritability; gross tremulousness; diaphoresis; severe headaches; insomnia; intermittent tinnitus; blurred vision; auditory, olfactory, gustatory, and tactile hypersensitivity; mental confusion and visual sensory distortions; difficulty in initiating urination; and constipation. After the second four-day placebo phase, the administration of diazepam was not resumed. The abstinence syndrome continued for an additional 11 days and began to subside progressivly over the next 11 days. During the second placebo phase, the plasma elimination half-life of diazepam was 47 hr and that of its major metabolite, desmethyldiazepam, was 75 hr. These values are in the range for healthy persons and are indicative of the slow metabolism and/or excretion of diazepam, which is comparable to that of chlordiazepoxide, 48 hr (Hollister et al., 1961). It is remarkable, therefore, that in the case reported by Winokur et al. (1980), diazepam abstinence phenomena began during the second day of drug withdrawal, whereas in the case reported by Pevnick et al. (1978), the onset of diazepam abstinence phenomena was delayed for five days, as might be expected from the data on the chlordiazepoxide abstinence syndrome of Hollister et al. (1961).

In principle, the treatment of dependence on barbiturates, nonbarbiturate sedatives, and "minor" tranquilizers involves the substitution of pentobarbital for any of these drugs in doses and frequency of administration sufficient to suppress all signs of barbiturate-type abstinence and to produce a *very mild* degree of barbiturate-type continuous intoxication; after "stabilization" on such a daily dosage of pentobarbital, the *daily* dose of pentobarbital is reduced *very slowly, at a rate not exceeding 100 mg/day*. If even mild barbiturate-type abstinence phenomena appear on such a dose reduction schedule, the dose reduction is temporarily suspended, until the abstinence phenomena disappear; then the dose reduction of pentobarbital is resumed, perhaps at a slower rate (e.g., 50 mg/day), until the patient is completely detoxified (Wikler, 1968).

Alcohol Dependence

The signs of chronic intoxication with alcohol are remarkably similar to those produced by intoxicating doses of barbiturates, namely, ataxia, dyssynergia, slurring of speech, and impairment of judgment and of the sensorium. Unlike the barbiturates, which produce a mixture of rhythmic fast and slowed alpha activity in the electroencephalogram, only slowing of frequencies is observed during the acute or chronic administration of alcohol (Wikler *et al.*, 1956). Two types of tolerance develop during experimental chronic intoxication with high daily levels of alcohol consumption (Wikler *et al.*, 1956): (1) initially, at a constant daily intake of alcohol (up to a limit), degrees of behavioral intoxication, blood levels of alcohol, and slowing of electroencephalographic frequencies decrease ("metabolic" or "dispositional" tolerance); (2) with a small increase in daily intake of alcohol, the subject becomes reintoxicated, blood levels of alcohol rise, and electroencephalographic frequencies slow, but as drinking at this level continues, the degree of behavioral intoxication and of slowing of electroencephalographic frequencies declines to a moderate extent, despite the continued maintenance of high blood alcohol concentrations ("tissue" or "functional" tolerance). On abrupt withdrawal of alcohol from such high daily levels of alcohol consumption, an abstinence syndrome emerges that, except for time course, is similar to the barbiturate abstinence syndrome and, like the latter, can be divided into "minor" and "major" withdrawal phenomena. The "minor" withdrawal phenomena begin within a few hours after the last drink and increase in intensity during the first abstinence day and beyond. They consist of severe anxiety, tremulousness, weakness, profuse perspiration, hyperpnea, increase in arterial pH, decrease in serum magnesium, tachycardia, elevation of blood pressure, hyperreflexia, insomnia, transitory visual and/or auditory hallucinations, fever, nausea, and vomiting. Generalized seizures, a "major" withdrawal phenomenon, can occur during the first abstinence day, while the other "major" withdrawal phenomenon, delirium tremens (disorientation, visual and auditory hallucinations, fever, dilated pupils, diaphoresis, delusions, and agitation), generally begins on the third or fourth day of alcohol abstinence (Victor & Adams, 1953, Isbell *et al.*, 1955; Wikler *et al.* 1956). Remarkably, Wikler *et al.* (1956) found no specific changes in the electroencephalograms of three patients during the alcohol abstinence syndrome except for brief high-voltage, bifrontal discharges that occurred only between the 15th and 19th hours after abrupt withdrawal of alcohol, when blood alcohol concentrations had fallen to zero; this limited time period for electroencephalographic paroxysmal discharges is consonant with the finding of Victor and Brausch (1967) that the peak incidence of spontaneous convulsions after the last drink of alcohol in chronic alcoholics was between 15 and 21 hr. Generally, delirium tremens lasts less than 72 hr, but it may go on for as long as 6 days (Victor & Adams, 1953). While full-blown delirium tremens is relatively common, it is potentially fatal. In a series of 101 cases of alcoholic delirium tremens, 15 had a fatal outcome (Victor & Adams, 1953).

Treatment of "minor" alcohol withdrawal phenomena (during the first two days of alcohol abstinence) may be accomplished by the substitution of pentobarbital (stabilization on a daily dosage of pentobarbital that suppresses all alcohol abstinence phenomena and produces very mild chronic pentobarbital intoxication for a few days), followed by *slow* progressive reduction of the daily dosage of pentobarbital according to the method described by Wikler (1968) for the treatment of drug dependence of the barbiturate type. Or chlordiazepoxide may be given every six hours instead of pentobarbital, in doses producing comparable effects, yet permitting the patient to be ambulant and to feed himself. Phenothiazines are contraindicated at this stage because they lower the convulsive threshold and may precipitate seizures (as already noted, the peak incidence of spontaneous alcohol withdrawal seizures is between the fifteenth and twenty-first hours of alcohol abstinence). If pentobarbital or chlordiazepoxide substitution is carried out early enough in the "minor" withdrawal stage, "major" withdrawal phenomena (generalized seizures and delirium tremens) will probably be prevented. However, if the patient is not seen until full-blown delirium tremens has developed, treatment should be aimed at heavy sedation and vigorous general medical supportive therapy. For adequate sedation of the extremely agitated patient, pentobarbital may be dangerous because of the narrow margin between its heavy sedative and respiratory–circulatory depressant effects. Chlordiazepoxide and paraldehyde are safer; phenothiazines may also be used, since the peak incidence of spontaneous alcohol-withdrawal seizures has passed by the time delirium tremens develops. A comparison of pentobarbital, chlordiazepoxide, paraldehyde, and perphenazine with details of dosages in the treatment of delirium tremens has been published by Kaim and Klett (1972). For treatment of severe delirium tremens, Thompson *et al.* (1975) found repeated intravenous injections of diazepam more effective than repeated rectal doses of paraldehyde. In addition to heavy sedation, fluids should be given intravenously (initially, 1000 ml of normal saline solution, then 5% glucose in water up to 5000 ml/day). Specific electrolyte imbalances may require special correction. A water-soluble vitamin B and C preparation should be added to the intravenous infusions. Hypotension should be controlled with metaraminol by intravenous drip or with methoxamine administered intramuscularly. Blood transfusions and/or plasma expanders may be needed. Infection (e.g., pneumonitis) should be treated with appropriate antibiotics. Hyperpyrexia (a rectal temperature of 104°F or more) in the absence of infection is an ominous sign and should be combatted with ice packs or a cooling mattress. In the treatment of other chronic alcoholic syndromes (Wernicke's disease, Korsakoff's psychosis, alcoholic neuropathy), high doses of thiamine hydrochloride parenterally and other B vitamins, together with the resumption of a normal diet as soon as possible, are especially important (Victor, 1976).

Amphetamine Dependence

Formerly widely prescribed for its appetite-reducing effects, amphetamine (*d*-amphetamine or its racemate, *d,l*-amphetamine) and certain of its congeners (methamphetamine, phenmetrazine) have become "street drugs." In low doses (orally or intravenously), they produce increased alertness, a sense of well-being (euphoria), overconfidence, increased capacity for physical exertion, elevation of blood pressure with reflex bradycardia, suppression of rapid eye movement (REM) sleep, and anorexia. Higher doses produce "jitteriness," fine tremors, irritability, anxiety, insomnia, sometimes cardiac irregularities, and in very high doses, toxic delirium. The toxic delirium caused by very high doses of amphetamine should be distinguished from the paranoid psychosis resembling that of paranoid schizophrenia that often develops during *chronic* amphetamine intoxication with as little as 50 mg/day and that, unlike toxic delirium, is characterized by a clear sensorium and full orientation (Connell, 1958). Tolerance develops over a period of a few weeks to the euphoric, anorexic, and REM-sleep-suppressant actions of amphetamine, but no tolerance appears to develop to the "stimulant" effects of high doses. After abrupt withdrawal of amphetamine, the toxic delirium or the paranoid psychosis, if they developed during chronic amphetamine intoxication, disappears within two or three weeks without treatment. Also, an abstinence syndrome emerges that is characterized by prolonged sleep (with REM rebound), followed by hyperphagia and mild affective depression. A special pattern of abuse, most often with methamphetamine ("speed") in the United States and phenmetrazine (Preludin) in Sweden, consists of intravenous self-injection of increasing doses every two or three hours in "runs" for a week or so, which are said to produce intense orgastic experiences. As this pattern continues, the user exhibits stereotyped useless activities (e.g., shining shoes all day long, taking radios or television sets apart and reconstructing them). Eventually, intense anxiety and/or psychosis develops, and the user ceases, or is persuaded to cease, self-administration of methamphetamine or phenmetrazine, after which prolonged sleep, hyperphagia, and depression occur (abstinence syndrome, or "crash"). Then, the cycle of the methamphetamine or phenmetrazine "run," followed by the "crash" is resumed, or the user tries heroin for relief of depression, sometimes becoming a heroin addict (Kramer et al., 1967; Carey & Mandel, 1969).

In treatment, amphetamine and its congeners should be withdrawn abruptly. Amphetamine psychoses respond well to phenothiazines (e.g., Chlorpromazine), but if the differential diagnosis between amphetamine paranoid psychosis and paranoid schizophrenia is uncertain, phenothiazines should be withheld and nonspecific sedative drugs should be prescribed as needed, until the different diagnosis is clarified. If the psychosis is indeed due solely to amphetamine, it will disappear without treatment within two or three weeks; if the patient is treated with phenothiazines and the psychosis attenuates within the same period, the differential diagnosis will remain uncertain. No treatment is required for withdrawal hypersomnolence or hyperphagia, but withdrawal depression may require treatment with tricyclic antidepressant drugs.

Cocaine Dependence

In the United States, cocaine is usually taken intranasally ("snorting") or intravenously, while among the Indians in the high Andes in South America, coca leaves (mixed with alkaline ash) are chewed and ingested. In placebo-controlled studies in man, Resnick et al. (1977) found that by the intravenous route, 10 or 25 mg of cocaine produced a "high" remarkably like that produced by amphetamine; similar highs were produced by 25 or 100 mg of cocaine intranasally. By the intravenous route, both doses of cocaine elevated heart rate and systolic blood pressure; in addition, diastolic blood pressure was elevated by 100 mg of cocaine intranasally. The onset of these effects occurred within 2 min of cocaine administration and peaked earlier (5–10 min) after intravenous than after intranasal (15–20 min) administrations. Of the 19 subjects in this study, 6 reported dysphoric effects after the highs wore off; in street terminology, such dysphoric effects are known as *postcoke blues* or *crashing,* and in this study, they were characterized by anxiety, depression, fatigue, and wanting more cocaine. Though expressed in behavioral rather than physiological terms, such dysphoric reactions following the termination of the high produced by the drug, which were not present before the cocaine was administered, constitutes an abstinence syndrome. Whether this abstinence syndrome is indicative of "psychic" or "physical" dependence depends on one's definintion of *psychic* as opposed to *physical* (to the extent that such a distinction can be made). Chronic intravenous or intranasal use of cocaine may produce perceptual distortions, including formications ("cocaine bugs"), "snow lights," and visual hallucinations of objects moving swiftly in the peripheral visual field or of geometric patterns (resembling entoptic phenomena or migraine hallucinations), as well as auditory, tactile, and olfactory hallucinations (Siegel, 1978). The daily dosage and duration of chronic use necessary to produce such perceptual distortions and hallucinations have not been determined. In the author's experience, one experimental subject was given cocaine intravenously, beginning with 20 mg at 30-min intervals, increasing to 50 mg at 5 to 10-min intervals over a period of 12 hr. As the dosage increased, the subject became tremulous; had hyperactive tendon reflexes, mydriasis, and elevated blood pressure; and sweated profusely. When he had received a total of 2 g of cocaine, he began following a nonexistent butterfly in the air, "caught" it, and handed it to the examiner. Then he plucked a nonexistent insect from the skin of his arm and handed it also to the examiner. He was also very paranoid, racing up and down the ward corridor and jumping away from a nonexistent "detective" who, he claimed, was peeping at him through every door. These physiological and behavioral changes subsided and eventually disappeared spontaneously after administration of the cocaine ceased. Cocaine abusers in the United States often try to prevent the perceptual distortions and psychotomimetic effects of cocaine by combining cocaine with heroin; such "speedballs" are also said to enhance the euphoric effects of the heroin content. Repeated use of speedballs produces heroin dependence. In treatment of cocaine dependence, the drug should be withdrawn abruptly; postcoke blues are short-lived and generally require no special treatment, but if necessary, tricyclic antidepressant drugs may be given.

Hallucinogen Dependence

Because it has been so thoroughally investigated experimentally in man (Isbell *et al.*, 1956; Isbell, 1959; Isbell *et al.*, 1961; Wolbach *et al.*, 1962a,b), LSD-25 (D-lysergic acid diethylamide) serves here as the prototype drug for hallucinogen dependence, while other hallucinogenic agents are mentioned more briefly. Depending on the dose ($0.5\mu g/kg$– $3.0\mu g/kg$), LSD-25 produces light-headedness, giddiness, nausea, euphoria and/or anxiety, distortion of visual perception and of body image, increased sensitivity to sound, synesthesias (stimuli in one sensory modality evoke sensations in another modality), colored visual hallucinations of geometric, symmetrically arranged objects ("entopic" hallucinations) moving across the visual field, and true hallucinations (formed objects, landscapes, and animal or human faces that are often grotesque). Auditory hallucinations are less common. Ideas of reference and paranoid delusions are more frequent. Familiar surroundings seem strange (derealization), and weird alterations of self-awareness (depersonalization) occur. Orientation and memory are surprisingly intact, though they may be difficult to test because of the user's preoccupation with his inner feelings and with trivial objects in his environment. Suggestibility is enhanced. The subjective changes produced by LSD-25 are minimized by engaging the user in attention-demanding tests (e.g., psychological test batteries). Physiologically, LSD-25 produces sympathomimetic activity: pupillary dilation (with intact light reflex), mild tachycardia, elevation of blood pressure, and increased sweating. Body temperature is elevated and the knee jerk threshold is lowered. Occasionally, tremors are seen, and catalepsy may occur. The dose–effect relationship of mescaline and psilocybin are very similar to that of LSD-25. However, LSD-25 is about 100 times as potent as psilocybin and 3500–4000 times as potent as mescaline, on a $\mu g/kg$ basis. On oral administration, the onset of the effects of LSD-25 and mescaline is about 20 min; peak effects are reached in 60–90 min, remain at peak level for 2.0–2.5 hr and then subside over 8–10 hr. The onset of the effects of orally administered psilocybin is within a few minutes, peak effects are reached in 30 min, and the syndrome subsides completely in less than 4 hr. "Flashbacks" may occur weeks or months after a single dose of LSD-25 (it has been observed that smoking marijuana may induce "flashbacks" in persons who have used LSD-25 previously). On daily administration of LSD-25, a very marked degree of tolerance develops, especially to the pupillary and subjective effects. The same is true also of mescaline and psilocybin. Persons tolerant to LSD-25, mescaline, or psilocybin are cross-tolerant to the other two hallucinogens. No abstinence syndrome follows abrupt withdrawal of LSD-25, mescaline, or psilocybin, despite the prior development of tolerance. Treatment of dependence on these hallucinogens includes abrupt withdrawal of the drug. Psychotic reactions may respond to phenobarbital or, if they do not, to a phenothiazine. Patients do best in a quiet room (not soundproof), in the presence of relatives or friends.

Other hallucinogens with properties similar to LSD-25 are DMT (*N,N,*-dimethyltryptamine) and DOM (2,5-dimethoxy-4-methylamphetamine), also known as *STP* on the street. DMT is about one three-hundredth, and DOM one thirtieth as potent as LSD-25 on a μg/kg basis. Abuse of phencyclidine (PCP, "angel dust") is usually by smoking leafy substances sprinkled with the powder, or through nasal application ("snorting"), or by oral self-administration. At low doses, agitation and excitement, catatonic rigidity, multidirectional nystagmus, hypertension, impairment of peripheral sensation, diaphoresis, salivation, psychoses resembling toxic delirium or paranoid schizophrenia, muscle twitches, convulsions, and coma may supervene (Petersen & Stillman, 1978). Treatment of phencyclidine toxicity depends on the clinical manifestations. Acidification of the urine to promote its urinary excretion and removal of pheneyclidine from the stomach by gastric suction will facilitate recovery. Severe hypertension can be combated by intravenous injection of diazoxide (Hyperstat). Convulsions may be controlled by intravenous injections of diazepam or phenytoin (Dilantin). For control of aggressive, assaultive behavior, removal to a quiet environment under the watchful eye of several husky men and perhaps sedation with diazepam or chlordiazepoxide may be required. For treatment of phencyclidine psychosis, haloperidol, rather than phenothiazine, is recommended, because the central anticholinergic action of the latter may aggravate the psychosis produced by phencyclidine (Allen and Young, 1978).

Abuse of anticholinergic agents (atropine, scopolamine, stramonium, jimsonweed, antihistamines) may lead to the production of a toxic delirium with disorientation, confusion, impairment of memory and cognitive abilities, incoherence of speech, blurred vision, perceptual distortions, visual and auditory hallucinations, delusions, weakness, giddiness, incoordination, agitation, or coma. Physiologically, the pupils are dilated and react sluggishly or not at all to light and in accommodation; the skin is dry, flushed, and hot; the mouth is dry; the cardiac rate and blood pressure are increased; and the rectal temperature is elevated (progressive hyperpyrexia is an ominous sign). The pupillary changes are presistent and usually outlast the behavioral changes. Some degree of tolerance to anticholinergic agents has been demonstrated experimentally in man (Isbell *et al.*, 1964). No abstinence syndrome appears after abrupt withdrawal of anticholinergic agents in man, but in the mouse, it has been demonstrated that central nervous system supersensitivity to pilocarpine develops during chronic oral administration of scopolamine; such supersensitivity declines after the withdrawal of scopolamine over a time course consistent with an abstinence syndrome, which is masked by the prolonged duration of action of scopolamine (Friedman & Jaffe, 1969; Friedman *et al.*, 1969). In the treatment of anticholinergic syndromes, the drug is withdrawn abruptly. Hyperpyrexia can be controlled by alcohol sponges, ice packs, or the use of a cooling mattress. For sedation, pentobarbital, diazepam, or chlordiazepoxide should be used; phenothiazines should be avoided because of their anticholinergic properties. Physostigmine (eserine) is a specific anticholinergic antagonist and may be given in a dose of 1 or 2 mg intravenously or 3.5 mg intramuscularly, repeated as often as necessary, with due attention to possible peripheral actions of physostigmine (excessive salivation and other hypersecretions), which may require reductions in the dose.

Cannabis (Marijuana, Hashish) Dependence

The effects of cannibis products are related mainly to the properties of ($-$)Δ^9-trans-tetrahydrocannabinol (THC), the most active principle in marijuana, hashish, and other cannabis preparations. The THC content of marijuana grown in the United States is relatively low; it is higher in marijuana grown in Mexico, South America, and Asia, and highest in hashish. Marijuana is prepared for smoking from the upper leaves of the plant *Cannabis sativa*; hashish (also known as *kif, ganja, charas,* and *dagga*) is prepared for smoking or chewing from the flowering tops of the female plant and consists mainly of the resin. Depending on the dose of THC absorbed through the lungs or from the gastrointestinal tract, the effects of marijuana or hashish include euphoria and/or anxiety, impairment of immediate memory, disruption of the logical sequence of thoughts leading toward a goal (especially manifested in speech), alteration of time sense (as if an internal, biological clock were speeded up), outbursts of pointless laughter, ideas of reference, paranoid delusions, and, after higher doses, visual illusions, hallucinations, and depersonalization (Wikler, 1974). Physiologically, THC produces dose-related tachycardia, a tendency toward postural hypotension, diuresis, reddening of the eyes (chemosis, regardless of the route of administration of THC), and, in some cases, an appetite for sweets. Tolerance to some functions impaired by marijuana smoking and a "reverse tolerance" to the high produced by marijuana have been reported (Wikler, 1976). Lemberger *et al.* (1970, 1971) found that unlike naive subjects, experienced marijuana users reported subjective effects reminiscent of marijuana after intravenous injections of a "nonpharmacological" dose of radioactivity labeled THC; these authors also observed that the half-life of the slower phase of disappearance of the drug from the plasma was 57 hr in naive subjects and only 28 hr in experienced marijuana users; in both groups, the active metabolite, 11-hydroxy-Δ^9-THC, appeared in the plasma within 10 min after intravenous injection of the "nonpharmocological" dose of THC, but quantitative differences were not reported. In an experimental study on the oral administration of THC every 4 hr in man over a period of approximately two to three weeks (final dose, 30 mg every 4 hr), Jones *et al.* (1976) found that tolerance developed to THC-induced mood changes, tachycardia, orthostatic hypotension, skin temperature decrease, body temperature increase, salivary flow decrease, intraocular pressure decrease, electroencephlographic slowing, evoked-potential changes and sleep-tracing changes, sleep time and quality changes, eye-tracking changes, and psychomotor task-performance impairment. Abrupt withdrawal of THC resulted in a cannabis abstinence syndrome that ran its course in 72–96 hr and was reversible by smoked or oral doses of marijuana or THC. The abstinence syndrome included mood changes, disturbed sleep, decreased appetite, restlessness, irritability, perspiration, chills, feverish feelings, nausea, abdominal distress, tremulousness, hyperactivity, hiccups (rare), nasal congestion (rare), weight loss, hemoconcentration, salivation, tremor, loose bowel movements, increase in body temperature, REM-rebound (in sleep), waking electroencephalographic changes, and increase in intraocular pressure. Evidently, tolerance and physical dependence on cannabis can develope in chronic, high-dose THC intoxication. Whether or not physical dependence develops in moderately "heavy" marijuana smokers is unknown. Soueif (1967) has described an "oscillation of temperament" in hashish users that is characterized by social ease, a desire to mix, acquiescence, elation, and agreeableness when under immediate drug effect, and seclusiveness, negativism, depression of mood, and pugnacity when deprived of hashish. Soueif (1967) considered such "oscillation of temperament" evidence of psychic dependence, but in as much as it appears to be a *consequence* of long-continued hashish smoking and not an antecedent, "oscillation of temperament" would seem to be evidence of physical dependence, even though its characteristics are expressed in behavioral terms.

Tolerance and physical dependence have been described in monkeys (Deneau & Kaymakcalan, 1971; Kaymakcalan, 1973) and in rats (Kaymakcalan *et al.*, 1977) after multiple daily doses of THC. In monkeys that received automatic intravenous injections of THC every 6 hr for one month in doses that increased from 0.1 and 0.4 mg/kg, tolerance developed to the initial effects (ptosis, blank staring, scratching, and docility). When injections of THC were abruptly terminated, the following abstinence signs appeared, beginning at about 12 hr and continuing for about 5 days: yawning, anorexia, piloerection, hyperirritability, increase in aggressiveness, scratching, biting and licking fingers, pulling hair, tremors, twitches, penile erection and masturbation with ejaculation, eating feces and other unusual things, slapping on cage walls, staring in circles, and grasping as if catching flies (hallucinations?). Before commencement of this study (Deneau & Kaymakcalan, 1971; Kaymakcalan, 1973), none of the six monkeys used would self-administer THC, but during the THC-abstinence syndrome, two did initiate and maintain intravenous self-injections of THC. In rats that received THC subcutaneously twice daily in increasing doses (up to 40 mg/kg/dose) for five weeks (Kaymakcalan *et al.*, 1977), tolerance developed to the hypothermic effect of THC. After abrupt withdrawal of THC, an abstinence syndrome emerged that peaked at 48 hr and consisted mainly of ptosis, teeth chattering, piloerection, defecation, urination, complete palpebral closure, and dyspnea. Remarkably, the "pure" opioid antagonist, naloxone, in single doses of 1 and 4 mg/kg intraperitoneally, given to THC-tolerant rats, precipitated similar abstinence syndromes (this phenomenon had been reported earlier by Hirschhorn & Rosecrans, 1974).

Since in man, the cannabis-abstinence syndrome, if it develops, lasts no more than 72 hr (Jones *et al.*, 1976), detoxification may be accomplished in most cases by abrupt withdrawal of the drug, (marijuana, hashish). If definite TCH-abstinence phenomena appear, and they are distressing, they may be ameliorated by an occasional dose of THC (if legal authorization to do so can be obtained) during the first 72 hr of cannabis abstinence, or perhaps by the administration of nonspecific "minor tranquilizers" (diazepam, chlordiazepoxide).

Tobacco Dependence

What is known about the pharmacological aspects of tobacco dependence has been reviewed by Jarvik (1979) and by Shiffman (1979). In nonsmokers and after a period of abstinence from tobacco (cigarettes) in smokers, smoking one or two cigarettes produces tachycardia, increased blood pressure and cardiac output, stroke volume, velocity of contraction of the heart, myocardial contractile force, coronary blood flow, myocardial oxygen consumption, arrhythmic induction, and changes in the electrocardiogram. These changes are attributed to the pharmacological effects of low doses of nicotine, which stimulate both sympathetic and parasympathetic ganglia and release epinephrine and norepinephrine from chromaffin cells in the adrenal medulla, heart, blood vessels, and skin. After intravenous injection of 1 mg of nicotine, none of the smokers reported nausea, but all nonsmokers reported it in various degrees (Beckett et al., 1971). According to Jones and Farrell (1978), tolerance develops rapidly in both smokers and nonsmokers (more in smokers) to the tachycardia produced initially by the intravenous injection of nicotine (700 μg in smokers, 300 μg in nonsmokers), when such injections are repeated three times at intervals of approximately 1 hr. Apparently, such tolerance is lost rapidly after a period of abstention from cigarettes, since Knapp et al. (1963) stated that tolerance develops to nausea but not to the cardiovascular effects of smoking. Some of the effects of nicotine may be appetitively reinforcing, since Jarvik (1979) stated that smokers increased cigarette consumption under a mecamylamine blockade of central and ganglionic nicotine receptors. The reinforcing effects of nicotine *may* be relative to increased arousal, or at least to maintenance of a normal state of arousal, since Itil et al. (1971) reported that after cigarette deprivation for 24 hr, there was an increase in 3- to 5-Hz and 7-Hz activity in the electroencephalograms of smokers. Similarly, Knott and Venables (1977) found that after 13–15 hr of cigarette deprivation, there was significant slowing of the alpha frequency in the electroencephalograms of smokers, and that smoking two cigarettes restored the alpha frequency to that of nonsmokers and nondeprived smoker-control groups. These studies indicate that brief abstention from tobacco is associated with *hypoarousal* in smokers, and that resumption of smoking restores the arousal state to normal. Perhaps the initial effects of nicotine have been to produce *hyperarousal*, but tolerance develops to such arousing effects and the smoker becomes dependent on nicotine for maintenance of the "normal" arousal state. Besides such evidence of "tissue" (or "functional") tolerance, there is evidence of "metabolic" (or "dispositional") tolerance to tobacco. Thus, after a 1 mg dose of nicotine intravenously (Beckett et al., 1971), smokers excrete nicotine significantly faster than nonsmokers. Also, benzodiazepines, propoxyphene, pentazocine, phenacetin, and xanthines are metabolized to a greater extent in smokers than in nonsmokers (Jarvik, 1979).

In addition to the hypoarousal already described, decreases in heart rate and blood pressure are observed consistently early in the tobacco-abstinence syndrome (Knapp et al., 1963; Shiffman, 1979). Also, in tobacco-deprived smokers, performance is impaired on psychomotor tasks requiring vigilance and/or tracking (Shiffman, 1979). Over a longer period of time (e.g., 1–2 months), weight gain is common. Abstinent smokers complain of "emptiness," "gnawing," or "hungry" feelings in the stomach, and some complain of a feeling of "loss" (Knapp et al., 1963), nausea, headache, constipation, diarrhea, drowsiness, fatigue, insomnia, irritability, anxiety, and inability to concentrate. These symptioms generally last 3–14 days, but they are very variable and may last much longer. By far the most common and clinically important tobacco-withdrawal symptom is craving for tobacco, which may still be reported among former smokers who have been abstinent from tobacco for 5–9 years (Shiffman, 1979).

Treatment of tobacco dependence obviously requires permanent abstention from tobacco, but Hunt and Matarazzo (1973) have reported that of those who successfully cease smoking, only about 25% are likely to remain abstinent for more than six months. Shiffman (1979) has reviewed evidence that abrupt withdrawal from tobacco (cigarettes) may be preferable to gradual withdrawal, since the latter *prolongs* the tobacco-abstinence syndrome; he pointed out that more research is needed on the relationship between degree of tobacco deprivation and the emergence of withdrawal symptoms.

REFERENCES

Abelson, H. I., Fishburne, P. M., and Cisin, I. H., 1977, *National Survey on Drug Abuse, 1977: A Nationwide Study—Youth, Young Adults and Older Adults.* Response Analysis Corporation, Princeton.

Aivazian, G. H., 1964, Clinical evaluation of diazepam, *Dis. Nerv. System* 25:491–496.

Allen, R. M., and Young, S. J., 1978, Phencyclidine-induced psychosis. *Amer. J. Psychiat.* 135:1081–1084.

Austin, G. A., Macari, M. A., and Lettieri, D. J. (Eds.), 1978, *International Drug Use*, NIDA Research Issues 23, DHEW Publication No. (ADM) 79–809. Superintendent of Documents, U.S. Government Printing Office, Washington, D.C.

Ball, J. C., and Chambers, C. D. (Eds.), 1970, *The Epidemiology of Opiate Addiction in the United States.* Charles C Thomas, Springfield, Ill.

Beckett, A. H., Gorrod, J. W., and Jenner, P., 1971, The effect of smoking on nicotine metabolism *in vivo* in man, *J. Pharmacy Pharmacol.* 23 (Suppl.):62–67.

Belleville, R. E., and Fraser, H. F., 1957, Tolerance to some effects of barbiturates, *J. Pharmacol. Exp. Ther.* 120:469–474.

Capel, W. C., Goldsmith, B. G., Waddell, K. J., and Stewart, G. T., 1972, The aging narcotic addict: An increasing problem for the next decades, *J. Gerontol.* 27:102–106.

Carey, J. T., and Mandel, J., 1969, A San Francisco Bay area "speed scene" in *Drug Dependence*, No. 2., pp. 20–29. National Clearinghouse for Mental Health Information, National Institute of Mental Health, Bethesda, Md.

Center for New York City Affairs of the New School for Social Research, 1972, *City Almanac 6:2*.

Cherubin, C., McCusker, J., Baden, M., Kavaler, F., and Amsel, Z., 1972, The epidemiology of death in narcotic addicts, *Amer. J. Epidemiol. 96:11–22.*

Cohen, L., 1966, Stiff-man syndrome. Two patients treated with diazepam, *J. Amer. Med. Ass. 195:222–224.*

Connell, P. H., 1958, *Amphetamine Psychosis.* Chapman and Hall, London.

Deneau, G. A., and Kaymakcalan, S., 1971, Physiological and psychological dependence to synthetic Δ⁹-tetrahydrocannabinol (THC) in rhesus monkeys, *Pharmacologist 13:246.*

DuPont, R. L., 1978, International challenge of drug abuse: A perspective from the United States, in *The International Challenge of Drug Abuse* (R. C. Petersen, Ed.), NIDA Research Monogr. 19, DHEW Publication No. (ADM) 78–654, pp. 3–4. Superintendent of Documents, U.S. Government Printing Office, Washington, D.C. 20402.

Essig, C. F., 1964, Addiction to nonbarbiturate sedative and tranquilizing drugs, *Clin. Pharmacol. Ther. 5:334–343.*

Essig, C. F., and Fraser, H. F., 1958, Electroencephalographic changes in man during use and withdrawal of barbiturates in moderate dosage, *Electroenceph. Clin. Neurophysiol. 10:649–656.*

Fraser, H. F., Wikler, A., Essig, C. F., and Isbell, H., 1958, Degree of physical dependence induced by secobarbital or pentobarbital, *J. Amer. Med. Ass. 166:126–129.*

Friedman, M. J., and Jaffe, H. J., 1969, A central hypothermic response to pilocarpine in the mouse, *J. Pharmacol. Exp. Ther. 167:34–44.*

Friedman, M. J., Jaffe, J. H., and Sharpless, S. K., 1969, Central nervous system supersensitivity to pilocarpine after withdrawal of chronically administered scopolamine, *J. Pharmacol. Exp. Ther. 167:45–55.*

Grinspoon, L., 1971, *Marihuana Reconsidered*, p. 246. Harvard University Press, Cambridge, Mass.

Haertzen, C. A., and Hooks, N. T., 1969, Changes in personality and subjective experience associated with the chronic administration of opiates, *J. Nerv. Ment. Dis. 148:606–614.*

Haizlip, T. M., and Ewing, J. A., 1958, Meprobamate habituation. A controlled clinical study, *New Engl. J. Med. 258:1181–1186.*

Hirschhorn, I. D., and Rosecrans, J. A., 1974, Morphine and Δ⁹-tetrahydrocannabinol: Tolerance to the stimulus effects, *Psychopharmacologia 36:243–253.*

Hollister, L. E., Motzenbecker, F. P., and Degan, R. O., 1961, Withdrawal reactions from chlordiazepoxide (Librium), *Psychopharmacologia 2:63–68.*

Hollister, L. E., Bennett, J. L., Kimbell, I., Savage, C., and Overall, J. E., 1963, Diazepam in newly admitted schizophrenics, *Dis. Nerv. System 24:746–750.*

Hunt, W. A., and Matarazzo, J. D., 1973, Three years later: Recent developments in the experimental modification of smoking behavior, *J. Abnorm. Psychol. 82:107–114.*

Isbell, H., 1959, Comparison of the reactions produced by psilocybin and LSD-25 in man, *Psychopharmacologia 1:29–38.*

Isbell, H., Altschul, S., Kornetsky, C. H., Eisenman, A. J., Flanary, H. G., and Fraser, H. F., 1950, Chronic barbiturate intoxication. An experimental study. *Arch Neurol. Psychiat.* (Chicago) *64:1–28.*

Isbell, H., Fraser, H. F., Wikler, A., Belleville, R. E., and Eiseman, A. J., 1955, An experimental study of the etiology of "rum fits" and delirium tremens. *Quart. J. Stud. Alcohol* *16*:1–33.

Isbell, H., Belleville, R. E., Fraser, H. F., Wikler, A., and Logan, C. R., 1956, Studies on lysergic acid diethylamide (LSD-25). I. Effects in former morphine addicts and development of tolerance during chronic intoxication, *Arch. Neurol. Psychiat. (Chicago)* *76*:468–478.

Isbell, H., Wolbach, A. B., Wikler, A., and Miner, E. J., 1961, Cross tolerance between LSD and psilocybin, *Psychopharamacologia* *2*:147–159.

Isbell, H., Rosenberg, D. E., Miner, E. J., and Logan, C. R., 1964, Tolerance and crosstolerance to scopolamine, N-ethyl-3-piperidyl benzylate (JB 318) and LSD-25, in *Neuropsychopharmacology*, Vol. 3 (P. B. Bradley, F. Flügel, and P. Hoch, Eds.), pp. 440–446. Elsevier, Amsterdam.

Itil, T. M., Ulett, G. A., Hsu, W., Klingenberg, H., and Ulett, J. A., 1971, The effects of smoking withdrawal on quantitatively analyzed EEG, *Clin. Electroencephalog.* *2*:44–51.

Jarvik, M. E., 1979, Biological influences on cigarette smoking, in *The Behavioral Aspects of Smoking* (N. A. Krasnegor, Ed.), NIDA Research Monogr. No. 26, DHEW Publication No. (ADM) 79–882, pp. 7–45. Superintendent of Documents, U.S. Government Printing Office, Washington, D.C.

Jones, R. R., and Farrell, T. R., 1978, Tobacco smoking and nicotine tolerance, in *Self-Administration of Abused Substances: Methods for Study* (N. A. Krasnegor, Ed.), NIDA Research Monogr. No. 20, pp. 202–208. Alcohol, Drug Abuse and Mental Health Administration, Printing and Publications Management Branch, Rockville, Maryland.

Jones, R. T., Benowitz, N., and Bachman, J., 1976, Clinical studies of cannabis tolerance and dependence, in *Chronic Cannabis Use. Annals of the New York Academy of Sciences*, Vol. 282 (R. L. Dornbush, A. M. Freedman, and M. Fink, Eds.), pp. 221–239. The New York Academy of Sciences, New York.

Kaim, S. C., and Klett, G. J., 1972, Treatment of delirium tremens. A comparison of four drugs, *Quart. J. Stud. Alcohol* *33*:1065–1072.

Kaymakcalan, S., 1973, Tolerance to and dependence on cannabis, *U.N. Bull. Narcotics* *25*:39–47.

Kaymakcalan, S., Ayhan, I. H., and Tulunay, F. C., 1977, Naloxone-induced or postwithdrawal abstinence signs in Δ^9-tetrahydrocannabinol-tolerant rats, Psychopharmacology 55:243–249.

Knapp, P. H., Bliss, C. M., and Wells, H., 1963, Addictive aspects in heavy cigarette smoking, *Amer. J. Psychiat. 119*:966–972.

Knott, V. J., and Venables, P. H., 1977, EEG alpha correlates of nonsmokers, smokers, smoking and smoking deprivation, *Psychophysiology 14*: 150–156.

Kramer, J. C., Fischman, V. S., and Littlefield, D. C., 1967, Amphetamine abuse: Pattern and effects of high doses taken intravenously, *J. Amer. Med. Ass. 201*:305–309.

Kreek, M. J., 1973, Medical safety and side effects of methadone in tolerant individuals, *J. Amer. Med. Ass. 223*:665–668.

Kurtz, S., 1969, *The New York Times Encyclopedic Almanac 1970*, p. 205. Book and Educational Division, The New York Times, New York.

Lemberger, L., Silberstein, S. D., Axelrod, J., and Kopin, I. J., 1970, Marihuana: Studies in the disposition of Δ^9-tetrahydrocannibinol in man, *Science 170*:1320–1322.

Lemberger, L., Tamarkin, N. R., Axelrod, J., and Kopin, I. J., 1971, Δ^9-tetrahydrocannabinol: Metabolism and disposition in long-term marihuana smokers, *Science 173*:72–74.

McGlothlin, W. H., 1979, Drugs and crime, in *Handbook on Drug Abuse* (R. I. DuPont, A.

Goldstein, and J. O'Donnell, Eds.), pp. 357–364. Superintendent of Documents, U.S. Government Printing Office, Washington, D.C.

McGlothlin, W. H., Anglin, M. D., and Wilson, B. D., 1977, *An Evaluation of the California Civil Addict Program*, NIDA Services Research Monogr. Series, DHEW Publ. No. (ADM) 78–558. U.S. Government Printing Office, Washington, D.C.

Martin, W. R., Jasinski, D. R., Haertzen, C. A., Kay, D. C., Jones, B. E., Mansky, P. A. and Carpenter, R. W., 1973, Methadone—a reevaluation, *Arch. Gen. Psychiat.* 28:782–791.

Miles, C. P., 1977, Conditions predisposing to suicide: A review, *J. Nerv. Ment. Dis.* 164:231–246.

Nurco, D. N., and DuPont, R. L., 1977, A preliminary report on crime and addiction within a community-wide population of narcotic addicts, *Drug Alcohol Dependence* 2:109–121.

O'Donnell, J. A., Voss, H. L., Clayton, R. R., Slatin, G. T., and Room, R. G., 1976, *Young Men and Drugs—A Nationwide Survey*, NIDA Research Monogr. Series 5, DHEW Publication No. (ADM) 76–311. National Technical Information Service, Springfield, Va. 22161.

Parry, H. J., 1979, Sample surveys of drug abuse, in *Handbook on Drug Abuse* (R. I. DuPont, A. Goldstein, and J. O'Donnell, Eds.), pp. 381–394. Superintendent of Documents, U.S. Government Printing Office, Washington, D.C. 20402.

Paton, W. D. M., 1968, Drug dependence: A sociopharmacological assessment, *Advan. Sci.* 25:200–212.

Petersen, R. C. (Ed.), 1978, *The International Challenge of Drug Abuse*, NIDA Research Monogr. No. 19, DHEW Publication No. (ADM) 78–654. Superintendent of Documents, U.S. Government Printing Office, Washington, D.C.

Petersen, R. C., and Stillman, R. C., 1978, Phencyclidine: An overview, in *Phencyclidine (PCP) Abuse: An Appraisal* (R. C. Petersen and R. C. Stillman, Eds.), NIDA Research Monogr. No. 21, pp. 1–17. U.S. Government Printing Office, Washington, D.C.

Pevnick, J. D., Jasinski, D. R., and Haertzen, C. A., 1978, Abrupt withdrawal from therapeutically administered diazepam, *Arch. Gen. Psychiat.* 35:995–998.

Pillard, R. C., 1970, Medical progress: marihuana, *New Engl. J. Med.* 283:294–303.

Pillard, R. C., 1971, Book review: *Marihuana Reconsidered* by L. Grinspoon, *New Engl. J. Med.* 285:416–417.

Resnick, R. B., Kestenbaum, R. S., and Schwartz, L. K., 1977, Acute systemic effects of cocaine in man: A controlled study by intranasal and intravenous routes, *Science* 195:696–698.

Robbins, P. R., and Nugent, J. F., 1975, Perceived consequences of addiction: A comparison between alcholics and heroin-addicted patients, *J. Clin, Psychol.* 31:367–369.

Robins, L. N., 1979, Addict careers, in *Handbook on Drug Abuse* (R. I. DuPont, A. Goldstein, and J. O'Donnell, Eds.), pp. 325–336. Superintendent of Documents, U.S. Government Printing Office, Washington, D.C.

Sapira, J. D., 1968, The narcotic-addict as a medical patient, *Amer. J. Med.* 45:555–588.

Sells, S. B., Chatham, L. R., and Retka, R. L., 1972, A study of differential death rates and causes of death among 9276 opiate addicts during 1970–1971, *Contemp. Drug Probl.* 1:665–706.

Shiffman, S. M., 1979, The tobacco withdrawal syndrome, in *Cigarette Smoking as a Dependence Process* (N. A. Krasnegor, Ed.), NIDA Research Monogr. Series No. 23, DHEW Publ. No. (ADM) 79–800, pp. 158–184. Alcohol, Drug Abuse, and Mental Health Administration, Printing and Publications Management Branch, Rockville, Maryland.

Siegel, R. K., 1978, Cocaine hallucinations, *Amer. J. Psychiat.* 135:309–314.

Soueif, M. I., 1967, Hashish consumption in Egypt, with special reference to psychosicial aspects, *U.N. Bull. Narcotics* 19:1–12.

Soueif, M. I., 1971, The use of cannabis in Egypt: A behavioural study, *U.N. Bull. Narcotics* 23:17–28.

Terry, C. E., and Pellens, M., 1928, *The Opium Problem.* Bureau of Social Hygiene, New York.

Thompson, W. L., Johnson, A. D., Maddrey, W. L., and the Osler Medical Housestaff, 1975, Diazepam and paraldehyde for treatment of severe delirium tremens. A controlled trial, *Ann. Int. Med.* 82:175–180.

Victor, M., 1976, Alcoholism, in *Clinical Neurology* (A. B. Baker and L. H. Baker, Eds.), Vol. 2, Chap. 22, pp. 1–43. Harper & Row, New York.

Victor, M., and Adams, R. D., 1953, The effect of alcohol on the nervous system, in *Metabolic and Toxic Diseases of the Nervous System* (H. H. Merritt and C. C. Hare, Eds.), Res. Publ. Ass. Nerv. Ment. Dis., Vol. 32, pp. 526–573. Williams & Wilkins, Baltimore.

Victor, M., and Brausch, C., 1967, The role of abstinence in the genesis of alcohol epilepsy, *Epilepsia (Amsterdam)* 8:1–20.

Wikler, A., 1952, A psychodynamic study of a patient during self-regulated readdiction to morphine, *Psychiat. Quart.* 26:270–293.

Wikler, A., 1968, Diagnosis and treatment of drug dependence of the barbiturate type, *Amer. J. Psychiat.* 125:758–765.

Wikler, A., 1974, The marijuana controversy, in *Marijuana. Effects on Human Behavior* (L. L. Miller, Ed.), Academic Press, New York.

Wikler, A., 1976, Aspects of tolerance and dependence on cannabis, in *Chronic Cannabis Use. Annals of the New York Academy of Sciences*, Vol. 282 (R. L. Dornbush, A. M. Freedman, and M. Fink, Eds.), pp. 125–147. The New York Academy of Sciences, New York.

Wikler, A., Williams, E. G., Douglass, E. D., Emmons, C. W., and Dunn, R. D., 1942, Mycotic endocarditis: Report of a case, *J. Amer. Med. Ass.* 119:33–36.

Wikler, A., Williams, E. G., and Wiesel, C. S., 1943, Monilemia associated with toxic purpura, *Arch. Neurol. Psychiat.* (Chicago) 50:661–668.

Wikler, A., Pescor, F. T., Fraser, H. F., and Isbell, H., 1956, Electroencephalographic changes associated with chronic alcoholic intoxication and the alcohol abstinence syndrome, *Amer. J. Psychiat.* 113:106–114.

Winokur, A., Rickels, K., Greenblatt, D. J., Snyder, P. J., and Schatz, N. J., 1980, Withdrawal reaction from long-term, low-dosage administration of diazepam, *Arch. Gen. Psychiat.* 37:101–105.

Wolbach, A. B., Miner, E. J. and Isbell, H., 1962a, Comparison of psilocin with psilocybin, mescaline and LSD-25, *Psychopharmacologia* 3:219–223.

Wolbach, A. B., Isbell, H., and Miner, E. J., 1962b, Cross tolerance between mescaline and LSD-25, with a comparison of the mescaline and LSD reactions, *Psychopharmacologia* 3:1–14.

World Almanac and Book of Facts, 1979. Newspaper Enterprise Association, Inc., New York.

Wulff, M. H., 1959, The barbiturate withdrawal syndrome. A clinical and electroencephalographic study, *Electroenceph. Clin. Neurophysiol.* Suppl. 14:1–173.

CHAPTER 2

The Etiology of Opioid Dependence

DEFINITIONS AND DYNAMICS

The World Health Organization Expert Committee on Addiction-Producing Drugs (1964) defined drug dependence as

> ... a state of psychic or physical dependence, or both, on a drug, arising in a person following administration of that drug on a periodic or continuous basis. The characteristics of such a state will vary with the agent involved, and these characteristics must always be made clear by designating the particular type of drug dependence in each specific case; for example, drug dependence of the morphine type, of cocaine type, of cannabis type, of barbiturate type, of amphetamine type, etc.

Common to all of these types of drug dependence is the concept of "psychic" or "psychological" dependence, which is defined as a drive that requires administration of the drug to produce pleasure or to avoid discomfort (Eddy et al., 1970). Psychic dependence is usually distinguished from "physical" dependence, which is inferred from the appearance of drug-specific, transient abstinence phenomena (autonomic and behavioral) when the drug is withdrawn abruptly. However, as Eddy et al. (1970) pointed out, physical dependence is a powerful factor in reinforcing the influence of psychic dependence. It would seem that the main distinction between psychic and physical dependence is that the former is a vaguely defined cluster of inferences derived from subjective reports of the subject, while the latter is inferred from objective changes in his autonomic nervous system and his behavior. In an attempt to avoid this subjective–objective dichotomy, Wikler (1971) defined drug dependence as drug acquisitive behavior, that is, nonmedical drug-seeking and drug-using behavior that is contingent on pharmacological reinforcement and is resistant to extinction or suppression. Sources of pharmacological reinforcement are classified as *direct* and *indirect*. Direct pharmocological reinforcement (including some of the usages of psychic dependence) consists of interactions between the drug and organismic variables that have *not* been generated by the drug itself, such as the effects of morphine on certain appetitively reinforcing areas in the brain (median forebrain bundle, locus ceruleus) that the human drug-user interprets as a "high" (Wikler, 1973b; Esposito & Kornetsky, 1977; Kornetsky, 1979), and a reduction of presumably antecedent hypophoria and anxiety (Wikler, 1973a, 1975). Indirect pharmacological reinforcement (including the current usage of physical dependence) consists of interactions between the drug and organismic variables that *have* been generated by the drug itself. Thus, distressing drug-withdrawal syndromes are promptly alleviated by renewed administration of the drug in question, and it is presumed that such "need reduction" has powerful, appetitively reinforcing effects (Wikler, 1973a,b, 1975). Physical dependence has long been recognized as a feature of dependence on opioids, barbiturates (also nonbarbiturate sedatives and "minor tranquilizers"), and alcohol; with heavy, long-continued use, physical dependence can also develop to marijuana and other cannabis preparations, to amphetamines, and to tobacco; whether or not physical dependence develops to cocaine is a question partly dependent on one's definition of *physical*; apparently, no physical dependence develops to the hallucinogen LSD. Also reinforcing may be the arousal state induced by these drugs (stimulants, hallucinogens, tobacco, and, to some extent, low doses of opioids, short-acting barbiturates, and alcohol) before physical dependence has developed, as well as the arousal state associated with "hustling" for illegal drugs after the user has become physically dependent (Wikler, 1977). Another feature of drug dependence is the phenomenon of tolerance, which is the progressive decrease in the effects of a given dose of a drug upon repeated administration of that dose, and the necessity of increasing the doses (up to a limit) in order to regain all or some of the original effect. For the same drug, tolerance may develop at different rates and to different degrees for different effects. *Reverse tolerance* refers to sensitization to a given drug upon repeated administration. Given appropriate drug–environmental stimulus contingencies, psychic dependence, physical dependence, arousal, "hustling," and tolerance may be exteroceptively and/or interoceptively conditioned (see below).

A variety of animal species including man can become physically dependent on morphine and other opioids by receiving the drug *passively* in sufficient amounts over a sufficient period of time, and they display abstinence phenomena when the drug is withheld (Krueger *et al.*, 1941, 1943). However, such passive recipients of opioids may or may not display *opioid-acquisitive behavior* (the common characteristic of all drug dependencies), despite the presence of opioid-abstinence phenomena. In hospitals, many patients receive morphine or other opioids for relief of temporary pain and have abstinence phenomena (which are usually unrecognized as such) when the analgesic drug is discontinued; the majority of these patients do not seek opioids, although some of them do (Rayport, 1954). Lindesmith (1947) has contended that the human opioid user becomes an "addict" and regards himself as such when he makes a cognitive connection between administration of the drug and relief of his withdrawal distress. Apparently, the chimpanzee can also make such a "cognitive connection," since Spragg (1940) reported that although initially it evinced no interest in morphine given intramuscularly by the experimenter, it spontaneously assumed the posture for injection of the drug when the latter was withheld and the chimpanzee was displaying abstinence phenomena. Most beagle dogs will not self-administer morphine through an implanted intravenous catheter when they are not physically dependent, but after they have been made physically dependent by repeated passive intravenous injections of morphine and are displaying abstinence phenomena when the drug is withheld, they will learn to self-administer morphine intravenously and maintain their addiction; after removal from the experimental cage and subsidence of the morphine-abstinence syndrome, return to the experimental cage up to six months later results in prompt relapse to intravenous self-administration of morphine (Jones & Prada, 1973). Opioid-acquisitive behavior is manifested by rats and monkeys equipped for intravenous self-administration of drugs even in the absence of overt opioid-abstinence phenomena (Schuster & Villareal, 1968; Schuster & Thompson, 1969). Such drug-acquisitive behavior in animals is manifested also for certain nonopioid drugs such as amphetamine, cocaine, nicotine, pentobarbital, and alcohol, indicating that these drugs, like opioids, are appetitively reinforcing; on the other hand, animals will not self-administer mescaline, nalorphine, or chlorpromazine (Schuster & Thompson, 1969). In the case of opioids, Esposito and Kornetsky (1977) have reported that in the rat, the threshold for electrical self-stimulation of appetitively reinforcing areas in the brain is lowered by morphine, and that no tolerance to this effect develops during chronic morphine administration. Equating the lowering of the threshold for appetitive electrical reinforcement in rats with the subjective report of pleasure (euphoria) in man, Kornetsky (1979) has argued that human opioid dependence (as well as some other drug dependencies) is based on the long-continued hedonistic effects of the drug. However, most heroin addicts state that the effects of the *first* dose of heroin they ever took were unpleasant (nausea, vomiting, dizziness, fainting), and that only after repeated self-administration under "peer" pressure did they become euphoric (Wikler, 1975). With the development of tolerance and physical dependence, the prevailing mood of the opioid addict becomes *dysphoric* (Wikler, 1952; Haertzen & Hooks, 1969; Martin *et al.*, 1973), although he may continue to experience a transient "thrill" or "rush" following intravenous self-injection of heroin (Wikler, 1952; McAuliffe & Gordon, 1974). Therefore, the long-persistent lowering of the threshold for appetitive electrical reinforcement in the rat can be dissociated from the less persistent hedonic effects of opioids in man. As already noted, physical dependence on opioids can provide a source of "indirect" pharmacological appetitive reinforcement of opioid-acquisitive behavior through prevention or suppression of abstinence phenomena, in addition to "direct" pharmacological reinforcement through excitation of appetitively reinforcing areas in the brain.

Equally important in maintaining drug-acquisitive behavior is *operant conditioning*, the essential requirements for which have already been mentioned, namely, self-administration of the drug and the appetitively reinforcing pharmacological effects of the latter. In the United States, the vast majority of opioid addicts begin and continue their use of the drug (usually heroin) by self-injection in emulation of their drug-using peers in the "street-corner society" (Clausen, 1957a,b; Brown *et al.*, 1971). It should be noted that heroin self-injection is only one of innumerable behaviors that have been and are reinforced, appetitively and aversively, in the developing heroin addict. He does things to obtain food and other necessities, to gain approval by his friends, to avoid the police, etc. Though these behaviors are not under experimental control, they may be viewed as instances of operant conditioning, with particular (sometimes varying) reinforcement schedules of their own. Just what such reinforcement schedules may be and how they may affect the reinforcers are unknown, but it is conceivable that despite the initially aversive pharmacological effects of heroin (nausea, etc.), the drug may be transformed into an appetitive reinforcer through interactions among schedules of reinforcement, quite independently of its "direct" and "indirect" appetitively reinforcing pharmacological properties. Thus, McKearney (1968) found that monkeys can be trained to respond for delivery of electric shock to the skin on a 10-min fixed-interval schedule by superimposing this schedule on a previous electric-shock-postponement schedule and subsequently eliminating the latter. Kelleher and Morse (1968, Experiment III) reported that in a monkey previously trained on a 2-min variable-interval food reinforcement schedule, concurrent imposition of a 10-min fixed-interval electric shock presentation schedule followed immediately by a 1-min fixed-ratio 1 schedule (in which each response produced electric shock) resulted, after elimination of the 2-min food reinforcement schedule and allowing the monkey free access to food in its living cage, in accelerated responding for delivery of electric shock in the 10-min fixed-interval schedule and in suppression of responding during the immediately following 1-min fixed-ratio 1 schedule. In other words, the same stimulus, electric shock, could act as an appetitive reinforcer and as an aversive reinforcer concurrently in the same animal, depending on the history of schedules of reinforcement and on the reinforcement schedules operating at any given time. If the monkey could talk, it would come as no surprise to hear it say that electric shock was "painful" (during the electric-shock-postponement or 1-min fixed-ratio 1 schedule) and also that it was "pleasurable" (during the 10-min fixed-ratio schedules). Perhaps such a transformation of reinforcing properties through operant conditioning also helps explain the persistent self-administration (through various routes) of hallucinogens, including phencyclidine, in man, though the "rewards" of the psychoses they produce are a mystery.

Self-administration of heroin (or other opioids) in man is associated in a unique and frequent manner with certain environmental variables, such as drug-using peers, "pushers," and the relative availability of illegal drugs. In time, these environmental variables acquire the properties of discriminative stimuli in operant conditioning, providing occasions for renewed self-administration of the drug. At the same time, the same environmental variables are uniquely and frequently paired with the pharmacological effects of heroin, which, after physical dependence has developed, become cyclic, early abstinence phenomena following the initial narcotic action. In consequence of such repeated pairings, the pharmacological effects of heroin become *classically conditioned* to these environmental stimuli, which, in time, acquire the property of eliciting fragments of heroin narcotic action and of the heroin abstinence syndrome, long after the unconditioned effects of heroin, including the heroin abstinence syndrome, have been dissipated. It might be remarked that both operant and classical conditioning proceed without awareness in the opioid addict. These conditioning processes, the evidence pertaining thereto, and their relation to relapse will be discussed more fully in Chapter 7. As a result of such conditioning processes, opioid dependence in the "street addict" (in whom these conditioning factors are most likely to operate) is not merely a "symptom" of disturbed personality and/or social environment but constitutes a "disease, *sui generis,*" or an "artificially induced drive" (Bejerot, 1972), generated by complex interactions involving the pharmacological actions of the drug, the personality of the drug user, the self-administration of the drug, and the environmental features that are associated with procuring and self-administering the drug.

PERSONALITY STUDIES

Hill *et al.* (1960) found that the great majority of long-detoxified opioid addicts at the USPHS Hospital in Lexington, Kentucky, showed significant elevations on the psychopathic and neurotic scales of the Minnesota Multiphasic Personality Inventory (MMPI). At the same institution, addict physicians also exhibited elevations, though less marked, on the psychopathic and neurotic scales, whereas the MMPIs of an extrainstitutional control group of nonaddict physicians were within the normal range (Hill *et al.*, 1968). Applying the Lexington Personality Inventory in a study on detoxified opioid addicts at the clinical research centers in Lexington, Kentucky, and Fort Worth, Texas, Monroe *et al.* (1971) found evidence of characterological disorder (psychopathy or sociopathy) in 42%, emotional disturbance in 29%, and thinking disorder in 22%; only 7% were asymptomatic. However, personality studies on groups other than detoxified opioid addicts have revealed similar abnormalities. Thus, Hill *et al.* (1962) found significant elevations on the psychopathic scale of the MMPI in institutionalized chronic alcoholics and in institutionalized juvenile delinquents who were neither opioid addicts nor alcoholics. In their nationwide survey of young men and drugs (*all classes*), O'Donell *et al.* (1976) found that high scores on a "Total Drug Use Index" were associated with lower age, failure to complete a started education (whether high school or college), lack of a stable marital situation, criminal activities, and acceptance of unconventional behavior. Similarly, in a study on Vietnam veterans, Robins *et al.* (1977) found that a "Youthful Liability Scale," composed of items ascertainable before the soldiers went to Vietnam, was well correlated with heroin use in Vietnam ($r = 0.47$): the men who used heroin were just those especially exhibiting adjustment problems even before they used heroin. Apparently, deviant behavior at an early age is characteristic not only of the half million or so heroin users but also of the millions of nonopioid drug users in the United States.

Martin *et al.* (1977) have proposed that detoxified opioid addicts and long-abstaining chronic alcoholics have increased "need states" that give rise to impulsivity, egocentricity, and feelings of hypophoria. In a study of these two experimental groups and a control group consisting of students or faculty members of a religious college and seminary, it was found that compared with the control group, the experimental groups had significantly elevated plasma levels of luteinizing hormone and testosterone (but not of follicle-stimulating hormone), as well as significantly elevated scores on the psychopathic deviate, hypomania, and depression scales of the MMPI, and on the impulsivity, egocentricity, need, and sociopathy subscales of a maturation scale that the investigators devised. All items in the maturation scale where phrased in the present tense. The need subscale consisted of items referring to sexual desire, hunger, body health, pain, and general wanting; the impulsivity subscale to thoughtlessness and uninhibited behavior; the egocentricity subscale to selfishness, inability to love, and callousness; and the hypophoria subscale to a generally negative perception of life, poor self-image, feelings of inefficiency or ineptness, withdrawal from competition, worry, anger, and feelings of being disrespected, disapproved of, and unappreciated. In connection with Martin *et al.*'s (1977) hypothesis that detoxified opioid addicts (as well as abstaining chronic alcoholics) have increased needs, it is interesting to note that plasma testosterone levels *decline* during chronic heroin use (Mendelson and Mello, 1975) and during methadone maintenance (Cicero *et al.*, 1975); and that actively addicted opioid addicts report decreased sexual desire and poor sexual performance due to delayed ejaculation, failure to ejaculate, or impotence (Cicero *et al.*, 1975). It would seem that if chronic use of heroin is indeed a response to an increased need (for sexual intercourse), it overfulfills its purpose.

SOCIOENVIRONMENTAL STUDIES

Sociological studies (Clausen, 1957a,b; Chein *et al.*, 1964) have revealed that the great majority of adolescent opioid users live in metropolitan slum areas characterized by the lowest socioeconomic status, large minority populations, instability of family life, and high incidence of other social problems. In such areas, illegal drugs of all sorts are more readily available than elsewhere. More of the youthful population are members of the street-corner society, the antisocial attitudes of which include permissiveness or even encouragement of drug use. In a study by Brown *et al.* (1971), the "influence of friends" was the major reason given by juvenile male addicts for their first use of heroin; "curiosity" was also mentioned prominently; and "relief of personal disturbances" and "seeking a high" were mentioned much less often. In contrast, "friends" had nothing to do with initial or subsequent attempts to discontinue heroin self-administration. The main reasons for initial withdrawal from heroin were drug-related physical problems and the intention to change their overall life patterns, which had become self-demeaning and futile. Brown *et al.* (1971) concluded that heroin addiction may be more of a response to meet the pathology of the community than the pathology of the individual.

As Clausen (1957a,b) and Chein *et al.* (1964) pointed out, the social orientation of metropolitan slum-dwellers, with its rejection of conventional middle-class standards, distrust of the police and other law-enforcement officers, and less condemnatory attitudes toward drug abuse, applies to the nonaddict population as well as to addicts. Gerard and Kornetsky (1955) found that half of a control (nonaddict) sample from a New York slum area showed evidence of psychiatric disorder, though the addict sample was more severely disturbed. These findings raise the question of appropriate controls for the personality studies reviewed above. Ideally, such controls should consist of the *nonaddict siblings* of addicts, born of the same parents and reared in the same environment. To the author's knowledge, no such studies have been published.

MODE OF SPREAD OF OPIOID DEPENDENCE

As Bejerot (1972) has emphasized, opioid and other drug addictions starting in the street-corner society are "contagious"; that is, one or more addicts introduce another person or persons into addiction, and the newly recruited addicts do likewise. This process gives rise to "epidemic addictions" that spread throughout the country and internationally. The high profits in the illegal drug trade assure a supply for the increased demand. Increased efforts on the part of authorities to curtail the drug supply may temporarily reduce the size of the epidemic, but it cannot be eliminated as long as the mode of contagion continues unchanged. Bejerot (1972) has proposed that chronic street addicts be removed to an area remote from large cities and be given their drug under medical supervision as long as they remain there, or voluntarily undergo drug withdrawal. Epidemic addiction is distinguished from occasional use of nonmedically indicated chemical agents, from single addictions occurring in medical treatment for relief of pain in patients with incurable illnesses or in dying patients, from addictions inadvertently but rarely caused by medical treatment, from self-established addictions in persons whose professions give them easy access to drugs, and from "endemic addictions" that are socially accepted, such as alcoholism in Europe and the United States, cannabis use in parts of Asia and North Africa, and coca chewing among South American Indians.

PROGNOSIS

Winick (1962, 1965) reported that the rate at which names were dropped from the file of active addicts maintained by the former Federal Bureau of Narcotics increased sharply between the ages of 35 and 40 years; this finding suggests that, in some cases at least, "maturation" may lead to abstention from opioid drugs with or without formal treatment and despite earlier relapses. Winick (1965) estimated that the average total addiction period was 8.6 years, only 7% of opioid addicts having records extending over a period of 15 years or more. In a test of this maturation hypothesis, Ball and Snarr (1969) found that of 108 males residing in Puerto Rico who had been treated for heroin addiction as the USPHS Hospital in Lexington, Kentucky, 23 had abstained from opioids during the 3-year period before they were interviewed, while 85 were either in prison or using opioids continually or intermittently. The mean age at interview was 38.8 years for those who had abstained from opioid use, and it was 39.3 years for the others. Ball and Snarr (1969) concluded that the maturation hypothesis might be valid for 23 of the 108 patients. The prognosis was worst in those who began opioid use at 16 or 17 years of age, while cure was most likely in those who began opioid use at age 32 years (Zahn & Ball, 1972).

A better prognosis appears to apply to Vietnam war veterans who were addicted to heroin in Vietnam. (Robins et al., 1977; Robins, 1979). A sample of 900 veterans were interviewed by Robins et al. (1977), 8–12 months after their return from Vietnam, and 617 were reinterviewed three years after their return from Vietnam. About 20% of the original sample reported themselves to have been addicted to heroin in Vietnam, but only 1% reported readdiction during the first year, and 2% in the second or third year, after returning from Vietnam. Of all the men addicted to heroin in Vietnam, only 12% had relapsed to heroin addiction at any time during the three years following their return (however, Figure 4 in Robins et al., 1977, shows an additional 23% "used heroin regularly" during the same period). Robins, and her co-workers (1977) pointed out that heroin users are polydrug users of an extreme kind, smoking marijuana and taking amphetamines and barbiturates as well as self-administering heroin, and that despite heroin's reputation as a rapidly addicting drug, heroin users, after their return from Vietnam, were able to take the drug without becoming dependent and to discontinue taking it at will.

The relatively low incidence of relapse to heroin among returning Vietnam veterans who were addicted to heroin in Vietnam may be a consequence of their detoxification *in Vietnam* just before they were returned to the United States—a procedure prescribed by the Department of Defense under the urging of the head of the Special Action Office, Jerome H. Jaffe, M.D. (Robins *et al.*, 1977). The removal of the detoxified soldiers from Vietnam ensured also the removal of the conditioned reinforcers and other environmental stimuli to which heroin self-administration and the cyclic pharmacological effects of heroin had become conditioned. In the United States, the already-detoxified soldiers had no need to come into contact with drug-associated environmental stimuli such as addicts, active or under treatment, or drug-abuse treatment facilities. Hence, the probability of their relapse would be minimized, except to the extent that they had formed such relationships *before* they were inducted into the armed forces and sent to Vietnam. In connection with this explanation, it is interesting to note that in the study of Robins *et al.* (1977), it is mentioned that the Youthful Liability Scale correlated fairly well ($r = 0.28$) with heroin use in the last two years of the three-year period following the return of the soldiers from Vietnam. It would also be interesting to know the relationship between nonuse of heroin after return from Vietnam and Youthful Liability Scale scores among soldiers who had been addicted to heroin in Vietnam.

REFERENCES

Ball, J. C., and Snarr, R. W., 1969, A test of the maturation hypothesis with respect to opiate addiction, *U. N. Bull. Narcotics* 21:9–13.

Bejerot, N., 1972, *Addiction: An Artifically Induced Drive.* Charles C Thomas, Springfield, Ill.

Brown, B. S., Gauvey, S. K., Meyers, M. B., and Stark, S. D., 1971, In their own words: Addicts' reasons for initiating and withdrawing from heroin, *Int. J. Addictions, 6:635–645.*

Chein, I., Gerard, D. L., Lee, R. S., and Rosenfeld, E., 1964, *The Road to H. Narcotics, Deliquency and Social Policy.* Basic Books, Inc., New York.

Cicero, T. J., Bell, R. D., Wiest, W. G., Allison, J. H., Polakoski, K., and Robins, E., 1975, Function of the male sex organs in heroin and methadone users, *New Engl. J. Med.* 292:882–887.

Clausen, J. A., 1957a, Social and psychological factors in narcotic addiction, *Law and Contemporary Problems* 22 (*Winter*):34–51.

Clausen, J. A., 1957b, Social patterns, personality and adolescent drug use, in *Explorations in Social Psychiatry* (A. H. Leighton, J. A. Clausen, and R. N. Wilson, Eds.), pp. 232–272. Basic Books, Inc., New York.

Eddy, N. B., Halbach, H., Isbell, H., and Seevers, M. H., 1970, Drug dependence: Its significance and characteristics in *Drug Abuse: Data and Debate* (P. H. Blachly, Ed.), Appendix A, pp. 259–282. Charles C Thomas, Springfield, Ill.

Esposito, K., and Kornetsky, C., 1977, Morphine lowering of self-stimulation thresholds: Lack of tolerance with chronic administration, *Science* 195:189–191.

Gerard, D. L., and Kornetsky, C., 1955, Adolescent opiate addiction: A study of control and addict subjects, *Psychiat. Quart.* 29:457–489.

Haertzen, C. A., and Hooks N. T., 1969, Changes in personality and subjective experience associated with the chronic administration and withdrawal of opiates, *J. Nerv. Ment. Dis.* 148:606–614.

Hill, H. E., Haertzen, C. A., and Glaser, R., 1960, Personality characteristics of narcotic addicts as indicated by the MMPI, 1960, *J. Gen. Psychol.* 62:127–139.

Hill, H. E., Haertzen, C. A., and Davis, H., 1962, An MMPI factor analytic study of alcoholics, narcotic addicts and criminals, *Quart. J. Stud. Alcohol* 23:411–431.

Hill, H. E., Haertzen, C. A., and Yamahiro, R. S., 1968, The addict physician: A Minnesota Multiphasic Personality Inventory of the interaction of personality characteristics and availability of narcotics, in *The Addictive States*, Res. Publ. Ass. Nerv. Ment. Dis. Vol. 46 (A. Wikler, ed.), pp. 321–332. Williams & Wilkins, Baltimore.

Jones, B. E., and Prada, J. A., 1973, Relapse to morphine use in dog, *Psychopharmacologia* 30:1–12.

Kelleher, R. T., and Morse, W. H., 1968, Schedules using noxious stimuli. III. Responding maintained with response-produced electric shocks, *J. Exp. Anal. Behav.* 11:819–838.

Kornetsky, C., 1979, Intracranial self-stimulation thresholds: A model for the hedonic effects of drugs of abuse, *Arch. Gen. Psychiat.* 36:289–292.

Krueger, H., Eddy, N. B., and Sumwalt, M., 1941, *The Pharmacology of the Opium Alkalokds*, Part 1, Supplement No 165 to the Public Health Reports. Superintendent of Documents, U.S. Government Printing Office, Washington, D.C.

Krueger, H., Eddy, N. B., and Sumwalt, M., 1943, *The Pharmacology of the Opium Alkaloids*, Part 2, Supplement No. 165 to the Public Health Reports. Superintendent of Documents, U.S. Government Printing Office, Washington, D.C.

Lindesmith, A. R., 1947, *Opiate Addiction*. Principia Press, Bloomington, Ind.

Martin, W. R., Jasinski, D. R., Haertzen, C. A., Kay, D. C., Jones, B. E., Mansky, P. A., and Carpenter, R. W., 1973, Methadone—A reevaluation, *Arch. Gen. Psychiat.* 28:286–295.

Martin, W. R., Hewett, B. B., Baker, A. J., and Haertzen, C. A., 1977, Aspects of the psychopathology and pathophysiology of addiction, *Drug and Alcohol Dependence* 2:185–202.

McAuliffe, W. E., and Gordon, R. W., 1974, A test of Lindesmith's theory of addiction: The frequency of euphoria among long-term addicts, *Amer. J. Sociol.* 79:795–840.

McKearney, J. W., 1968, Maintenance of responding under a fixed-interval schedule of electric shock presentation. *Science* 160:1249–1251.

Mendelson, J. H., and Mello, N. K., 1975, Plasma testosterone levels during chronic heroin use and protracted abstinence: As study of Hong Kong addicts, *Clin. Pharmacol. Ther.* 17:529–533.

Monroe, J. J., Ross, W. R., and Berzins, J. I., 1971, The decline of the addict as "psychopath": Implications for community care, *Int. J. Addictions* 6:601–608.

O'Donnell, J. A., Voss, H. L., Clayton, R. R., Slatin, G. T., and Room, R. G., 1976, *Young*

Men and Drugs—A Nationwide Survey, NIDA Research Monogr. Series 5, DHEW Publication No. (ADM) 76-311. National Technical Information Service, Springfield, Virginia 22161.

Rayport, M., 1954, Experience in the management of patients medically addicted to narcotics, *J. Amer. Med. Ass. 156*:684–691.

Robins, L. N., 1979, Addict careers, *in Handbook on Drug Abuse* (R. I. DuPont, A. Goldstein, and J. O'Donnell, Eds.), pp. 325–336. Superintendent of Documents, U.S. Government Printing Office, Washington, D.C.

Robins, L. N., Helzer, J. E., Hesselbrock, M., and Wish, E., 1977, reported to the Committee on Problems of Drug Dependence at its 39th annual scientific meeting in Cambridge, Massachusetts.

Schuster, C. R., and Thompson, T., 1969, Self-administration of and behavioral dependence on drugs, *Annual Rev. Pharmacol. 9*:483–502.

Schuster, C. R., and Villareal, J. E., 1968, The experimental analysis of opioid dependence, *in Psychopharmacology: A Review of Progress 1957–1967* (D. H. Efron, Ed.), pp. 811–828. Public Health Service Publication No 1836, Superintendent of Documents, U.S. Government Printing Office, Washington D.C.

Spragg, S. D. S., 1940, *Morphine Addiction in Chimpanzees*, Comparative Psychology Mongr. No. 15, pp. 1–238. Johns Hopkins Press, Baltimore, Maryland.

WHO Expert Committee on Addiction-Producing Drugs, 1964, World Health Organization Technical Report Series, No. 273:1–20, Geneva (p. 9).

Wikler, A., 1952, A psychodynamic study of a patient during self-regulated readdiction to morphine, *Psychiat. Quart. 26*:270–293.

Wikler, A., 1971, Present status of the concept of drug dependence, *Psychol. Med. (London) 1*:377–380.

Wikler, A., 1973a, Conditioning of successive adaptive responses to the initial effects of drugs, *Conditional Reflex 8*:193–210.

Wikler, A., 1973b, Dynamics of drug dependence: Implications of a conditioning theory for research and treatment, *Arch. Gen. Psychiat. 28*:611–616.

Wikler, A., 1975, Opioid antagonists and deconditioning in addiction treatment, *in Drug Dependence–Treatment and Treatment Evaluation* (H. Boström, T. Larsson, and N. Ljungstedt, Eds.), Symposium October 15–17, 1974, pp. 157–182. Skandia International Symposia, Almqvist and Wiksell International, Stockholm.

Wikler, A., 1977, Footnote No. 2 to presentation of paper, *in Common Processes in Habitual Substance Use: A Research Agenda. Appendix C: Proceedings, Conference on Commonalities in Substance Abuse and Habitual Behavior*, pp. 395–397. National Academy of Sciences, Washington, D.C.

Winick, C., 1962, Maturing out of narcotic addiction, *U.N. Bull. Narcotics 14*:1–7.

Winick, C., 1965, Epdemiology of narcotics use, *in Narcotics* (D. M. Wilner and G. G. Kassebaum, Eds.) McGraw-Hill, New York.

Zahn, M. A., and Ball, J. C., 1972, Factors related to cure of opiate addiction among Puerto Rican addicts, *Int. J. Addictions 7*:237–245.

CHAPTER 3

Opioid Analgesics and Opioid Antagonists

OPIOID ANALGESICS

By *opioid* is meant any drug, regardless of chemical structure, that acts like morphine. The term *opioid* is preferred to the older term, *opiate*, for two reasons: first, because *opiate* implies presence in or derivation from opium, which indeed contains the analgesic drugs morphine and codeine but also contains thebaine, a strong stimulant (convulsive) drug with minimal analgesic properties, and also papaverine and noscapine, which have no analgesic actions; and second, because of a host of purely synthetic drugs with actions qualitatively similar to those of morphine and codeine that, unlike the analgesics found in opium or derived therefrom, lack the phenanthrene nucleus (e.g., methadone, meperidine, *d*-propoxyphene). Opium is prepared from the sap of the poppy *Papaver somniferum* and contains about 10% by weight of morphine and about 0.5% by weight of codeine. Analgesic compounds that are derived from morphine and that retain the phenanthrene nucleus and are classed as opioids include heroin (diacetylmorphine), hydromorphone (Dilaudid), oxymorphone (Numorphan), and oxycodone (Percodan). Purely synthetic analgesic compounds that lack the phenanthrene nucleus but are classed as opioids include methadone (Dolophine), meperidine (Demerol), *d*-propoxyphene (Darvon), levorphanol (Levo-Dromoran), and phenazocine (Prinadol). In man, the analgesic potencies of these drugs relative to morphine (all drugs given *subcutaneously*) are codeine, one-twelfth; heroin, 2–3 times; hydromorphine, 6–8 times; oxymorphone,

7–10 times; oxycodone, two-thirds to equipotent; methadone, equipotent; meperidine, one-tenth to one-eighth; levorphanol, 2–3 times; and phenazocine, 3 times. By the oral route, 65 mg of d-propoxyphene is equivalent to 32–45 mg of codeine for analgesia, but 32 mg of d-propoxyphene may be no more effective than placebo. A newer synthetic compound, pentazocine (Talwin), exerts some morphinelike effects (analgesia, respiratory depression, sedation) in doses of 30–50 mg given parenterally (equivalent to 10 mg of morphine) or of 50 mg given orally (equivalent to 60 mg of codeine); at higher doses, pentazocine also produces dysphoric and psychotomimetic effects that can be reversed by naloxone, but not by nalorphine. In addition, pentazocine has weak opioid-antagonistic actions and can precipitate abstinence phenomena in morphine-dependent individuals. Though not in clinical use, etorphine (Immobilon), an opioid derived from oripavine and ultimately from thebaine, is of interest because of its extreme potency. In man, it is about 400 times as potent as morphine, though its duration of action is much shorter; in animals, its potency is even greater than in man, and it is used for immobilizing large game animals (Harthoorn & Bligh, 1965). Although of all these opioid analgesics, heroin is the most widely abused in the United States, its pharmacological effects (including the development of tolerance and physical dependence) do not differ *qualitatively* from those of morphine. The same is true also of hydromorphone, oxymorphone, oxycodone, levorphanol, phenazocine, and methadone, but the pharmacological effects of meperidine, d-propoxyphene, and pentazocine present more prominent differences with regard to "toxicity" and/or physical dependence. The pharmacological effects of morphine serve here as a prototype of the actions of opioids in general, and deviations from this prototype are noted for some particular opioid analgesics.

Morphine

Effects of Single Doses in the Nontolerant State

In nontolerant human subjects, single doses of morphine (10–15 mg) typically produce analgesia, with variable changes in mood, pupillary constriction (miosis), slowing of respiratory rate and minute volume, lowering of rectal temperature, decrease in systolic and diastolic blood pressure, bradycardia, nausea, emesis and faintness (partially on arising suddenly from the recumbent position), spasm of smooth muscle sphincters and delayed peristalsis (resulting in constipation), inhibition of diuresis, and mild hyperglycemia. In some persons, morphine produces a feeling of "mental clouding" (Smith & Beecher, 1959), with little impairment of performance on psychometric tests, except those in which speed is required (Smith *et al.*, 1962). Rarely, some individuals exhibit an atypical reaction to morphine (and other opioids): widely dilated pupils (mydriasis) and excitement and delirium (so-called cat reaction). In drug-free former opioid addicts ("postaddicts"), single doses of morphine produce the typical effects already noted; in addition, some special features have been observed that may or may not be exhibited by nonaddicted individuals. Postaddicts (not in pain) uniformly report "a sense of unusual well-being" and affirm the items in the Morphine–Benzedrine Group (MBG) Scale (Jasinski, 1973) that express "euphoric" reactions common to morphine and amphetamine. In some postaddicts, such "euphoria" is accompanied by nausea, vomiting, and ghastly pallor, which may alarm the observer, but the subjects refer to these apparently distressing reactions as "a good sick." Some subjects may "go on the nod" (sitting in a chair or lying in bed, gazing at a newspaper or telecast while dozing and rousing in alternation), while others may "drive" (talking incessantly, boasting, and busying themselves with "things that need to be done"); or they may "nod" and "drive" alternately, depending on the social situation. Itching of the skin, with attendant rubbing and scratching (e.g., of the nose), is a common effect and is regarded as pleasurable by postaddicts. When morphine is administered intravenously, postaddicts report two additional sensations: a "pins-and-needles" sensation, accompanying intense flushing of the skin, and a "thrill" lasting a minute or so, which they often compare with sexual orgasm, though it is referred to the abdomen rather than to the genitalia and is not accompanied by ejaculation. Male postaddicts report that in the nontolerant state, single doses of morphine delay ejaculation but do not impair penile erection, though sexual desire may be inhibited (Wikler, 1952a). In postaddicts, single doses of morphine produce occasional slow waves and slight slowing of alpha frequencies in the waking electroencephalogram (Andrews, 1943; Wikler, 1954); during nocturnal sleep, the number and duration of rapid eye movement (REM) periods is decreased, those of spontaneous awakenings and light sleep (Stages 1 and 2) are increased, and those of deep sleep (Stages 3 and 4) are decreased (Kay *et al.*, 1969).

The nature of the analgesia and mood alteration produced by single doses of morphine as well as the mechanisms involved therein are discussed in detail in Chapter 5. In brief, morphine analgesia appears to be part of a more general effect, namely, production of "indifference" to or "detachment" from the anticipated consequences of ongoing internal and external stimuli; the more variable mood-altering effects appear to depend on the presence or absence of pain and, in the latter circumstance, on whether the expectancies of the subjects are, on the whole, punitive or rewarding. Results of animal investigations indicate that morphine exerts analgesic actions at specific sites in the spinal cord, the brain stem, and the cerebral cortex.

In young monkeys, morphine augments the grasp reflex; since this reflex becomes less active as the monkey matures, it is inferred that its augmentation in young monkeys by morphine is due to depression of a cortical inhibitory reflex (Richter & Paterson, 1932). Wikler (1950) observed that morphine impairs tactile placing and hopping reactions in intact dogs and ascribed this effect to a cortical depressant action of the drug, inasmuch as Brooks and Peck (1940) found that cortical lesions impaired the development of placing and hopping reactions in rats. Allen *et al.* (1945) reported that in the intact dog, morphine produces marked bradycardia, which may be due to a cortical depressant effect, since a similar degree of bradycardia occurs in nonmorphinized decerebrated dogs, in which morphine produces no further slowing of cardiac rate, though such slowing can be achieved by intravenous injection of neosynephrine. Despite such (indirect) evidence of cortical depression, low doses of morphine (10–15 mg/kg) do not alter cortical responsivity to electrical stimulation in rabbits, though they do produce marked central depressant effects (Tainter *et al.*, 1943).

The actions of morphine on the hypothalamus and indirectly on the pituitary gland are quite complex. Morphine does not alter autonomic responses or "sham rage" elicited by direct electrical stimulation of the hypothalamus in the cat (Masserman, 1939), but it does depress or abolish sham rage elicited by nociceptive stimulation in decorticated cats (Wikler, 1944) and decorticated dogs (Wikler, 1952b), indicating that morphine blocks afferent nociceptive impulses to the sham-rage-integrating center of the hypothalamus. DeBodo (1944) observed that morphine inhibited water (but not saline) diuresis in the dog, and that this antidiuretic effect, which was similar to that produced by pitressin, could be abolished by ablation of the neurohypophysis but not by removal of the adenohypophysis; he concluded that morphine antidiuresis is produced by a stimulant action on the hypothalamus, resulting in increased secretion of antidiuretic hormone by the neurohypophysis. The hyperglycemic effect of morphine likewise appears to be due to a stimulant action of the drug on the hypothalamus. Thus, DeBodo and Brooks (1937) showed that in the cat, morphine hyperglycemia was abolished by transection of the spinal cord at the sixth cervical segment, indicating a supraspinal site for this action. Hambourger (1940) reported that morphine produced hyperglycemia in decorticated as well as in intact cats, thus eliminating the cerebral cortex as necessary for morphine hyperglycemia. Finally, Brooks *et al.* (1941) found that morphine hyperglycemia was abolished by large lesions in the posterior hypothalamus. Though dependent on the integrity of the posterior hypothalamus, morphine hyperglycemia is mediated by descending sympathetic pathways ultimately innervating the adrenal glands (CoTui *et al.*, 1937). The hypothermic effect of morphine appears to be due to lowering of the "set point" of the thermoregulatory center in the anterior hypothalamus, thus facilitating heat loss or inhibiting heat gain mechanisms. Thus, in the dog, morphine lowers the threshold for panting (heat loss) in response to artificially induced increases in body temperature (Hemingway, 1938). In the rat, Lotti *et al.* (1965b) found that intravenous injection of morphine, 1 and 5 mg/kg, produced no change or a rise in core temperature, but 10 mg/kg consistently caused a drop in core temperature that increased with the dose up to a maximum at 35–50 mg/kg. Microinjection of 50 μg of morphine sulfate into the region of the preoptic–anterior hypothalamic nuclei likewise caused a drop in core temperature, whereas microinjections of morphine elsewhere in the hypothalamus were ineffective, and microinjections of morphine into the mammillary nuclei produced hyperactivity and hyperthermia. Lotti *et al.* (1965b) speculated that morphine may render the cells of the thermoregulatory center insensitive to the stimulus of the input from cold receptors in the skin, which are sensitive to small temperature changes. In another study, Lotti *et al.* (1965a) found the microinjection of the opioid antagonist *N*-allylnormorphine (nalorphine) into the anterior hypothalamic nuclei not only antagonizes the hypothermia produced by intravenous injection of morphine or microinjection of morphine into the anterior hypothalamic nuclei but also, in the latter case, produced hyperthermia. Lotti *et al.* (1965a) believed that morphine exerts both hypothermic and hyperthermic actions in the rat, and that microinjection of nalorphine into the anterior hypothalamus antagonizes only the hypothermic effect (thereby unmasking the hyperthermic effect). Further studies (Lotti *et al.*, 1966) revealed that tolerance to the hypothermic effect of intravenous morphine (15 and 20 mg/kg) or morphine microinjected into the anterior hypothalamus (10–15 μg) began with the second dose, and some rats displayed hyperthermic reactions to this and subsequent doses (doubling or tripling the dose of morphine restored the hypothermic effect in these rats). Lotti *et al.* (1966) pointed out that their findings can be explained by assuming, in accordance with the "dual action" hypothesis of Seevers and Woods (1953), that tolerance develops only to the depressant effects of morphine (i.e., the hypothermic actions in the anterior hypothalamus), leaving unmasked the stimulant effect (i.e., hyperthermic actions) on the thermoregulatory center in the anterior hypothalamus. In regard to the release of adenohypophysial hormones through actions on the hypothalamus, morphine acts both as a "stressor" and as a blocking agent. George and Way (1955a,b, 1959) reported that in the rat, single doses of morphine acted as stressors since they decreased the ascorbic acid content ot the adrenal glands; this effect was abolished by hypophysectomy or lesions of the median eminence of the hypothalamus but not by adrenal demedullation. Similarly, Lotti *et al.* (1969) found that microinjection of 50 μg of morphine sulfate into the medial (but not the rostral or caudal) region of the hypothalamus caused a significant fall in adrenal ascorbic acid; microinjection of 5 μg of morphine sulfate into the same region caused a rise in plasma corticosterone level. In consonance with George and Way (1959), Lotti *et al.* (1969) concluded that the pituitary–adrenal activation resulting from systemic administration of morphine in rats is mediated by an action of the drug on the mid-region of the hypothalamus. On the other hand, single doses of morphine block the release of luteinizing hormone (LH) that occurs in the rat on the first day of proestrus; this effect coincides with electroencephalographic evidence of depression of the reticular activating system, the activity of which may be necessary for "a central timing mechanism or afferent stimulation to excite hypothalamic centers controlling adenohypophyseal function" (Sawyer *et al.*, 1955). Briggs and Munson (1954) found that in rats anesthetized with pentobarbital, or "accustomed" to morphine by daily administration of the drug for four days, single doses of morphine no longer released ACTH but blocked ACTH release in response to histamine or vasopressin. The effects of ACTH and of adrenocortical hormones are of special interest in relation to opioid dependence since Winter and Flataker (1951) found that in rats, single doses of ACTH or cortisone antagonized the analgesic effect of morphine, whereas deoxycorticosterone augmented morphine analgesia. Also, Eisenman *et al.* (1969) reported changes in adrenocortical metabolites in man (postaddicts) that suggested that hypothalamic-adenohypophysial function is depressed by chronic administration of morphine and increases transiently above control levels during the acute morphine-abstinence period (see below).

Morphine miosis appears to be due to an action of the drug on centers in the midbrain that control pupilloconstrictor tone. McCrea *et al.* (1942) found that in both man and dog, morphine miosis varies directly with the intensity of light falling on the retina, and they concluded that morphine accentuates the normal light reflex; however, morphine miosis in man occurs even in almost complete darkness (Fraser *et al.*, 1954), indicating that morphine miosis is not due only to enhancement of the pupillary light reflex. That morphine miosis may be due to direct or indirect augmentation of pupilloconstrictor tone, mediated by cholinergic (muscarnic) parasympathetic fibers in the oculomotor nerve, and not to depression of sympathetic pupillodilator tone was demonstrated by Wikler (1953) in studies on man. Thus, after dilating the pupil maximally by repeated and continued instillation of paredrine (a local sympathomimetic agent), procaine block of the cervical sympathetic chain in the vicinity of the stellate ganglion failed to constrict the pupil, but miosis was readily observed after subcutaneous injection of morphine. On the other hand, morphine did not constrict the pupil when the latter was maximally dilated by conjunctival instillation of atropine (producing muscarinic blockade) or by a lesion of the ipsilateral oculomotor nerve (localized hemorrhage due to an aneurysm of the posterior communicating artery). In the dog, Lee and Wang (1975) confirmed that morphine miosis depends on the integrity of the oculomotor nerve, and they showed that morphine, 0.2 mg/kg intravenously, in creased the frequency of firing of pupilloconstrictor neurons in the visceral nuclei of the oculomotor nuclear complex, whereas the light-evoked response was diminished; the effects of morphine were antagonized by the opioid antagonist levallorphan, 0.05 mg/kg intravenously. The site of action of morphine in producing morphine miosis in the dog was further elucidated very recently by Sharpe and Pickworth (1980). These investigators found that microinjection of morphine into the Edinger–Westphal nucleus depresses presynaptic inhibitory terminals, the postsynaptic pathways of which activate the ciliary ganglion synaptically; postganglionic fibers from the ciliary ganglion activate the circular (pupilloconstrictor) smooth muscles of the eye, thereby producing miosis. The presynaptic inhibitory terminals in the Edinger–Westphal nucleus are muscarinic, so that microinjection of atropine into the Edinger–Westphal nucleus produces miosis, not mydriasis. The postsynaptic pathways from the Edinger–Westphal nucleus that synapse with the ciliary ganglion, as well as the postganglionic fibers from the ciliary ganglion to the circular smooth muscles, are likewise muscarinic, but blockade of them through instillation of atropine into the conjunctional sac produces mydriasis, not miosis.

The respiratory, vasomotor, electroencephalographic, and emetic effects of morphine can be ascribed, in whole or in part, to actions in the pons and the medulla. Morphine reduces the sensitivity of the respiratory center to CO_2 (Martin et al., 1968; see also review by Wikler, 1950) and enhances vagal respiratory reflexes (Henderson and Rice, 1939), chemoreceptor (sinoaortic and carotid body) reflex respiratory control mechanisms (Schmidt, 1940; Dripps & Dumke, 1943), and carotid sinus pressoreceptor respiratory reflexes (Marri & Hauss, 1939). According to Fischlewitz (1948), vagal respiratory and sinoaortic chemoreceptor reflexes may be released from inhibition by an action of morphine on the caudal pons. Drew *et al.* (1946) found that in man, 10–30 mg of morphine produced no significant changes in pulse rate, blood pressure, or cardiac output, but that sudden tilting from the previously horizontal position to the upright position resulted in fainting or evidence of circulatory collapse in many subjects. After morphine, the cardioaccelerator response to tilting remained intact and the Hering–Breuer respiratory reflex appeared to be enhanced; hence Drew *et al.* (1946) concluded that the circulatory disturbances on tilting after morphine were due to a peripheral vasodilating action of the drug. However, Himmelsbach (1944) reported that in a patient with unilateral dorsal sympathectomy, morphine increased blood flow in the contralateral (intact) hand but not in the ipsilateral (denervated) hand, though in the latter, blood flow could be increased by direct warming. It appears, therefore, that morphine depresses sympathetic outflow through a central action. Huggins *et al.* (1949) found that in the dog, elevation of the hind legs or the head resulted in a significant reduction of blood flow to the part raised, and they concluded that morphine may produce partial inhibition of the vasoconstrictor center. On the other hand, morphine enhances the cardiac slowing and fall in blood pressure produced by stimulation of pressor receptors in the carotid sinus (Rovenstine and Cullen, 1939). In the dog, low doses of morphine (2–5 mg/kg) produce slow activity in the occipital region and bursts of 8- to 12-sec waves alternating with slower activity in the frontal and parietal regions (Wikler & Altschul, 1950). These changes resemble those produced in the cat by destruction of the brain-stem activating mechanism (Lindsley *et al.*, 1949) or mesencephalic transection (Bremer, 1937), indicating that the effects of low doses of morphine on the electroencephalogram may be due to depression of the reticular activating system in the pons and the medulla. Low doses of barbiturates also depress the reticular activating system (Arduini & Arduini, 1954), but Silvestrini and Longo (1956) found in the rabbit that whereas morphine depresses arousal responses to painful stimuli more than to tactile or auditory stimuli, the reverse is true for pentobarbital. Morphine-produced nausea and emesis appear to be due to an excitatory (dopaminergic) action of the drug on the medullary chemoreceptor trigger zone (Wang and Glaviano, 1954).

In addition to these actions, morphine affects spinal reflexes both directly and through supraspinal inhibitory and facilitatory actions, which are considered in detail in Chapter 5. For example, two standard analgesic tests, the tail flick in the rat (D'Amour & Smith, 1941) and the skin twitch in the dog (Andrews & Workman, 1941), are depressed by morphine in the spinal animal and to a greater extent in the intact animal (Irwin *et al.*, 1951; Houde & Wikler, 1951). Also, Leimdorfer (1948) reported that in white mice, transection of the spinal cord abolishes the augmentation of the Straub tail response to morphine, which is produced by pressure over the lumbodorsal spine, indicating a supraspinal site of action of morphine for such augmentation.

Tolerance and Physical Dependence

In man, the effects of the first injection of morphine (10–15 mg) wear off after 4–6 hr. The effects of the drug are reinstituted by a second dose, but with continued repetition of the same doses at intervals sufficient to prevent cumulative actions, progressive attenuation of its analgesic, respiratory-depressant, hypothermic, hypotensive, emetic, and antidiuretic actions occurs, with little alteration of its miotic and constipating actions. Increasing the size of the dose partially restores the original effects, but they become progressively attenuated with continued administration at the new dose level. The rate at which such tolerance develops in nonaddicts is not known precisely. In postaddicts who have been abstinent from all opioids for six months or more, Fraser and Isbell (1952) found no evidence of "residual" tolerance to the effects of single dose of morphine (20 mg) on pupil size, respiratory and cardiac rates, or systolic blood pressure, but drop in rectal temperature was significantly less than in nonaddicts and vomiting occurred less often than in nonaddicts. Yet, in postaddicts, it was possible to attain a daily dose of morphine of 500 mg without serious complications by progressively increasing the dose over a period of 10 days from an initial schedule of 25 mg four times daily (Fraser *et al.*, 1957). In tolerant addicts, up to 5000 mg of morphine have been administered in one day without dangerous effects (Williams & Oberst, 1946). In addicts, the transient "thrill" after intravenous injection of morphine apparently continues unabated, but the longer-lasting initial euphoric effects eventually disappear and the prevailing modd becomes dysphoric and hypochondriacal (Wikler, 1951a; Haertzen & Hooks, 1969). Tolerance develops to the occasional slow-wave activity and increased synchrony initially produced by morphine in the waking electroencephalogram (Andrews, 1943), and partial tolerance develops to the sleep disturbance initially produced by morphine (shift in sleeping electroencephalographic patterns toward lighter stages of sleep and increased spontaneous awakenings) concomitantly with an increased number of "delta bursts" (Kay, 1975a). Tolerance to morphine is accompanied by hyperirritability of the autonomic nervous system since pressor response to cold stimuli are en-chanced, compared with responses in control subjects (Himmelsbach, 1941). In an experimental study of morphine readdiction in man (post-addicts), Martin and Jasinski (1969) found that in comparison with pre-addiction values, mean values of systolic and diastolic blood pressure, cardiac rate, and rectal temperature were elevated, while pupillary diameter was smaller and cardiac rate was slower, when measured just before the morning dose of morphine after the subjects had become tolerant to 240 mg/day (60 mg four times daily). Depression of respira-tory rate was associated with decreased sensitivity of the respiratory center to CO_2, although administration of a large dose of morphine (60 or 120 mg) produced little or no additional respiratory depression (Mar-tin *et al.*, 1968). Eisenman *et al.* (1969) found that when postaddicts were stabilized on morphine, urinary norepinephrine excretion and urine volumes were significantly elevated over control values, while urinary excretion of epinephrine and 17-hydroxycorticoids as well as of urinary dopamine and creatinine remained unchanged. In an earlier study, Eisenman *et al.* (1961) reported that adrenocorticoid hormone secretion (as measured by 17-hydroxycorticoid excretion and plasma 17-hydroxycorticoid levels) decreased in the morphine-tolerant state com-pared with control values, although the responsivity of the adrenal gland to injected ACTH and the catabolism of infused hydrocortisone were the same as in the control period. This finding suggests that re-peated doses of morphine exert an inhibitory effect on hypothalamic–adenohypophysial function. All of these findings—behavioral, physiological, and biochemical—indicate that the morphine-tolerant in-dividual is not "normal." However, there is little change in basal metabolism, blood electrolytes, and cell constituents, except for mild secondary anemia (Williams & Oberst, 1946; Isbell, 1947).

Physical dependence is inferred from the appearance of an absti-nence (or withdrawal) syndrome when the administration of morphine is discontinued. The morphine-abstinence syndrome proceeds in two phases: an early (or acute, or primary) phase lasting 4–10 weeks, and a protracted (or chronic, or secondary) phase that emerges during the latter part of the early phase and continues for 26–30 weeks or longer (Martin & Jasinski, 1969). The intensity of the abstinence syndrome (early phase) that follows abrupt withdrawal of morphine is related to previous dosage, duration of addiction, and the degree of tolerance that has been developed (Andrews & Himmelsbach, 1944). After abrupt withdrawal of morphine, the earliest abstinence sign is restlessness, beginning about 4 hr after the last dose. Gross early phase abstinence phenomena appear about 8 hr after the last dose, and subside asympto-tically by the 10th day after morphine withdrawal; some abstinence signs, including continued increased pressor responses to cold stimuli, do not stabilize for up to 6 months (Himmelsbach, 1942a). Roughly in order of their appearance, the gross abstinence phenomena of the early phase are anxiety, yawning, lacrimation, rhinorrhea, mydriasis, piloerection (gooseflesh), sweating, weakness, tremors, muscle twitches (particularly in the lower extremities), extreme restlessness, hot and cold flashes, leukocytosis, hemoconcentration, elevation of blood glucose, precipitous drop in eosinophil count, anorexia, nausea and vomiting, loss of body weight, and rise in blood pressure, cardiac rate, rectal temperature, and respiratory rate (with increased sensitivity of the respiratory center to CO_2). Curiously, alpha activity, if present in prewithdrawal electroencephalograms, continues during the early abstinence period in spite of manifest anxiety (Andrews, 1943). Urinary excretion of norepinephrine, epinephrine, and dopamine are within the preaddiction control range, while urine volumes and excretion of creatinine are statistically decreased (Eisenman et al., 1969). On the other hand, plasma levels and urinary excretion of 17-hydroxycorticoids increase significantly during the early abstinence period (Eiseman et al., 1961, 1969); this increase may be interpreted as a "rebound" from the depressive effects of repeated doses of morphine on adrenal secretion (Eisenman et al., 1961). The addict in early morphine abstinence typically expresses a craving for sweets but an aversion to tobacco, and he often prefers to lie on a hard, cold surface (such as the floor) in a "curled-up," lateral recumbent position, with a blanket drawn over his head, even on a hot summer day. In addition to these "nonpurposive" abstinence phenomena, the addict typically displays "purposive" abstinence phenomena, consisting of verbal demands for drugs to relieve his distress and more individualized patterns of behavior designed to achieve the same end (threatening violence or suicide, assuming bizarre postures, repeated self-induced vomiting, etc.).

Whereas the early morphine-abstinence syndrome evolves with increasing intensity over a period of about two days after abrupt withdrawal of the drug, it may be "precipitated" within minutes in a morphine-tolerant addict by subcutaneous—or with even less delay by intravenous—injection of an opioid antagonist, such as nalorphine or naloxone (see Chapter 8).

The protracted phase of morphine abstinence, first described in the rat (Martin et al., 1963), differs qualitatively from early abstinence, being characterized by small but persistent decreases in blood pressure, cardiac rate, body temperature, and pupillary diameter and sensitivity of the respiratory center to CO_2 (Martin & Jasinski, 1969; Martin et al., 1968). Urinary excretion of epinephrine increased significantly during the 7th and 17th weeks after complete withdrawal of morphine, indicating that protracted abstinence is a stressful state or that subjects in protracted abstinence are hyperresponsive to stress (Eisenman *et al.*, 1969).

Details of the mechanisms involved in tolerance to and physical dependence on morphine are considered in Chapter 6. Here are mentioned only that bilateral prefrontal lobotomy, carried out for relief of intractable phantom limb pain in a patient tolerant to large doses of morphine (which no longer exerted analgesic effects), did not alter the nonpurposive early abstinence phenomena after abrupt withdrawal of morphine but did abolish the purposive abstinence phenomena. At the same time, the previously intractable pain was greatly relieved by the neurosurgical procedure (Wikler *et al.*, 1952). Evidently, the integrity of frontothalamic and frontolimbic circuits is not critical for the expression of nonpurposive morphine-abstinence phenomena, but it would seem to be critical for purposive behaviors, such as demanding drugs and threatening suicide, which the patient exhibited on attempted morphine withdrawal before bilateral prefrontal lobotomy; however, at that time, he also complained of unbearable phantom limb pain. It is difficult to judge whether the absence of purposive abstinence phenomena after bilateral prefrontal lobotomy was due to interruption of neural circuits involved only in the amplification of pain or also in goal-directed behavior, namely, seeking relief from distressful states of any sort, including nonpurposive morphine-abstinence phenomena.

Heroin

In equivalent doses, the effects of heroin (diacetylmorphine) differ in no essential way from those of morphine. In single doses, the two drugs produce comparable subjective effects (Smith & Beecher, 1959) and effects on psychometric performance (Smith *et al.*, 1962). Experienced addicts can often distinguish heroin from morphine after *intravenous* injection, presumably because of the greater intensity of the pins-and-needles sensation after morphine that occurs when the two drugs are administered by this route (Martin & Fraser, 1961). However, there are no qualitative or quantitative differences between heroin and morphine as regards the rate of development of tolerance on repeated administration or the characteristics of the abstinence syndrome that ensues after abrupt drug-withdrawal (Martin & Fraser, 1961).

Methadone

When the two drugs are given by the oral route, methadone is more effective than morphine, though parenterally, the potency of methadone and morphine for analgesia are the same. Given *intravenously,* single doses of methadone produce the same effects as morphine, including intense euphoria in postaddicts (Isbell, 1948a). Given orally four times each day, the effects of methadone—particularly respiratory depression, sedation, and diffuse slowing of the electroencephalogram —tend to be cumulative, because of the drug's relatively long duration of action (Isbell *et al.,* 1948b). In the sleep electroencephalogram, the number of spontaneous awakenings decreases and delta bursts increase (Kay, 1975a). However, partial tolerance, notably to the respiratory depressant and sedative effects, does develop eventually. After abrupt withdrawal of methadone, no objective abstinence phenomena are observed for two to three days; then relatively mild abstinence signs appear that last several days. However, the patient complains of lassitude, anorexia, insomnia, and aching of the bones and muscles for many weeks after abrupt withdrawal of methadone (Isbell *et al.,* 1948b). In the sleep electroencephalogram, the methadone-abstinence syndrome is characterized by increased rapid eye movement (REM) sleep and delta-stage sleep (Kay, 1975a). Contrasting with the delayed onset and relatively mild intensity of the abstinence syndrome that follows abrupt withdrawal of methadone is the immediate appearance of an intense abstinence syndrome that can be "precipitated" in methadone-tolerant subjects by parenteral administration of an opioid antagonist (Wikler *et al.,* 1953).

Because methadone is effective by the oral route, has a relatively long duration of action, and can substitute for other opioids in suppressing abstinence syndromes resulting from withdrawal of them, and because the abstinence syndrome following withdrawal of methadone is mild (though long-persisting), substitution of methadone for morphine heroin, and similar opioids over a few days followed by gradual withdrawal has become the method of choice for detoxification of opioid addicts (Isbell *et al.,* 1948b). The use of methadone for "maintenance" of addicts is more controversial (see Chapter 8).

Meperidine

Though in comparison with morphine, the analgesic potency of meperidine is less (one-eighth to one-tenth) and its duration of action is shorter (2–4 hr), the effects of single doses and the general features of tolerance to and physical dependence on meperidine in man are qualitatively similar to those of morphine (Himmelsbach, 1942b, 1943). However, there are some notable quantitative differences. As already noted, the duration of action of meperidine is relatively short, and as tolerance develops, it becomes still shorter. Concomitantly, abstinence phenomena—consisting mainly of extreme restlessness, muscle twitching, sweating, and anxiety—appear earlier after the last does. In consequence, the meperidine addict is impelled both to increase the dose and to self-administer the drug at shorter intervals. The dose threshold for convulsions is soon reached in the presence of tolerance to the respiratory-depressant effects of meperidine, so that at a daily dose level of 2000–3000 mg, myoclonic jerks and/or generalized seizures may occur (Wikler & Pescor, 1954). In the presence of myoclonic jerks without generalized seizures, the physician may have difficulty in deciding whether the patient is suffering from meperidine toxicity (due to overdosage) or from early meperidine abstinence phenomena (due to underdosage), or perhaps from both, since the patient may shift rapidly from toxicity to abstinence or vice versa. Clinical experience indicates that such a situation can be handled by reducing the daily dosage of meperidine to a subconvulsive level but increasing the frequency of drug injection (e.g., to every two hours). Subsequently, the patient may be detoxified by rapid reduction of the daily dose of meperidine, or by substitution and eventual withdrawal of methadone (see Chapter 8).

Codeine

By the intravenous route, codeine (methylmorphine) often produces intense flushing of the skin, edema of the face, and sometimes severe hypotension. For this reason, codeine is usually given subcutaneously, intramuscularly, or orally. Though its analgesic potency is only one-twelfth that of morphine, codeine suppresses morphine abstinence phenomena in doses about five times as great as morphine. In adequate multiple daily doses continued for sufficient periods of time, codeine can produce physical dependence; however, the abstinence syndrome that follows abrupt withdrawal of codeine is much milder than, though qualitatively similar to, that of morphine (Himmelsbach *et al.*, 1940; Fraser *et al.*, 1961). Abuse of elixirs containing codeine (e.g., elixir of terpin hydrate with codeine) may lead to physical dependence on both codeine and the alcohol content of the elixir.

d-Propoxyphene

Though structurally related to methadone, the analgesic potency of *d*-propoxyphene (Darvon) is somewhat less than that of codeine (Drug and Therapeutic Information, 1970). Initial investigations of its addiction liability indicated that in this respect, too, physical dependence on *d*-propoxyphene was somewhat less than that on codeine (Fraser & Isbell, 1960). More recently, however, the Food and Drug Administration (FDA Drug Bulletin, 1979) has warned that both physical and psychological dependence of the morphine type can occur after chronic administration of as little as 500–800 mg/day of d-propoxyphene hydrochloride or 800–1200 mg/day of d-propoxyphene napsylate (a water-insoluble salt, designed to prevent addicts from bypassing the usual oral route through intravenous self-injection of the water-soluble salt, d-propxyphene hydrochloride, marketed for oral use as Darvon). The Food and Drug Administration (FDA Drug Bulletin, 1979) also reported that 1000–2000 deaths a year are associated with d-propoxyphene alone or in combination with other drugs (alcohol, tranquilizers, sedative–hypnotics) and that d-propoxyphene ranks second only to barbiturates as the leading prescription drug associated with drug fatalities. Other complications of overdosage with d-propoxyphene are toxic psychoses and/or convulsions (Karliner, 1967). In 1977, d-propoxyphene was placed under Schedule IV of the Controlled Substances Act (FDA Drug Bulletin, 1979).

Pentazocine

In some patients, pentazocine produces psychotomimetic effects, principally visual hallucinations (De Noraquo, 1969), which can be antagonized by the "pure" opioid antagonist naloxone, but not by the mixed agonist–antagonist drug nalorphine. Overdosage with pentazocine can produce stupor or coma, which likewise can be antagonized by naloxone, but not by nalorphine. Tolerance develops to pentazocine on repeated administration, and after its abrupt withdrawal, a mild, atypical abstinence syndrome appears, consisting mainly of abdominal cramps, diarrhea, nausea, vomiting, restlessness, dizziness, chills, and fever. In patients tolerant to pentazocine, an abstinence syndrome can be "precipitated" by naloxone, but not by nalorphine (Fraser & Rosenberg, 1964). While the addiction liability of pentazocine has been rated relatively low, individual case reports of pentazocine abstinence phenomena have been reported in adults (Sandoval & Wang, 1969) and in neonates born of pentazocine-dependent mothers (Goetz & Bain, 1974; Scanlon, 1974). The Food and Drug Administration has reported that abuse of pentazocine is rising and that the state of Illinois has placed pentazocine under Schedule II (FDA Drug Bulletin, 1978–1979).

OPIOID ANTAGONISTS

The history of specific opioid antagonists (see Figure 1) begins with the report of Pohl (1915) on the antagonistic action of the N-allyl derivative of norcodeine on the respiratory depressant effects of morphine or

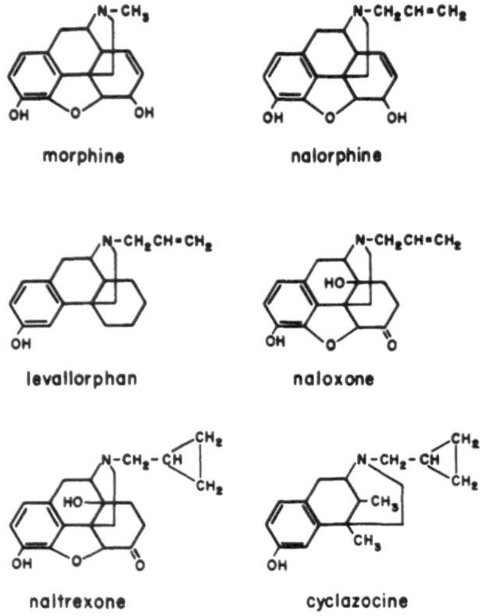

FIGURE 1. Structural formulas of some opioid antagonists (nalorphine, levallorphan, naloxone, naltrexone, and cyclazocine) compared with that of an opioid agonist (morphine).

heroin in the rabbit and the dog. If given first, N-allylnorcodeine prevented the respiratory-depressant effects of morphine or heroin. In the rabbit, the respiratory-depressant effect of chloral hydrate was also antagonized by N-allylnorcodeine, but only to a moderate extent. Pohl (1915) speculated that morphine and N-allylnorcodeine have similar "side-chains" and are therefore taken up by the same cells in the respiratory center; in essence, this hypothesis remains the same in current theories about the mechanisms of antagonistic interactions between opioids and opioid antagonists (see Chapter 4). The antagonistic actions of N-allylnorcodeine on morphine-produced narcosis and respiratory depression in the rabbit were confirmed by Meissner (1923). Otherwise, Pohl's (1915) findings received little attention until N-allylnormorphine (nalorphine) was synthesized by McCawley *et al.* (1941) and by Weijlard and Erickson (1942). During the next two decades, extensive investigations were made of the animal and human pharmacology of nalorphine and of levallorphan, the N-allyl derivative of levorphanol, a morphinan compound. These two drugs were found to have mixed "agonist-antagonist" properties; that is, in drug-free animals or man, they exerted some morphinelike and also psychotomimetic actions (most obviously in man), while they antagonized the depressant effects of large doses of morphine. More recently, numerous other opioid antagonists have been synthesized, notably cyclazocine, which likewise is a mixed opioid agonist–antagonist, and naloxone and naltrexone, which have little or no agonistic actions and, for practical purposes, are regarded as "pure" opioid antagonists.

Nalorphine

Effects of Single Doses in the Drug-Free State

In drug-free postaddicts, Wikler (1951, 1954), Wikler et al. (1953), Isbell (1956), and Fraser et al. (1956) observed that subcutaneous injection of 5–15 mg of nalorphine produced autonomic changes resembling those of morphine but variable effects on state of consciousness, the sensorium, mood, and content of thought. Thus, respiratory minute volume was decreased to a degree comparable to that produced by equivalent doses of morphine; pupillary size was reduced, although to a lesser extent than after morphine; and slight but significant slowing of cardiac rate and lowering of rectal temperature occurred. Some subjects were euphoric but noted that this euphoria was not morphinelike, resembling more the state produced by small doses of short-acting barbiturates or alcohol. Other subjects were definitely dysphoric and complained of giddiness, nausea, sweating, and disturbing "daydreams." In a few, visual hallucinations, generally of a pleasant sort, were reported. After subcutaneous injection of 30–75 mg of nalorphine, the autonomic changes resembled even more clearly those produced by morphine, including miosis, pseudoptosis, and marked drop in rectal temperature. Concomitantly, a few of the subjects became more relaxed and drowsy, but most of them exhibited panic states and complained of uncontrollable "thoughts racing through the head," daydreams of "nightmarish" quality, and sensations of movement in the lower extremities with eyes closed (proprioceptive hallucinations?). At all times, however, the subjects remained well oriented and responded logically to questions. The electroencephalogram remained unchanged in some subjects despite marked changes in behavior; in others, increased synchronization with slight slowing of frequencies occurred in association with relaxation and drowsiness, and the reverse with anxiety and/or daydreams and hallucinations.

Other investigators reported that in drug-free human subjects, nalorphine can produce postural hypotension (Eckenhoff et al., 1952), has antitussive actions (Bickerman and Barach, 1954), has antispasmodic effects on the gastrointestinal tract in contrast to the spasmogenic actions of morphine (Gray & Beckman, 1956), decreases respiratory sensitivity to CO_2 (Tenney & Mithoefer, 1953), impairs psychomotor performance (Bauer and Pearson, 1956), and produces analgesia comparable to that produced by morphine, although its clinical usefulness as an analgesic is impaired by its psychotomimetic effects (Lasagna and Beecher, 1954; Keats and Telford, 1956). The analgesic potency of nalorphine in man was surprising because in the majority of studies with standard analgesic tests in animals (e.g., tail flick in the rat and skin twitch in the dog), nalorphine was found to have very low analgesic potency (Woods, 1956); however, Nilsen (1961) and Perrine *et al.* (1972) reported that like morphine, nalorphine does elevate the threshold of electrical stimulation of the tail for evocation of squeaking in the mouse, and Pearl *et al.* (1969) found that nalorphine protects the mouse against the "writhing" effects of intraperitoneal injection of phenyl-*p*-quinone.

Tolerance and Physical Dependence

In postaddicts, Isbell (1956) noted that tolerance to the hallucinatory effects of nalorphine developed on a dose schedule of 10 mg every 6 hr, increasing to 25–35 mg every 6 hr over a period of 14 days, and continuing at the same level for an additional 14 days; no definite abstinence phenomena were observed after abrupt withdrawal of nalorphine. However, Schrappe (1959) reported mild, but definite morphinelike abstinence phenomena in one of two patients with affective disorders (nonaddicts) after abrupt withdrawal of nalorphine, 150 mg/day following 40 days of drug administration. The question was reinvestigated by Martin and Gorodetzky (1965), who administered nalorphine subcutaneously to seven postaddicts in doses progressing from 1 mg/70 kg to 40 mg/70 kg six times daily (6 mg/70 kg to 240 mg/70 kg daily) over a period of 40–45 days, continuing at the same sevel for an additional 25–32 days. The subjects developed a high level of tolerance to the subjective effects of nalorphine and to its respiratory-depressant and hypothermic effects, but only partial tolerance to its miotic effects; during chronic administration of nalorphine, caloric intake increased and there was a marked gain in body weight. Eight hours after substitution of placebo, scratching, itching, and "shocks" associated with myoclonic jerks appeared; later in the first and second day after abrupt withdrawal of nalorphine (and substitution of placebo), yawning, lacrimation, rhinorrhea, perspiration, tachycardia, hyperthermia, and anorexia developed. Diarrhea occurred on the third or fourth day of nalorphine abstinence, but mydriasis did not become maximal and significant until the eighth day, and respiratory rate did not become markedly elevated until the ninth day. At no time during the nalorphine-abstinence period did the subjects display purposive abstinence phenomena (demanding opioid drugs for relief of their distress). Martin and Gorodetzky (1965) concluded that the nalorphine-abstinence syndrome was early in onset and mild, though relatively prolonged, and that it differed from the morphine-abstinence syndrome, resembling more the cyclazocine-abstinence syndrome (see below).

Opioid-Antagonistic and Opioid-Blocking Actions in the Nontolerant State

The effects of nalorphine on the actions of morphine in nontolerant animals have been reviewed by Woods (1956). In brief, nalorphine antagonizes or prevents morphine-produced narcosis, analgesic test responses, and respiratory depression in the mouse, rat, rabbit, dog, and monkey; miosis, bradycardia, hypotension, and hypothermia in the dog; excitation phenomena in the cat; but not convulsions in the mouse and rat. In man, Fraser *et al.* (1956) found that when nalorphine (3, 6, or 10 mg) was given simultaneously with 30 mg of morphine, or when 10 mg of nalorphine was given one and three-quarters hr after 30 mg of morphine to postaddicts, the euphoric and miotic effects of morphine were blocked or diminished. However, respiratory depression and lowering of rectal temperature by this dose of morphine were not antagonized by nalorphine. Similarly, 10 mg of nalorphine given simultaneously with 10 mg of heroin antagonized the miotic but not the respiratory–depressant effect of heroin. The failure of nalorphine to antagonize *mild* respiratory depression produced by morphine contrasts sharply with the spectacular antagonistic action of nalorphine on *severe* respiratory depression produced by overdoses of opioid analgesics (Eckenhoff *et al.*, 1951, 1952; Fraser *et al.*, 1952). The dependency of the antagonistic action of nalorphine on the dose of morphine is partly explained by the mixed agonist–antagonist properties of nalorphine (see Chapter 4).

Opioid-Antagonistic and Opioid-Blocking Actions in the Tolerant State

In postaddicts tolerant to morphine, methadone, or heroin, Wikler *et al.* (1953) found that single doses of nalorphine not only antagonized the agonistic effects of these opioids but also "precipitated" abstinence syndromes that resembled those following abrupt withdrawal of morphine or heroin, except that the precipitated abstinence syndrome began within 1 or 2 min after subcutaneous injection of nalorphine, reached a peak after about 45 min, and disappeared after about 2 hr (this was true also of the subject tolerant to methadone). Mild but definite signs and symptoms of abstinence could be precipitated by subcutaneous injection of 15 mg of nalorphine in subjects who had received 15–30 mg of morphine, 10 mg of methadone, or 15 mg of heroin four times daily for 2–5 days. As the doses of these opioids increased, the dose of nalorphine needed to precipitate abstinence decreased; for example, at a dose level of 240 mg/day of morphine, 2–5 mg of nalorphine precipitated an abstinence syndrome fully as severe as that precipitated by 15 mg of nalorphine earlier, when the dose level of morphine was 60 mg/day or 120 mg/day. On the other hand, 15 mg of nalorphine failed to precipitate abstinence syndromes when administered 3 days after all clinical evidence of abstinence changes had disappeared following rapid withdrawal of morphine; instead, nalorphine now produced effects identical with those observed before experimental readdiction to morphine was begun. Very similar observations were made by Wikler and Carter (1953) on the hind-limb reflexes of chronic spinal dogs. Single doses of nalorphine could precipitate hyperactivity of the flexor reflex and "running movements" of the hind limbs (signs of morphine abstinence) after a single large dose of morphine in some experiments, and regularly after repeated doses of morphine, even before tolerance to the depressant of morphine on the flexor reflex had developed. Interestingly, the subcutaneous injection of morphine did not reverse the abstinence phenomena precipitated by nalorphine. The theoretical significance of these observations is discussed in Chapter 6. Nalorphine—and more recently, the "pure" opioid antagonist naloxone—has been used for both theoretical and practical purposes in the diagnosis of physical dependence on opioids (see Chapter 8).

When chronically administered together, nalorphine can attenuate or abolish the development of tolerance to and physical dependence on opioids. Thus, Orahovats et al. (1953) found that concomitant administration of nalorphine and morphine prevented the development of tolerance to the analgesic action of morphine in the rat. Wikler (1954, cited by Martin, 1967, p. 492) observed that during concomitant administration of nalorphine (1.25 mg/kg) and morphine (3.75 mg/kg) every six hours, the development of tolerance to the depressant effects of morphine on the flexor reflex of chronic spinal dogs was retarded; in other experiments, when nalorphine (5 mg/kg) was administered every 3 hr and morphine (2.5 mg/kg) every 6 hr, no effects of morphine on hind-limb reflexes occurred, and on abrupt withdrawal of both drugs, the abstinence syndrome that emerged was far less intense than would have been expected from the morphine dosage schedule alone. In contrast, single doses of nalorphine (5 mg/kg) precipitated severe abstinence syndromes in the hind limbs of chronic spinal dogs that had received morphine (2.5 mg/kg) every 6 hr for 1 week. Similar observations on the attenuation of tolerance to and physical dependence on morphine by concomitant administration of levallorphan in the monkey were reported by Seevers and Deneau (1963). In man (postaddicts), Isbell (1954, cited by Martin, 1967, pp. 491–492) found that administration of nalorphine–morphine mixtures in various ratios every 3–4 hr in increasing dosage for 28–30 days resulted in the appearance of profuse sweating and muscular twitching and jerking for about 20 min after each injection of the mixture (precipitated morphine-abstinence phenomena?) and dysphoria generally, despite continued evidence of morphine effects (miosis, respiratory depression, constipation); on abrupt withdrawal of the mixtures, the subjects showed mild morphine-abstinence phenomena that were much less severe than those exhibited by some of the subjects when morphine was abruptly withdrawn following replacement of the morphine content of the mixtures for the same period of time.

In addition to retarding the development of tolerance to and physical dependence on morphine, chronic administration of nalorphine alone can block certain agonistic effects of morphine, as was demonstrated by Martin et al. (1966). In postaddicts, nalorphine given subcutaneously every four hours in doses increasing to 240 mg/70 kg/day blocked the effects of a single dose of morphine (16 mg/70 kg), subjects' and observers' identification of morphine as a narcotic, and "liking" scores, even though a high degree of tolerance had developed to the subjective effects of nalorphine. These properties of nalorphine, which are shared by other opioid antagonists, are the basis of the use of orally effective, long-acting opioid antagonists (cyclazocine, naltrexone) in the postdetoxification treatment of opioid-dependent persons (see Chapter 8).

Cyclazocine

Cyclazocine (N-cyclopropylmethyl benzomorphan, or 2-cyclopropyl-methyl-2'-hydroxy-5,9-dimethyl-6,7-benzomorphan in the benzomorphan numbering system) was synthesized by Archer et al. (1962, 1964), and its animal pharmacology was investigated by Harris and Pierson (1964) and others. Like nalorphine, cyclazocine has mixed agonist–antagonist properties. The human pharmacology of cyclazocine was studied by Martin et al. (1965). In man (postaddicts), cyclazocine is 10–20 times as potent as morphine or nalorphine (all three drugs given parenterally) in producing opioidlike agonistic effects such as miosis, opioid signs and symptoms, and "liking." However, there were some differences: dose-effect curves for cyclazocine and nalorphine reached a "plateau," and maximal pupillary construction produced by these drugs was less than could be produced by morphine. Also, sleepiness and "drunkenness" were dose-related for cyclazocine, contrasting with the "coasting" and "soapboxing" (talkativeness) produced by morphine (sleepiness was also a prominent effect of nalorphine). Lower doses of cyclazocine and nalorphine were identified by both subjects and observers as narcotic analgesics, but higher doses of cyclazocine and nalorphine were identified as barbiturates, whereas large doses of morphine were identified as "dope." A high degree of tolerance developed to the opioidlike symptoms and certain of the opioidlike signs of cyclazocine effect during a 10- to 15-week period of chronic subcutaneous administration of cyclazocine four times daily, beginning with 0.4 mg/70 kg/day and increasing to a stabilization level of 13.2 mg/70 kg/day. The cyclazocine-tolerant subjects were cross-tolerant to nalorphine (though tolerance to the miotic effects of nalorphine could not be evaluated because of the large degree of residual miosis produced by cyclazocine). During chronic administration of cyclazocine, the drug was identified by the subjects as a barbiturate or as an amphetaminelike agent, and they expressed indifference to it. Three of the six subjects had no adverse effects; one became excessively sedated at times, another had episodes of depression and was disturbed by thoughts of violence, and the other reported episodes of dyspneic breathing when trying to fall asleep. On abrupt withdrawal of cyclazocine, an abstinence syndrome appeared, beginning on the third or fourth day after drug withdrawal, reaching maximal intensity on the seventh day, and persisting in attenuated form for up to six weeks. In general, the cyclazocine abstinence syndrome, though delayed in onset and longer lasting, resembled the nalorphine-abstinence syndrome more than the morphine-abstinence syndrome. Its features included rhinorrhea, lacrimation, mydriasis, hyperthermia, tachycardia, decrease in caloric intake, weight loss, and complaints of "shocks in the head" or "shocks" in the base of the neck or chest that radiated upward into the head; as in the nalorphine-abstinence syndrome, the subjects in cyclazocine abstinence made few complaints and did not demand drugs for relief of their distress.

Like nalorphine, single doses of cyclazocine also exert opioid-antagonistic actions. Thus, Martin *et al.* (1965) reported that both nalorphine in doses of 3.0 mg/70 kg and cyclazocine in doses of 0.75 and 1.0 mg/70 kg precipitated abstinence syndromes in subjects tolerant to morphine, 240 mg/70 kg/day. In another study, Martin *et al.* (1966) found that 1.0 mg/70 kg of cyclazocine given subcutaneously partially blocked the effects of a single dose of morphine, 25 mg/70 kg for 12–24 hr. During chronic *oral* administration of cyclazocine, similar morphine-blocking effects were observed; for example, in subjects receiving cyclazocine, 2.0

mg/70 kg twice daily, the effects of single doses of morphine, 60 and 120 mg/70 kg, were equal to or less than those produced in the control, drug-free state by single doses of morphine, 10 and 30 mg/70 kg. Similar blocking effects were noted in subjects given single doses of heroin, up to 60 mg/70 kg. Five of the six subjects stabilized on cyclazocine, 2.0 mg/70 kg twice daily, had minor complaints, such as sedation, sleepiness, headaches, and constipation; the other subject had episodes of irritability, uncontrolled thoughts, and visual imagery with his eyes closed, sometimes reaching hallucinatory proportions, but eventually he developed tolerance to these psychotomimetic effects. After stabilization on orally administered cyclazocine (4.0 mg/70 kg/day) was achieved, the subjects were also given subcutaneous injections of morphine four times daily, beginning with a dose of 40 mg/70 kg/day, which was increased to 240 mg/70 kg/day over a period of 11 days and maintained at that level for an additional 9 days, when morphine was abruptly withdrawn (cyclazocine was continued at 4.0 mg/70 kg/day). During the chronic administration of morphine, the effects of morphine were mild to moderate; after abrupt withdrawal of morphine (cyclazocine continued), the abstinence syndrome that emerged was much milder than that seen in other studies on the unantagonized morphine-abstinence syndrome, and none of the subjects displayed drug-seeking behavior. Martin *et al.* (1966) concluded that because orally administered cyclazocine exerts long-lasting opioid antagonistic effects, blocking the euphoria produced by morphine or heroin and also reducing the degree of physical dependence developed by repeated doses of these drugs, it should be useful in the ambulatory management of detoxified opioid addicts.

Naloxone and Naltrexone

Unlike nalorphine and cyclazocine, naloxone (*N*-allynoroxymorphone) is a "pure" opioid antagonist, practically devoid of opioidlike agonistic actions (Blumberg *et al.*, 1961; Foldes *et al.*, 1963; Jasinski *et al.*, 1967). One possible exception to this generalization is the report of Lasagna (1965) that naloxone exerts some analgesic effects in man, maximal at 2 mg and less at higher and lower doses. Naloxone has been reported to facilitate nociceptive responses in otherwise untreated animals and in animals and man rendered analgesic by focal electrical stimulation of certain brain sites or by acupuncture, but such actions of naloxone are attributed to its antagonism of endogenous opioid peptides (see Chapters 4 and 5). The morphine-antagonistic actions of naloxone in man (postaddicts) were investigated by Jasinski *et al.* (1967). Single doses of naloxone (15 mg) given subcutaneously before morphine (30 mg) given by the same route blocked the effects of morphine for at least 9 hr after administration of naloxone, the degree of blockade generally diminishing as the time interval between administration of the two drugs increased. In subjects receiving naloxone subcutaneously every 4 hr in increasing doses over a period of 4 weeks to a stabilization level of 90 mg/day, which was maintained for an additional 2 weeks, persistence of morphine blockade was demonstrated; for example, the effects of single doses of morphine (90 mg) were equal to or less than those of morphine (10 mg) in the drug-free control period; however, the morphine-blocking effects decayed over the time period between scheduled doses of naloxone (every 4 hr). No physiological changes were observed during the entire 6-week period of chronic administration of naloxone, and no abstinence syndrome emerged after abrupt withdrawal of the drug, except for an increase in respiratory rate. In subjects tolerant to morphine, 240 mg/day, morphine-abstinence syndromes were precipitated by subcutaneous single doses of naloxone, 0.25 and 0.50 mg (seven times as potent as nalorphine). By the oral route, naloxone is much less effective as an opioid antagonist; Eddy and May (1973) estimated that naloxone is 100 times less effective orally than subcutaneously.

Naltrexone (N-cyclopropylmethyl-noroxymorphone), an analogue of naloxone, was found by Blumberg and Dayton (1972) to have slight opioid-agonist (limited analgesia in rats by the phenylquinone "writhing" test) and powerful opioid-antagonist activity, being about twice as potent as naloxone in this respect and longer lasting. In man (post-addicts), Martin et al. (1973) found that most of the 11 subjects who received single doses of naltrexone (0.01–80.0 mg/70 kg) subcutaneously identified it as a "blank." One subject displayed scratching, talkativeness, and "coasting" after naltrexone on two occasions, and observers thought he had received an opioid analgesic. Another subject who received naltrexone (70 mg/70 kg) became nauseated and irritable, had racing thoughts, and saw Disney-like characters when his eyes were closed. In precipitating abstinence in subjects tolerant to morphine (60 mg/day), naltrexone by the subcutaneous route was 17 times as potent as nalorphine and about 1.7 times as potent as naloxone. For comparison of the morphine-blocking actions of naltrexone and naloxone in nontolerant subjects, single doses of the two drugs were used that were calculated to be equipotent in precipitating abstinence in morphine-tolerant subjects. Given subcutaneously, naltrexone was more potent than naloxone, and the half-life of its antagonistic action was at least twice as long as that of naloxone in blocking the effects of morphine (25 mg) subcutaneously.

In drug-free subjects, naltrexone (30 mg) by the *oral* route significantly increased diastolic blood pressure and lowered rectal temperature; the pupils were slightly but not significantly constricted. A single oral dose of naltrexone (15 mg) produced blockade of the effects of morphine (30 mg) given subcutaneously; the blocking effect became evident 6 hr after the administration of naltrexone, became maximal by 12 hr, and persisted for 24 hr. During chronic administration of naltrexone orally, in doses of 15 mg and 25 mg twice daily (30 and 50 mg/day), the effects of morphine (100 mg subcutaneously) were less than those of 15 mg in the drug-free control period. Chronic administration of naltrexone orally was continued, while subcutaneous injections of morphine four times daily were begun, with doses of morphine increasing to 240 mg/day over a period of 6 days, after which the daily morphine level was maintained for an additional 11 days. During chronic administration of morphine, only one of the nine subjects identified this medication as a narcotic, and then on only two occasions; three of the others identified the medication as a barbiturate, amphetamine, chlorpromazine, meprobamate, or chlordiazepoxide. On abrupt withdrawal of the morphine (naltrexone continued), the expected abstinence syndrome was markedly attenuated, especially in those subjects who were receiving the larger daily oral doses of naltrexone (50 mg/day); in these subjects, the intensity and time course of the morphine-abstinence syndrome approximated those observed after abrupt withdrawal of morphine while continuing to receive cyclazocine orally (4 mg/day). After subsidence of the attenuated morphine-abstinence syndrome, naltrexone was abruptly discontinued; no abstinence syndrome emerged, regardless of the previous daily dosage of naltrexone (30 or 50 mg/day). Martin *et al.* (1973) concluded that because of naltrexone's much greater oral effectiveness, potency, and longer duration of action as an opioid antagonist, it has definite advantages over naloxone in the treatment of detoxified heroin addicts (see Chapter 8).

REFERENCES

Allen, C. R., Murphy, M. A., and Meek, W. J., 1945, The action of morphine in slowing the heart rate of unconditioned dogs, *Anesthesiology* 6:149–153.

Andrews, H. L., 1943, Changes in the electroencephalogram during a cycle of morphine addiction, *Psychosom. Med.* 5:143–147.

Andrews, H. L., and Himmelsbach, C. K., 1944, Relation to the intensity of the morphine abstinence syndrome to dosage, *J. Pharmacol. Exp. Ther.* 81:288–293.

Andrews, H. L., and Workman, W., 1941, Pain threshold measurements in the dog, *J. Pharmacol. Exp. Ther.* 73:99–103.

Archer, S., Albertson, N. F., Harris, L. S., Pierson, A. K., Bird, J. G., Keats, A. S., Telford,

J., and Papadopoulos, C. N., 1962, Narcotic antagonists as analgesics, *Science* 137:541–543.

Archer, S., Albertson, N. F., Harris, L. S., Pierson, A. K., and Bird, J. G., 1964, Pentazocine: Strong analgesics and analgesic antagonists in the benzomorphan series, *J. Med. Chem.* 7:123–127.

Arduini, A., and Arduini, M. G., 1954, Effect of drugs and metabolic alterations on brain stem arousal mechanism, *J. Pharmacol. Exp. Ther.* 110:76–85.

Bauer, R. O., and Pearson, R. G., 1956, The effects of morphine-nalorphine mixtures on psychmotor performance, *J. Pharmacol. Exp. Ther.*, 117:258–264.

Bickerman, A. A., and Barach, A. L., 1954, The experimental production of cough in human subjects induced by citric acid aerosis: Preliminary studies on the evaluation of antitussive agents, *Amer. J. Med. Sci.* 228:156–163.

Blumberg, H., and Dayton, H. B., 1972, Narcotic antagonist studies with EN–1639A (*N*-cyclopropylmethylnoroxymorphone hydrochloride), in *Fifth International Congress on Pharmacology, San Francisco, 23–28 July 1972, Abstracts of Volunteer Papers*, p. 23.

Blumberg, H., Dayton, H. B., George, M., and Rapaport, D. N., 1961, *N*-allylnoroxymorphone: A potent narcotic antagonist, *Fed. Proc.* 20:311.

Bremer, F., 1937, Différence d'action de la narcose éthérique et du sommeil barbiturique sur les réactions sensorielles acoustiques du cortex cérébral: Signification de cette différence en ce qui concerne la mécanisme du sommeil, *Compt. Rend. Soc. Biol. Paris* 124:848–852.

Briggs, F. N., and Munson, P. L., 1954, Suppression of the release of adrenocortictrophic hormone (ACTH) my morphine, *J. Pharmacol. Exp. Ther.* 110:7–8.

Brooks, C. McC., and Peck, M. E., 1940, Effect of various cortical lesions on development of placing and hopping reactions in rats, *J. Neurophysiol.* 3:66–72.

Brooks, C. McC., Goodwin, R., and Willard, H. N., 1941, The effect of various brain lesions on morphine induced hyperglycemia and excitement in the cat, *Amer. J. Physiol.* (Proc.) 133:226–227.

CoTui, F. W., DeBodo, R. C., and Bengalia, A. E., 1937, Morphine Hyperglycemia, *J. Pharmacol. Exp. Ther.* 61:48–57.

D'Amour, F. E., and Smith, D. L., 1941, A method for determining loss of pain sensation, *J. Pharmacol. Exp. Ther.* 72:74–79.

DeBodo, R. C., 1944, The antidiuretic of morphine and its mechanism, *J. Pharmacol. Exp. Ther.* 82:74–85.

DeBodo, R. C., and Brooks, C. McC., 1937, The effects of morphine on blood sugar and reflex activity in the chronic spinal cat, *J. Pharmacol. Exp. Ther.* 61:82–88.

De Noraquo, N., 1969, The hallucinatory effect of pentazocine (Talwin), *J. Amer. Med. Ass.* 210:502.

Drew, J. H., Dripps, R. D., and Comroe, J. H., 1946, Clinical studies on morphine. II. The effect of morphine upon the circulation of man and upon the circulatory and respiratory responses to tilting, *Anesthesiology* 7:4–61.

Dripps, R. B., and Dumke, P. R., 1943, The effect of narcotics on the balance between central and chemoreceptor control of respiration, *J. Pharmacol. Exp. Ther.* 77:290–300.

Drug and Theraputic Information, Inc. (New York), 1970, Propoxyphene hydrochloride (Darvon) and Darvon compounds, *The Medical Letter* 12(2), Jan. 23.

Eckenoff, J. E., Elder, J. D., and King, B. D., 1951, The effect of *N*-allylnormorphine in treatment of opiate overdose, *Amer. J. Med. Sci.* 222:115–117.

Eckenhoff, J. E., Elder, J. D., and King, B. D., 1952, *N*-allylnormorphine in the treatment of morphine or Demerol narcosis, *Amer. J. Med. Sci.* 223:191–197.

Eddy, N. B., and May, E. L., 1973, The search for a better analgesic, *Science* 181:407–414.

Eisenman, A. J., Fraser, H. F., and Brooks, J. W., 1961, Urinary excretion and plasma levels of 17-hydroxycorticosteroids during a cycle of addiction to morphine, *J. Pharmacol. Exp. Ther.* 132:226–231.

Eisenman, A. J., Sloan, J. W., Martin, W. R., Jasinski, D. R., and Brooks, J. W., 1969, Catecholamine and 17-hydroxycorico-steroid excretion during a cycle of morphine dependence in man, *J. Psychiat. Res.* 7:19–28.

Fischlewitz, J., 1948, Über den Angriffspunkt des Morphins am Atmungszentrum, *Helv. Physiol. Acta.* 6:455–461.

Foldes, F. F., Lunn, J. N., Moore, J., and Brown, I. M., 1963, N-allylnoroxymorphone: A new potent narcotic antagonist, *Amer. J. Med. Sci.* 245:23–30.

Food and Drug Administration, Pentazocine abuse rises—Schedule IV status proposed, 1978–1979, *FDA Drug Bull.* 8(6):34.

Food and Drug Administration, 1979, Fatalities due to propoxyphene, *FDA Drug Bull.* 9(1):2.

Fraser, H. F., and Isbell, H., 1952, Comparative effects of 20 mg., of morphine sulfate on non-addicts and former addicts, *J. Pharmacol. Exp. Ther.* 105:498–502.

Fraser, H. F., and Isbell, H., 1960, Human pharmacology and addiction liability of *dl*- and *d*-propoxyphene, *U. N. Bull. Narcotics* 12:9–14.

Fraser, H. F., and Rosenberg, D. E., 1964, Studies of human addiction liability of 2'-hydroxy-5, 9-dimethy-2-(3,3-dimethylallyl)-6,7-benzomorphan (WIN 20,228): Weak narcotic antagonist, *J. Pharmacol. Exper. Ther,* 143:149–156.

Fraser, H. F., Wikler, A., Eiseman, A. J., and Isbell, H., 1952, Use of N-allylnormorphine in treatment of methadone poisoning in man: Report of two cases, *J. Amer. Med. Ass.* 148:1205–1207.

Fraser, H. F., Nash, T. L., Van Horn, G. D., and Isbell, H., 1954, Use of miotic effect in evaluating analgesic drugs in man, *Arch. Int. Pharmacodyn. Ther.* 98:443–451.

Fraser, H. F., Van Horn, G. D., and Isbell, H., 1956, Studies on N-allylnormorphine in man: Antagonism to morphine and heroin and effects of mixtures of N-allylnormorphine and morphine, *Amer. J. Med. Sci.* 231:1–8.

Fraser, H. F., Isbell, H., and Van Horn, G. D., 1957, Effects of morphine as compared with a mixture of morphine and diaminphenylthiazole (Daptazole), *Anesthesiology* 18:531–535.

Fraser, H. F., Van Horn, G. D., Martin, W. R., Wolbach, A. B., and Isbell, H., 1961, Methods for evaluating addiction liability. (A) "Attitude" of opiate addicts toward opiate-like drugs. (B) A short-term "direct" addiction test, *J. Pharmacol. Exp. Ther.* 133:371–387.

George, R., and Way, E. L., 1955a, Adrenal cortical response of normal, adrenal demedullated and hypophysectomized rats to morphine and methadone, *J. Pharmacol. Exp. Ther.* 113:23.

George, R., and Way, E. L., 1955b, Studies on the mechanism of pituitary–adrenal activation by morphine, *Brit. J. Pharmacol. Chemother.* 20:260–264.

George, R., and Way, E. L., 1959, The role of the hypothalamus in pituitary–adrenal activation and antidiuresis by morphine, *J. Pharmacol. Exp. Ther.* 125:111–115.

Goetz, E. L., and Bain, R. V., 1974, Neonatal withdrawal symptoms associated with maternal use of pentazocine, *J. Pediatr.* 84:887–888.

Gray, G. W., and Beckman, H., 1956, Effects of certain analgesic and analgesic–antagonist drugs on intestinal motility, *J. Pharmacol. Exp. Ther.* 116:25.

Haertzen, C. A., and Hooks, N. T., 1969, Changes in personality and subjective experience associate with the chronic administration of opiates, *J. Nerv. Ment. Dis.* 148:606–614.

Hambourger, W. E., 1940, The excitant action of morphine on the cat, *J. Pharmacol. Exp. Ther.* (Abstract) *69*:287.

Harris, L. S., and Pierson, A. K., 1964, Some narcotic antagonists in the benzomorphan series, *J. Pharmacol. Exp. Ther. 143*:141–148.

Harthoorn, A. M., and Bligh, J., 1965, The use of a new oripavine derivative with potent morphine-like activity for the restraint of hoofed wild animals, *Res. Vet. Sci. 6*:290–299.

Hemingway, A., 1938, The effect of morphine on the skin and rectal temperatures of dogs as related to thermal polypnea, *J. Pharmacol. Exp. Ther. 63*:414–420.

Henderson, V. W., and Rice, H. V., 1939, The action of certain drugs on respiratory reflexes, *J. Pharmacol. Exp. Ther. 66*:336–349.

Himmelsbach, C. K., 1941, Studies on the relation of drug addiction to the autonomic nervous system: Results of cold pressor tests, *J. Pharmacol. Exp. Ther. 73*:91–97.

Himmelsbach, C. K., 1942a, Clinical studies on drug addiction. Physical dependence, withdrawal and recovery, *Arch. Int. Med. 69*:766–722.

Himmelsbach, C. K., 1942b, Studies of the addiction liability of "Demerol" (D-140), *J. Pharmacol. Exp. Ther. 75*:54–68.

Himmelsbach, C. K., 1943, Further studies of the addiction liability of Demerol (1-methyl-4-phenylpiperidine-4-carboxylic acid ethyl ester hydrochloride), *J. Pharmacol. Exp. Ther. 79*:5–9.

Himmelsbach, C. K., 1944, Studies on the relation of drug addiction to the autonomic nervous system: results of tests of peripheral blood flow, *J. Pharmacol. Exp. Ther. 80*:343–353.

Himmelsbach, C. K., Andrews, H. L., Felix, R. H., Oberst, F. W., and Davenport, L., 1940, Studies on codeine addiction, *Publ. Health Rep. Suppl. 158.*

Houde, R. R., and Wikler, A., 1951, Delineation of the skin-twitch response in dogs and the effects thereon on morphine, theiopental and mephenesin, *J. Pharmacol. Exp. Ther. 103*:236–242, 1951.

Huggins, R. A., Handley, C. A., and La Forge, M., 1949, Effects of morphine, codiene and dilaudid on blood flow, *J. Pharmacol. Exp. Ther. 95*:318–322.

Irwin, S., Houde, R. W., Bennett, D. R., Hendershot, L. C., and Seevers, M. H., 1951, The effects of morphine, methadone, and meperidine on some reflex responses of spinal animals to nociceptive stimulation, *J. Pharmacol. Exp. Ther. 101*:132–143.

Isbell, H., 1947, Effect of morphine addiction on blood, plasma and "extracellular" fluid volumes in man, *Pub. Health Reports 62*:1499–1513.

Isbell, H., 1956, Attempted addiction to nalorphine, *Fed. Proc. 15*:442.

Isbell, H., Eisenman, A. J., Wikler, A., and Frank, K., 1948a, The effects of single doses of 6-dimethylamino-4, 4-diphenyl-3-heptanone (Amidon, methadon, or "10820") on human subjects, *J. Pharmacol. Exp. Ther. 92*:83–89.

Isbell, H., Wikler, A., Eisenman, A. J., Daingerfield, M., and Frank, K., 1948b, Liability of addiction of 6-dimethylamino-4, 4-diphenyl-3-heptanone (methodon, amidone or "10820") in man, *Arch. Int. Med. 82*:362–396.

Jasinski, D. R., 1973, Assessment of the dependence liability of opiates and sedative hypnotics, in *Psychic Dependence* (L. Goldberg and F. Hoffmeister, Eds.), p. 164. Springer-Verlag, New York.

Jasinski, D. R., Martin, W. R., and Haertzen, C. A., 1967, The human pharmacology and abuse potential of N-allylnoroxymorphone (naloxone), *J. Pharmacol. Exp. Ther. 157*:420–426.

Karliner, J. S., 1967, Propoxyphene hydrochloride poisoning: Report of a case treated with peritoneal dialysis, *J. Amer. Ass. 199*:1006–1009.

Kay, D. C., 1975a, Human sleep and EEG through a cycle of methadone dependence, *Electroenceph. Clin. Neurophysiol. 38:35–43.*
Kay, D. C., 1975b, Human sleep during chronic morphine intoxication, *Psychopharmacologia* 44:117–124.
Kay, D. C., Eisenstein, R. B., and Jasinski, D. R., 1949, Morphine effects on human REM state, waking state and NREM sleep, *Psychopharmacologia* 14:404–416.
Keats, A. S., and Telford, J., 1956, Nalorphine, a potent analgesic in man, *J. Pharmacol. Exp. Ther.* 117:190–196.
Lasagna, L., 1965, Drug interaction in the field of analgesic drugs, *Proc. Roy. Soc. Med.* 58:978–983.
Lasagna, L., and Beecher, H. K., 1954, The analgesic effectiveness of nalorphine and nalorphine–morphine combinations in man, *J. Pharmacol. Exp. Ther.* 112:356–363.
Lee, H. K., and Wang, S. C., 1975, Mechanism of morphine-induced miosis in the dog, *J. Pharmacol. Exp. Ther.* 192:415–431.
Leimdorfer, A., 1948, An electroencephalographic analysis of the action of amidone, morphine and strychnine on the central nervous system. *Arch. Int. Pharmacodyn. Ther.* 76:153–162.
Lindsley, D. B., Bowden, J. W., and Magoun, H. W., 1949, Effect upon the EEG of acute injury to the brain stem activating mechanism, *Electroencephalog. Clin. Neurophysiol.* 1:475–485.
Lotti, V. J., Lomax, P., and George, R., 1965a, N-allylnormorphine antagonism of the hypothermic effect of morphine in the rat following intracerebral and systemic administration, *J. Pharmacol. Exp. Ther.* 150:420–425.
Lotti, V. J., Lomax, P., and George, R., 1965b, Temperature responses in the rat following intracerebral microinjection of morphine, *J. Pharmacol. Exp. Ther.* 150:135–139.
Lotti, V. J., Lomax, P., and George, R., 1966, Acute tolerance to morphine following systemic and intracerebral injection in the rat, *Int. J. Neuropharmacol.* 5:35–42.
Lotti, V. J., Kokka, N., and George, R., 1969, Pituitary–adrenal activation following intrahypothalamic microinjection of morphine, *Neuroendocrinology* 4:326–332.
Marri, R., and Hauss, W. H., 1939, Sinus carotidien et réflexes respiratoires: Influences de l'hypoxemie, de l'hypercapnie, de la saignée, de l'hyperthermie, de l'ésérine, de la morphine, du véronal et de l'évipan sur les réflexes respiratoires déclenchés par les variations de la pression sanguine au niveau du sinus carotidien, *Arch. Int. Pharmacodyn. Thér.* 63:449–469.
Martin, W. R., 1967, Opioid antagonists, *Pharmacol. Rev.* 19:463–521.
Martin, W. R., and Fraser, H. F., 1961, A comparative study of physiological and subjective effects of heroin and morphine administered intravenously in post-addicts, *J. Pharmacol. Exp. Ther.* 133:388–399.
Martin, W. R., and Gorodetzky, C. W., 1965, Demonstration of tolerance to and physical dependence on N-allylnormorphine (nalorphine), *J. Pharmacol. Exp. Ther.* 150:437–442.
Martin, W. R., and Jasinski, D. R., 1969, Physiological parameters of morphine dependence in man: Tolerance, early abstinence, protracted abstinence, *J. Psychiat. Res.* 7:9–17.
Martin, W. R., Wikler, A., Eades, C. G., and Pescor, F. R., 1963, Tolerance to and physical dependence on morphine in the rat, *Psychopharmacologia* 4:247–260.
Martin, W. R., Fraser, H. F., Gorodetzky, C. W., and Rosenberg, D. E., 1965, Studies of the dependence-producing potential of the narcotic antagonist 2-cyclopropylmethyl-2'-hydroxy-5, 9-dimethyl-6, 7 benzomorphan (cyclazocine, WIN-20, 740, ARC II-C-3), *J. Pharmacol. Exp. Ther.* 150:426–436.
Martin, W. R., Gorodetzky, C. W., and McClane, T. K., 1966, An experimental study in

the treatment of narcotic addicts with cyclazocine, *Clin. Pharmacol. Ther.* 7:455–465.

Martin, W. R., Jasinski, D. R., Sapira, J. D., Flanary, H. G., Kelly, O. A., Thompson, A. K., and Logan, C. R., 1968, The respiratory effects of morphine during a cycle of dependence, *J. Pharmacol. Exp. Ther.* 62:182–189.

Martin, W. R., Jasinski, D. R., and Mansky, P. A., 1973, Naltrexone, an antagonist for the treatment of heroin dependence, *Arch. Gen. Psychiat.* 28:784–791.

Masserman, J. H., 1939, Effects of morphine sulfate on hypothalamus of cat, *Proc. Soc. Exp. Biol. Med.* (N.Y.) 42:315–317.

McCawley, E. L., Hart, E. R., and Marsh, D. F., 1941, The preparation of N-allylnormorphine, *J. Amer. Chem. Soc.* 63:314.

McCrea, F. D., Eadie, G. S., and Morgan, J. E., 1942, The mechanism of morphine miosis, *J. Pharmacol. Exp. Ther.* 74:239–246.

Meissner, R. 1923, Ueber atmungserregende Heilmittel, *Z. gesamte Exp. Med.* 31:159–214.

Nilsen, O. L., 1961, Studies on algesimetry by electrical stimulation of the mouse tail, *Acta Pharmacol. Toxicol.* 18:10–22.

Orahovats, P. D., Winter, C. A., and Lehman, E. G., 1953, The effect of N-allylnormorphine upon the development of tolerance to morphine in the albino rat, *J. Pharmacol. Exp. Ther.* 109:413–416.

Pearl, J., Stander, H., and McKean, D. B., 1969, Effects of analgesics and other drugs on mice in phenylquinone and rotarod tests, *J. Pharmacol. Exp. Ther.* 167:9–13.

Perrine, T. D., Atwell, L., Tice, I. B., Jacobson, A. E., and May, E. L., 1972, Analgesic activity as determined by the Nilsen method, *J. Pharm. Sci.* 61:86–88.

Pohl, J., 1915, Über das N-allylnorcodein, einen Antagonisten des Morphins, *Z. exp. Path. Ther.* 17:370–382.

Richter, C. P., and Paterson, A. S., 1932, On the pharmacology of the grasp reflex, *Brain* 55:391–396.

Rovenstine, E. A., and Cullen, S. C., 1939, Anesthetic management of patients with hyperactive carotid sinus reflex, *Surgery* 6:167–176.

Sandoval, R. G., and Wang, R. I. H., 1969, Tolerance and dependence on pentazocine, *New Engl. J. Med.* 280:1391–1392.

Sawyer, C. H., Critchlow, B. V., and Barraclough, C. A., 1955, Mechanisms of blockage of pituitary activation in the rat by morphine, atropine and barbiturates, *Endocrinology* 57:345–354.

Scanlon, J. W., 1974, Pentazocine and neonatal withdrawal symptoms, *J. Pediatr.* 85:735–736.

Schmidt, C. F., 1940, Effect of carotid sinus and carotid body reflexes upon respiration, *Anesthesiol. Analgesia* 19:261–271.

Schrappe, O., 1959, "Physical dependence" nach chronischer Verabreichung von N-allylnormorphin, *Arzneim.-Forsch.* 9:130–132.

Seevers, M. H., and Deneau, G. A., 1963, Physiological aspects of tolerance and physical dependence, in *Physiological Pharmacology*, Vol. 1 (W. S. Root and F. G. Hofmann, Eds.), pp. 565–640. Academic Press, New York.

Seevers, M. H., and Woods, L. A., 1953, The phenomena of tolerance, *Amer. J. Med.* 14:546–557.

Sharpe, L. G., and Pickworth, W. B., 1980, Pharmacologic evidence for a tonic muscarinic inhibitory input to the Edinger–Westphal nucleus: Relation to morphine-induced miosis in the dog. (in preparation).

Silvestrini, B., and Longo, V. G., 1956, Selective activity of morphine on the "EEG arousal reaction" to painful stimul, *Experientia* 12:436–438.

Smith, G. M., and Beecher, H. K., 1959, Measurement of "mental clouding" and other subjective effects of morphine, *J. Pharmacol. Exp. Ther.* 126:50–62.

Smith, G. M., Semke, C. W., and Beecher, H. K., 1962, Objective evidence of mental effects of heroin, morphine and placebo in normal subjects, *J. Pharmacol. Exp. Ther.* 136:53–58.

Tainter, N. L., Tainter, E. G., Lawrence, W. A., Neura, E. N., Lackey, R. W., Ludnea, F. P., Kirland, H. B., and Gonzale, R. I., 1943, Influence of various drugs on the threshold for electrical convulsions, *J. Pharmacol. Exp. Ther.* 79:42–53.

Tenney, S. M., and Mithoefer, J. C., 1953, The respiratory depressant action of N-allylnormorphine in the normal subject and in patients with respiratory acidosis secondary to pulmonary emphysema, *New Engl. J. Med.* 249:886–890.

Wang, S. C., and Glaviano, V. V., 1954, Locus of emetic action of morphine and hydergine in dogs, *J. Pharmacol. Exp. Ther.* 111:329–334.

Weijlard, J., and Erickson, A. E., 1942, N-allylnormorphine, *J. Amer. Chem. Soc.* 64:869–870.

Wikler, A., 1944, Studies on the action of morphine on the central nervous system of the cat, *J. Pharmacol. Exp. Ther.* 80:176–187.

Wikler, A., 1950, Sites and mechanisms of action of morphine and related drugs in the central nervous system, *Pharmacol. Rev.* 2:435–506.

Wikler, A., 1951, Effects of large doses of N-allylnormorphine in man, *Fed. Proc.* 10:345.

Wikler, A., 1952a, A psychodynamic study of a patient during self-regulated re-addiction to morphine, *Psychiat. Quart.* 260:270–293.

Wikler, A., 1952b, Reactions of dogs without neocortex during cycles of addiction to morphine and methadone, *Arch. Neurol. Psychiat.* (Chicago) 67:672–684.

Wikler, A., 1953, *Opiate Addiction: Psychological and Neurophysiological Aspects in Relation to Clinical Problems*, pp. 27–28. Charles C Thomas, Springfield, Ill.

Wikler, A., 1954, Clinical and electroencephalographic studies on the effects of mescaline, N-allylnormorphine and morphine in man, *J. Nerv. Ment. Dis.* 120:157–175.

Wikler, A., and Altschul, S., 1950, Effects of methadone and morphine on the electroencephalogram of the dog, *J. Pharmacol. Exp. Ther.* 98:437–446.

Wikler, A., and Carter, R. L., 1953, Effects of single doses of N-allylnormorphine on hindlimb reflexes of chronic spinal dogs during cycles of morphine addiction, *J. Pharmacol. Exp. Ther.* 109:92–101.

Wikler, A., and Pescor, F. T., 1954, Clinical and electroencephalographic effects of drugs in man and dog, *Trans. Amer. Neurol. Ass.* 79th Annual Meeting, pp. 170–172.

Wikler, A., Pescor, M. J., Kalbaugh, E. M., and Angelucci, R. J., 1952, The effects of frontal lobotomy on the morphine abstinence syndrome in man: An experimental study, *Arch. Neurol. Psychiat.* (Chicago) 67:510–521.

Wikler, A., Fraser, H. F., and Isbell, H., 1953, N-allylnormorphine: Effects of single doses and precipitation of acute "abstinence syndromes" during addiction to morphine, methadone or heroin in man (post-addicts), *J. Pharmacol. Exp. Ther.* 109:8–20.

Williams, E. G., and Oberst, F. W., 1946, A cycle of morphine addiction. Part I. Biological investigations, *Pub. Health Reports* 61:1–25.

Winter, C. A., and Flataker, L., 1951, The effect of cortisone, desoxycorticosterone and adrenocorticotrophic hormone upon the responses of animals to analgesic drugs, *J. Pharmacol. Exp. Ther.* 103:93–105.

Woods, L. A., 1956, The pharmacology of nalorphine (N-allylnormorphine), *Pharmacol. Rev.* 8:175–198.

CHAPTER 4

Opioid Receptors and Endogenous Opioid Peptides

OPIOID RECEPTORS

According to Ariëns *et al.* (1964b), the concept of *receptors* was first proposed by J. N. Langley in 1905 to account for the actions of nicotine and curare at the myoneural junction, and by P. Ehrlich in 1906 to account for specific interactions between antigens and antibodies and for the selectivity of dyes for certain components of living cells. On the basis of his research, Ehrlich (1913) concluded that "If the law is true in chemistry that 'corpora non agunt nisi liquida,' then for chemotherapy the principle is true that 'corpora non agunt nisi fixata'" (substances do not act unless they are fixated). In modern drug–receptor interaction theory, *reversible* "fixation" of the drug to the receptor is held to produce the pharmacological effect, and drug–receptor interactions are viewed as analogous to substrate–enzyme interactions (Michaelis & Menten, 1913). In this view, subject to some qualifications expressed by Ariëns *et al.* (1956), the receptor concentration is regarded as if it were an enzyme concentration, the drug concentration as if it were a substrate concentration, and the pharmacological effect of the drug–receptor combination as if it were the initial reaction velocity of the enzyme-catalyzed substrate change. On the basis of these and some other assumptions, the dose–effect relationships of agonists, partial agonists, and antagonists, as well as their intrinsic activities (efficacies) and affinities, have been calculated. The term *agonist* implies that a given pharmacological effect of a drug increases with its dose (or its concentration) up to a maximum. The dose (or concentration) of the drug that produces a maximal effect is a measure of the efficacy or intrinsic activity of the drug–receptor combination (generally referred to as the *efficacy* or *intrinsic activity* of the drug), while the dose (or concentration) of the drug that produces a half-maximal effect is a measure of the *affinity* of the drug for the same receptor. For convenience, the effect is usually plotted against the logarithm of the dose (or concentration), yielding a sigmoid curve, or the reciprocal of the effect is plotted against the reciprocal of the dose (or concentration), yielding a straight line; in the latter case, the slope of the straight line indicates the drug's affinity, and the intercept of the straight line with the ordinate (reciprocal of effect) indicates its intrinsic activity. A *partial agonist* is a drug that exerts an effect qualitatively similar to that of an agonist but with lesser intrinsic activity; that is, the slope of its dose–effect curve is shallower, and its maximal effect is less than that of an agonist. Assuming that both a given agonist and a given partial agonist combine with the same receptor, the effect of the partial agonist will add to that of the agonist when the dose (or concentration) of the agonist is low, but it will antagonize the effect of the agonist (by competition for receptors) when the dose (or concentration) of the agonist is high. An *antagonist* is a drug with affinity for but no intrinsic activity at the receptor with which an agonist or a partial agonist combines; a measure of its antagonistic potency is the dose (or concentration) of the antagonist required to double the dose (or concentration) of the agonist or partial agonist needed to produce the same degree of pharmacological effect as in the absence of any antagonist. The mathematical equations for the interaction of one or more drugs with one receptor system and with different receptor systems are given in detail by Ariëns *et al*. (1956, 1964,b) and in more condensed form by Gero (1971).

It was long assumed that the morphine receptor was unitary and that the narcotic antagonist nalorphine interacted with the same receptor with greater affinity but lesser intrinsic activity, thus resulting in competitive dualism (assuming that the agonistic effects of morphine and nalorphine are exerted on the same receptor). However, Martin (1967) pointed out that this assumption is inconsistent with the biphasic dose–response curves for analgesic activity of mixtures of morphine and other opioids and nalorphine and other antagonists obtained by several investigators, and he postulated that there are two analgesic receptors, one where morphine acts as an agonist and nalorphine as a competitive antagonist (higher affinity, zero intrinsic activity), and the other where nalorphine acts as an agonist. This view was supported by the observations that subjects tolerant to the subjective effects of morphine are not cross-tolerant to the psychotomimetic effects of cyclazocine and that the nalorphine- and cyclazocine-abstinence syndromes are qualitatively different from the morphine-abstinence syndrome. Partly on the basis of studies on nondependent, morphine-dependent, and cyclazocine-dependent chronic spinal dogs (spinal cords transected at T-10), Martin *et al.* (1976) and Gilbert and Martin (1976) concluded that there are three receptors with which opioids and opioid antagonists may interact, namely, a μ (morphine) receptor, a κ (ketocyclazocine) receptor, and a σ (SKF-10,047, N-allylnormetazocine) receptor. In the chronic nondependent spinal dog, morphine, the prototype drug for the μ receptor, produced miosis, bradycardia, hypothermia, "indifference" to environmental stimuli, and dose-dependent depression of nociceptive responses (skin twitch, elicited above the level of spinal cord transection, and spinal flexor reflex). Ketocyclazocine, the prototype drug for the κ receptor, produced miosis and sedation (the dogs appeared to be asleep), with tremors above the level of spinal cord transection but no marked effects on body temperature, pulse rate, or respiration, and marked dose-dependent depressant effects on the spinal flexor reflex, while it was less effective than morphine in prolonging the latency of the skin twitch. SKF-10,047, the prototype drug for the σ receptor, produced mydriasis, tachypnea, tachycardia, and behavioral excitement suggestive of canine delirium, with slight depression of the spinal flexor reflex (dose-response curve much less steep than that of morphine) and no significant effect on the skin twitch. The effects of all three drugs could be antagonized by the "pure" antagonist, naltrexone, indicating that they are agonists. Further evidence of their agonistic properties was yielded by the observation that tolerance developed to the effects of morphine (μ), ketocyclazocine (κ), and SKF-10,047 (σ) upon chronic administration of these drugs. While morphine suppressed abstinence in the morphine-dependent dog, ketocyclazocine did not, indicating that ketocyclazocine had no intrinsic activity at the μ receptor; since ketocyclazocine, at best, precipitated only a liminal abstinence syndrome in the morphine-dependent dog, its affinity for the μ receptor was demonstrated to be low. Therefore, ketocyclazocine appears to be a relatively "pure" κ agonist. Ketocyclazocine could suppress abstinence signs in the cyclazocine-dependent dog, and the ketocyclazocine- and cyclazocine-abstinence syndromes were similar to each other but different from the morphine-abstinence syndromes, indicating that cyclazocine, too, was a κ agonist. Furthermore, 20 times as much naltrexone was needed to precipitate abstinence in cyclazocine-dependent dogs as was needed to precipitate abstinence in morphine-dependent dogs. However, unlike ketocyclazocine, cyclazocine could precipitate abstinence in the morphine-dependent dog, indicating that cyclazocine had a strong affinity for the μ receptor (but zero intrinsic activity). Also, in the nondependent dog, cyclazocine, besides depressing the spinal flexor reflex but not the skin twitch (κ receptor effects), produced mydriasis, tachycardia, tachypnea, and canine delirium, much as did SKF-10,047 (σ receptor effects). Hence, it was concluded that cyclazocine acts as a competitive antagonist at the μ receptor and as an agonist at the κ and σ receptors. Morphine suppressed the cyclazocine-abstinence syndrome, indicating that in addition to its agonistic action on the μ receptor, morphine has agonistic action on the κ receptor. Buprenorphine and propiram produced morphinelike effects in the nondependent dog, but the dose–effect curves for the skin twitch were less steep than those for morphine, and these drugs suppressed abstinence in low-dose morphine-dependent dogs but precipitated abstinence in high-dose morphine-dependent dogs. Hence it appeared that buprenorphine and propiram are partial agonists (high affinity, low intrinsic activity) at the μ receptor. In nondependent dogs, nalorphine produced miosis, lowering the body temperature, and depression of nociceptive reflexes, but the dose–effect curves reached a ceiling at less than maximal effect (compared with that of morphine). Nalorphine precipitated abstinence in morphine-dependent dogs but could suppress abstinence in low-dose cyclazocine-dependent dogs and precipitate abstinence in high-dose cyclazocine-dependent dogs. Therefore, it was concluded that nalorphine acts as a competitive antagonist at the μ receptor (high affinity, zero intrinsic activity), as a partial κ agonist (high affinity, low intrinsic activity), and (particularly because of its psychotomimetic effects in man) as a σ agonist. Analogous studies led to the conclusions that diprenorphine and oxilorphan, like nalorphine, are competitive antagonists at the μ receptor and partial agonists at the κ and σ receptors. Pentazocine appeared to be a competitive antagonist at the μ receptor and an agonist at the κ and σ receptors. Naloxone and naltrexone exhibited no intrinsic activity as any of the three postulated receptors, but high affinity for the μ receptor (competitive antagonism) and weaker affinities for the κ and σ receptors (weaker competitive antagonism).

Evidence for multiple opioid receptors in the *in vitro* guinea pig ileum and mouse vas deferens preparations, as well as in brain homogenates has been adduced by H. W. Kosterlitz and his collaborators. In studies on four benzomorphan derivatives that have potent antinociceptive activity in the mouse but do not suppress or precipitate abstinence in the monkey, Hutchinson *et al.* (1975) found that these compounds had greater agonist potencies relative to normorphine in the guinea pig ileum and the mouse vas deferens, but the ratio of potencies in mouse vas deferens to potencies in guinea pig ileum was about one-fourth that of the corresponding ratio for normorphine; also much higher concentrations of naloxone were required to antagonize their agonistic actions than to antagonize the agonistic actions of normorphine. The relative potencies of these benzomorphans to inhibit stereospecific ^{3}H-dihydromorphine binding by rat brain membrane fragments was more closely related to their relative agonist potencies in the mouse vas deferens than in the guinea pig ileum. Hutchinson et al. (1975) concluded that the benzomorphans investigated may act on a receptor different from the one that mediates the effects of agonists of the morphine type. In further studies, Lord et al. (1976) compared the actions of morphine, the endogenous opioid peptides (leucine-enkephalin, methionine-enkephalin, and β-endorphin) and two benzomorphan derivatives that had antinociceptive activity but did not suppress or precipitate abstinence in the morphine-dependent monkey, on the guinea pig ileum, on the mouse vas deferens, and on inhibition of ^{3}H-leucine-enkephalin binding in homogenates of guinea pig brain. The agonist potency of β-endorphin was approximately the same in the guinea pig ileum and the mouse vas deferens; the opioid pentapeptides (leucine-enkephalin and methionine-enkephalin) were much more potent on the mouse vas deferens than on the guinea pig ileum, while the reverse was true for morphine and the benzomorphans. The inhibition of ^{3}H-leucine-enkephalin binding was much weaker for morphine than for the opioid pentapeptides, and that for one of the benzomorphan compounds (Mr2034) was considerably weaker. In the mouse vas deferens, there was a directly proportional variation of the agonist potencies (relative to leucine-enkephalin) of all the agents tested with their potencies in inhibiting ^{3}H-leucine-enkephalin binding (relative to leucine-enkephalin). In the guinea pig ileum, however, the relative agonist potencies of morphine, Mr2034, and etorphine were much greater than in the mouse vas deferens at their respective relative potencies in inhibiting ^{3}H-leucine-enkephalin binding. Lord et al. (1976) concluded that in all three systems, there is a heterogenous population of opioid receptors. In the mouse vas deferens, the opioid pentapeptides have a high affinity for "δ-receptors" (from vas deferens); morphine, Mr2034, and etorphine may also combine with δ-receptors, but with low affinity. In the guinea pig ileum, the δ-receptors are in a minority; morphine and etorphine combine with μ-receptors, while Mr2034 may combine with κ-receptors. Lord et al. (1977) further showed that the concentration of naloxone required for doubling the concentration of agonist to produce the same pharmacological effect as in the absence of the antagonist was about 10 times higher for the endogenous opioid peptides than for normorphine in the mouse vas deferens, whereas it was only slightly higher for the endogenous opioid peptides than for normorphine in the guinea pig ileum. These findings indicate that in the mouse vas deferens, endogenous opioid peptides combine with δ-receptors, while normorphine combines with μ-receptors (and possibly with δ-receptors); in the guinea pig ileum, both the endogenous opioid peptides and normorphine combine with μ-receptors. Also, Lord *et al.* (1977) showed that in guinea pig brain homogenates, receptors for which ^{3}H-leucine-enkephalin has a high affinity are related to δ-receptors, while brain receptors for which ^{3}H-naloxone and ^{3}H-dihydromorphine have high affinities are related to μ-receptors.

Such differentiation of opioid receptors has received only little attention in the development of methods for demonstrating stereospecific binding sites of opioid agonists, partial agonists, and antagonists. Identification of the opioid receptor in neural and smooth muscle tissue is complicated by the fact that opioids are distributed not only at stereospecific binding sites where they exert their pharmacological actions, but also at nonspecific binding sites and, in a nonbound form, in surrounding lipids and/or water. In general, the levoisomers of opioid drugs are more active pharmacologically than their dextroisomers. Assuming that an excess of the dextroisomer of an opioid drug would mix freely with tracer amounts of the levoisomer in nonbinding sites and would displace the levoisomer from nonspecific binding sites but *not from stereospecific binding sites,* Goldstein *et al.* (1971) developed a method for measuring stereospecific binding of the opioid agonist levorphanol to subcellular fractions of mouse brain homogenates. Essentially, the method consists of subtracting the radioactivity of a tracer amount of radioactive levorphanol in the presence of a 100-fold excess of nonradioactive levorphanol from the radioactivity of the same tracer amount of radioactive levorphanol in the presence of a 100-fold excess of dextrorphan (Goldstein, 1973); the radioactivity remaining is due to the radioactive levorphanol stereospecifically bound to the presumed opioid receptor that was displaced by the excess of nonradioactive levorphanol but not by dextrorphan.

The radioactive tracer may be an opioid agonist like levorphanol in the technique of Goldstein *et al.* (1971), or it may be an opioid antagonist with high affinity for the opioid receptor. Employing ^{3}H-naloxone as the radioactive tracer in the presence of an excess of nonradioactive dextrorphan and in the presence of an excess of nonradioactive levorphanol, Pert and Snyder (1973) demonstrated stereospecific binding of ^{3}H-naloxone, mainly to mitochondria-synaptosomal fractions of homogenized brains of rats, mice, and guinea pigs and minced guinea pig intestine (no binding in Auerbach plexus-free guinea pig intestinal muscle). The distribution of stereoscopic specific bindings in the brain was uneven: highest density was in the corpus striatum, followed by midbrain, cerebral cortex, and brain stem, and very low density in the cerebellum. In other studies on the localization of opioid receptors in rat brain (by stereospecific ^{3}H-diprenorphine binding), Atweh and Kuhar (1977) demonstrated high densities of opioid receptors in the substantia gelatinosa of the spinal cord and of the spinal trigeminal nucleus, components of the vagal system, the nucleus ambiguous, and the area postrema. By substituting other nonradioactive opioid drugs (agonists and antagonists) for levorphanol in the stereospecific binding assay for ^{3}H-naloxone described above, Pert and Snyder (1973) were able to measure the concentration of the nonradioactive opioid drug required to inhibit by 50% the stereospecific binding of ^{3}H-naloxone (ED_{50}). A rough inverse parallelism was found for the known potencies of a variety of levo- and dextroisomers of opioid agonists and agonists with antagonist properties and their respective ED_{50}'s. In 1973, Pert et al. demonstrated that the stereospecific binding of radioactive opioid agonists in the absence of sodium ion (NaCl) was reduced in the presence of sodium ion, whereas that of opioid antagonists was increased in the presence of sodium ion. Similarly, the ED_{50}'s of nonradioactive "pure" opioid antagonists (naloxone, naltrexone, diprenorphine) was the same in the absence and in the presence of sodium ion, whereas the ED_{50}'s of nonradioactive opioid agonists (etorphine, meperidine, levorphanol, etc.) were much greater in the presence of sodium ion than in its absence. Thus, measurement of the effects of the absence or presence of sodium ion on stereospecific binding of radioactive opioids or on the inhibition of stereospecific binding of a radioactive opioid (^{3}H-naloxone) by nonradioactive opioid compounds (ED_{50}'s) affords a means of distinguishing opioid agonists from opioid antagonists in vitro. Interestingly, opioids with mixed agonist and antagonist properties (cyclazocine, levallorphan, nalorphine, pentazocine) showed effects of sodium ion on inhibition of stereoscopic binding of ^{3}H-naloxone that were similar to but much less than those of opioid agonists without antagonist properties.

In the same year, Simon et al. (1973) and Terenius (1973) independently reported stereospecific binding of radioactive opioid agonists to rat brain homogenates or synaptic plasma membrane fractions, using methods similar to those of Goldstein et al. (1971). The radioactive opioid agonist used by Simon et al. (1973) was ^{3}H-etorphine; they noted that its binding was inhibited by high sodium chloride concentrations and by various nonradioactive opioid agonists and antagonists. The radioactive opioid agonist used by Terenius (1973) was ^{3}H-dihydromorphine, and he noted that its binding was inhibited by nonradioactive nalorphine and naloxone but hardly at all by heroin and codeine.

ENDOGENOUS OPIOID PEPTIDES (ENKEPHALINS AND ENDORPHINS)

The discovery of stereospecific opioid receptors in neural tissues of the brain (including spinal cord) and of certain smooth muscles (guinea pig ileum and mouse vas deferens) and their localization at sites where morphine is known to act (though in man, the high density of stereospecific opioid receptors in the corpus stratum appears anomalous) suggested strongly that an endogenous morphinelike ligand must exist for these receptors. In a brief abstract published in 1974, Terenius and Wahlström reported the isolation of factors from rat brain and human cerebrospinal fluid that inhibited stereospecific binding of a radioactive opioid agonist. This report was more fully elaborated in two papers published by Terenius and Wahlström in 1975. In one (1975b), the factor was obtained from rat brain, had a molecular weight of 1000–1200 dalton (suggesting it might be a peptide), and inhibited the binding of ^{3}H-dihydromorphine to the opioid receptor in synaptic plasma membranes of rat brain and in the guinea pig ileum. In the other (1975a), the factor from human cerebrospinal fluid also had a molecular weight of 1000–1200 dalton and inhibited the binding of ^{3}H-dihydromorphine and of ^{3}H-naltrexone to synaptic plasma membrane preparations from rat brain; inhibition of ^{3}H-naltrexone binding was greater in the absence of sodium ion than in its presence, indicating that the factor had the properties of an opioid agonist, rather than an antagonist, hence the factor was termed *morphinelike factor* (MLF). Possibly of clinical significance was the finding that the level of MLF (measured as units/ml of receptor blocking activity) in the cerebrospinal fluid was 0.08–0.17 in seven patients with trigeminal neuralgia and 0.20–0.51 in four patients with intention tremor, cerebellar tumor, cerebral aneurysm, and cerebral tumor; however, one patient with trigeminal neuralgia had an MLF level of 0.24 units/ml.

Also in 1975, Pasternak *et al.* reported the isolation of a morphinelike substance (MLF) from rat and calf brains that was localized in synaptosomal fractions, that had a regional distribution correlating with that of opioid receptors, that had a molecular weight of about 1000, that could be degraded by carboxypeptidase A and leucine aminopeptidase (suggesting a peptide structure), and that inhibited ^{3}H-naloxone binding to a much greater extent in the absence of sodium ion than in its presence (and conversely in the absence and in the presence of manganese ion), indicating that this MLF was an endogenous opioid agonist.

In the same year, 1975, Hughes reported the extraction and purification of a substance of low molecular weight (700 or less dalton) from brains of pigs, rats, guinea pigs, and rabbits that inhibited, in a naloxone- and naltrexone-reversible manner, electrically stimulated contraction of mouse vas deferens and guinea pig ileum (which have opioid receptors in their neural layers) but not guinea pig or rabbit vas deferens (which do not have opioid receptors). The morphinelike substance was most highly concentrated in the corpus striatum, then in the midbrain, pons, and medulla; no activity was found in the cerebellum, liver, or lung. The substance was destroyed by carboxypeptidase and by leucine aminopeptidase, suggesting a peptide structure. Hughes *et al.* (1974b), studying a similar substance extracted from pig brain (molecular weight 800–1200), which they termed "enkephalin," showed that it acted like morphine on the electrically stimulated guinea pig ileum and mouse vas deferens, and that, as in the case of opioid agonists, levoisomer antagonists are much more potent than dextroisomer antagonists in reversing the inhibiting effects of enkephalin on the mouse vas deferens twitch; dose–effect curves for enkephalin and for normorphine were parallel, and the effects of mixtures of enkephalin and normorphine were additive. Further investigations by Hughes *et al.* (1975a) revealed that enkephalin consists of two pentapeptides, namely, H-tyrosine-glycine-glycine-phenylalanine-methionine-OH (methionine-enkephalin) and H-tyrosine-glycine-glycine-phenylalanine-leucine-OH (leucine-enkephalin). In pig brain, the ratio of methionine-enkephalin to leucine-enkephalin is about 3 or 4 to 1. Both pentapeptides have been synthesized. Methionine-enkephalin is about 20 times as potent as normorphine in inhibiting the twitch of the electrically stimulated mouse vas deferens, while leucine-enkephalin is half as potent as methionine-enkephalin. In inhibiting the twitch of the electrically stimulated guinea pig ileum, methionine-enkephalin is equipotent with normorphine, while leucine-enkephalin is one-fifth as potent. Methionine-enkephalin is 3 times more potent than morphine in inhibiting the stereospecific binding of ^{3}H-naloxone in sodium-free homogenates of guinea pig brain. The authors noted that the amino-acid sequence of methionine-enkephalin is present as residues 61–65 in β-lipotropin, isolated from pituitary glands of sheep by Li (1964), and they speculated that β-lipotropin may be a precursor for peptides with opioid agonist activity obtained from bovine pituitary (Teschemacher *et al.*, 1975) and crude ACTH (Cox *et al.*, 1975) as well as methionine-enkephalin.

In 1975, Teschemacher *et al.* and Cox *et al.* reported extraction and purification of a "pituitary opioid peptide 1" (POP-1) and crude ACTH from bovine and porcine pituitary glands that had morphinelike effects (reversible by naloxone) on the guinea pig ileum and the mouse vas deferens, respectively. Both substances inhibited the stereospecific binding of ^{3}H-etorphine and of ^{3}H-naloxone to synaptic membranes from guinea pig brain, and the inhibitory effect on ^{3}H-naloxone binding was reduced in the presence of sodium ion, indicating opioid agonist activity. POP-1 was found to be a trypsin- and chymotrypsin-sensitive peptide with a molecular weight of about 1750 dalton. These and other properties, as well as its origin, differentiated it from the "enkephalin" of Hughes *et al.* (1975a,b). Later, it appeared that this 1750-dalton peptide (POP-1) was a degradation product of a larger peptide (Goldstein & Cox, 1977) with opioid activity, which Li and Chung (1976) isolated from extracts of camel pituitary glands and designated "β-endorphin" (*endogenous morphine*). Analysis of the composition of β-endorphin revealed that it consists of a sequence of amino acids identical with amino acids 61–91 of the 1–91 amino-acid chain of β-lipotropin (β-LPH); hence, β-endorphin is also designated β-LPH$_{61-91}$. Interestingly, the amino-acid sequence 61–65 of β-endorphin and of β-lipotropin is the same as that of methionine-enkephalin, but whereas β-endorphin and methionine-enkephalin have opioid agonist activity, β-lipotropin has little or none; apparently, amino acid 61 (tyrosine) must occupy the NH$_2$-terminal position for the amino-acid sequence to possess opioid agonist activity (Cox *et al.*, 1976). Cox *et al.* reported that β-endorphin and methionine-enkephalin were equipotent but less active than normorphine in their inhibitory effects on the electrically stimulated guinea pig ileum. Stereospecific binding of ^{3}H-etorphine was more greatly inhibited by β-endorphin than by normorphine, but although methionine-enkephalin also inhibited ^{3}H-etorphine binding, such inhibition was less than by normorphine. In both the guinea pig ileum and the stereospecific binding tests, β-lipotropin had no effects or weak effects, the latter probably due to degradation of β-lipotropin to β-endorphin.

In the same year, 1976, Ling *et al.* isolated two other peptides from an extract of porcine hypothalamus–neurophypophysis that inhibited the twitch of the electrically stimulated guinea pig ileum in a naloxone-reversible manner and were named α-endorphin (β-LPH$_{61-76}$) and γ-endorphin (β-LPH$_{61-77}$). Also isolated from a similar extract (Guillemin, 1978) was still another compound, δ-endorphin (β-LPH$_{61-87}$), as well as β-endorphin (β-LPH$_{61-91}$).

It should be noted that although some authors, like Goldstein and Cox (1977), use the term *endorphins* to refer to all endogenous compounds with morphinelike activity, including the "enkephalins," only the latter have been found in the brain, except for nerve fibers in the median eminence and hypothalamus, where α-endorphin and β-endorphin have been demonstrated by immunocytochemical studies with highly specific antisera (Ling et al., 1976). In a study of the biosynthesis of ACTH and endorphins in an ACTH-secreting mouse pituitary tumor cell line, Mains et al. (1977) found that ACTH of high molecular weight (31,000 dalton) was the common precursor of lower molecular weight, physiologically active ACTH, β-lipotropin, and β-endorphin. It has long been known that ACTH is the primary pituitary hormone secreted in response to stress. Guillemin et al. (1977) have demonstrated that not only ACTH but also β-endorphin plasma levels rise steeply (correlation coefficient, 0.97) in response to stress (bone fracture) in rats; these responses to stress were abolished by prior hypophysectomy. However, Guillemin et al. (1977) pointed out that marked variations in the secretion of pituitary β-endorphin are not reflected in concomitant variations of brain levels of β-endorphin, and that the peripheral targets for stress-induced increased adenohypophysial secretion of β-endorphin are still unknown. In man, β-endorphin was not detectable in plasma under baseline conditions or after administration of vasopressin, which elevates β-lipotropin and ACTH; however, β-endorphin was present in the plasma of patients with endocrine disorders associated with elevated ACTH and β-lipotropin production (Suda et al., 1978).

POSSIBLE FUNCTIONS OF ENKEPHALINS AND ENDORPHINS

Analgesia

Pert et al. (1977) reported that in rats, the injection of partially purified "enkephalin" (PPE) into the periaqueductal gray matter produced transient excitation (lasting 15–45 sec) followed by sedation (about 10 min), with analgesic effects manifested by unresponsiveness to pinching of the extremities and tail and by prolongation of the tail flick response to radiant heat. The analgesic effect was more rapid in onset and much shorter in duration than after periaqueductal gray injection of morphine. Naloxone blocked the effects of both PPE and morphine. Surprisingly, PPE was much more potent than synthetic methionine-enkephalin or leucine-enkephalin, only the highest dose used of the former having a statistically significant effect on tail-flick latency. However, Belluzzi et al. (1976) found that synthetic methionine-enkephalin and leucine-enkephalin administered intraventricularly in the rat definitely prolonged tail-flick latencies; this effect developed rapidly, dissipated within 10–12 min, and could be abolished by naloxone (2 mg/kg subcutaneously). Loh *et al.* (1976) compared β-endorphin with morphine on analgesic tests in the mouse (hot plate, tail flick, and acetic acid writhing) following intracerebral injection. On a molar basis, β-endorphin was found to be 18–33 times more potent than morphine; in doses of 0.5–1.0 μg/mouse, β-endorphin produced analgesia lasting 60–90 min, and such analgesia was antagonized by naloxone, 1 mg/kg subcutaneously. Another opioid agonistlike action observed by Loh *et al.* (1976) was abolition of "wet dog" shakes induced by immersion of pentobarbital-anesthetized rats in ice water, by injection of β-endorphin into the periaqueductal gray matter; this effect was antagonized by naloxone, 5 mg/kg intraperitoneally. Likewise, the analgesic activity (elevation of threshhold for jaw-opening response to electrical stimulation of the tooth pulp, unresponsiveness to strong pinches of the skin) of β-endorphin and of morphine administered intraventricularly was demonstrated in the cat; on a molar basis, β-endorphin was 72–96 times more potent than morphine, and their analgesic effects were blocked by naloxone (Meglio *et al.*, 1977). Takagi *et al.* (1978) found that microinjection of methionine-enkephalin (0.2–20.0 μg) and leucine-enkephalin (1–20 μg) into the nuclei reticularis gigantocellularis and paragigantocellularis of the medulla oblongata produced dose-related and naloxone-antagonizable analgesia (tail-pinch test) in the rat; they pointed out that similar results had been obtained by microinjection of morphine into the nucleus reticularis gigantocellularis (Takagi *et al.*, 1977) and attributed the analgesic effects to augmentation of descending inhibition from the bulbar nuclei to lamina V cells in the dorsal horn of the spinal cord. Frederickson and Norris (1976) reported that methionine-enkephalin, applied microiontophoretically, depressed spontaneous and glutamate-induced firing of single neurons in the frontal cortex, caudate nucleus, and periaqueductal gray matter of the rat in a naloxone-reversible manner; these areas are rich in opioid receptors and enkephalin, and microiontophoretically applied enkephalin did not depress the firing of neurons in an area comparatively devoid of opioid receptors.

In man, electrical stimulation of periventricular brain sites (Akil *et al.*, 1978) or of the periaqueductal gray matter (Hosobuchi *et al.*, 1979) for relief of pain results in an increase in enkephalinlike activity (Akil *et al.*, 1978) or of immunoreactive β-endorphin (Hosobuchi *et al.*, 1979) in the ventricular cerebrospinal fluid. Akil *et al.* (1978) noted that "baseline" (preelectrical stimulation) levels of enkephalinlike activity in the cerebrospinal fluid of their patients were lower than normal—an observation recalling the finding of Terenius and Waldström (1975a) that the activity of their "morphinelike factor" was generally lower in the cerebrospinal fluid of patients with trigeminal neuralgia than with nonpainful neurological diseases. These findings suggest that if the endogenous opioid peptides play a role in the normal modulation of pain, their release must be only transitory and must be followed by relative depletion, although their release can be augmented artificially, for example, by focal electrical stimulation of the periaqueductal gray matter or the periventricular gray matter.

That release of endogenous substances with opioid agonist activity is involved in the production of analgesia by electrical stimulation of the periaqueductal or periventricular gray matter, in acupuncture analgesia, and in the modulation of certain responses to painful stimulation, is indicated by the effects of the "pure" narcotic antagonist naloxone on these phenomena.

Thus, Akil *et al.* (1972, 1976) reported that naloxone (1 mg/kg or higher doses) partially antagonized analgesia (prolongation of the tail-flick response to radiant heat) produced by electrical stimulation of the periaqueductal gray matter in the rat. Akil *et al.* (1976) suggested that the failure of naloxone to reverse the analgesia completely may be due to the contribution of non-opioid-releasing mechanisms in the analgesia produced by electrical stimulation of the periaqueductal gray matter. Adams (1976) found that naloxone (0.05–0.25 mg by intravenous drip) reversed the relief of pain produced by electrical stimulation of the periventricular gray matter in a patient with diabetic neuropathy.

In selected female mice giving a good squeak response to noxious heat from a slide lamp projector directed at the nose, Pomeranz and Chiu (1976) measured the latency of the squeak by triggering a microphone-oscilloscope recorder in synchrony with the lamp switch. An acupuncture needle was inserted into each foreleg at the "Hoku" point between the first and second metacarpal bones and stimulated electrically. "Sham acupuncture" was given through subcutaneous electrodes in the deltoid regions. Acupuncture or acupuncture with saline given subcutaneously produced significant increases in squeak latency at 40 min after start of acupuncture, while "sham acupuncture" or acupuncture with naloxone (0.9 mg/kg given subcutaneously) had no effect, the differences in squeak latencies in the latter two and in the former two procedures being highly significant. In mice not treated with acupuncture, naloxone (0.9 mg/kg subcutaneously) produced a 17% decrease in squeak latency (40 min after injection), which was significant in comparison with mice injected subcutaneously with saline or receiving no treatment at all. Pomeranz and Chiu (1976) concluded that endorphin is released at a low basal rate in normal mice, and at a much higher rate during acupuncture. In further studies on the mechanisms involved in acupuncture analgesia, Pomeranz *et al.* (1977) recorded, extracellularly, responses in lamina V of the L-7 dorsal horn to nonnoxious (pressure) and noxious (pinprick) stimuli applied to the toes in cats anesthetized with chloralose. Electroacupuncture was applied for 30 min through two needles in the ipsilateral hind leg at the "Futu" and "Yangling" points (corresponding to those used clinically for surgical operations on the foot). Mean reduction of responses to noxious stimuli was 28.3% for all 26 cells studied ($p < 0.0001$, t test), while responses of the same cells to nonnoxious stimuli remained unchanged ($p > 0.5$) during acupuncture. The onset of acupuncture effects was delayed for 10–15 min after the start of acupuncture, and recovery to control levels required 10–30 min after acupuncture needles were removed. The acupuncture effects were abolished by midcollicular decerebration or by spinal transection at C-1. In mice, Pomeranz *et al.* (1977) measured the voltage required to elicit squeaks on electrical stimulation near the intercostal nerves at T-6 to T-10 before and during electroacupuncture through needles in the "Hoku" and "Neikuan" points (thenar eminences and palmar surface of each forearm, 0.2 cm proximal to the wrist). Comparing mice hypophysectomized through a neck approach with sham-operated mice, Pomerantz *et al.* found that hypophysectomy abolished the acupuncture effect, suggesting that acupuncture stimulates sensory nerves that activate the pituitary gland to release morphinelike hormones. In their paper, Pomeranz *et al.* (1977) stated that preliminary results show that naloxone markedly reduced acupuncture effects in their cat and mouse (with intact hypophysis) models. In man, Mayer *et al.* (1977) measured the voltage required to elicit a report of "pain" on stimulating an intact tooth (usually upper canine) with a Pelton–Crane vitality tester. Acupuncture analgesia was induced by inserting a needle in each of the two "Hoku" points (between the thumb and the index finger at the approximate center of the interosseous dorsalis muscle) and twirling it for 2 min out of 5 min for 30 min. After 30 min, acupuncture elevated the mean pain threshold voltage 27.1%, compared to 6.9% in a no-acupuncture control group (difference, $p < 0.0003$, t test); a placebo-control group (no acupuncture but saline intravenously with the suggestion that it was a powerful analgesic) likewise showed a reliably smaller increase in mean pain threshold voltage (difference from acupuncture group $p < .01$, t test). In subjects whose mean pain threshold voltages were elevated more than 20% by acupuncture, naloxone (0.8 mg) or saline was given intravenously in a double-blind procedure. Five minutes after naloxone, the mean pain threshold voltage dropped from the acupuncture level to about the placebo-control level (difference, $p < 0.003$, t test), while saline had no effect. Mayer *et al.* (1977) concluded that naloxone antagonizes endorphins released (through acupuncture) in the periaqueductal gray matter and caudal diencephalon.

Jacob *et al.* (1974) observed that naloxone (0.1–1.0 mg/kg subcutaneously) shortened the latency to jumping in the hot-plate test in mice and rats; nalorphine, which has mixed agonist and antagonist properties, had no such effect. Grevert and Goldstein (1977b) likewise found that naloxone (0.1–10.0 mg/kg) shortened the latency of the jumping response in the hot-plate test in mice, and they also noted that after naloxone, mice took significantly longer to enter a dark box than saline controls. Bell and Martin (1977) reported that at intravenous doses too small to have nonspecific excitatory effects, naloxone and naltrexone greatly increased the C-fiber responses from the S-1 ventral root following electrical stimulation of the ipsilateral superficial peroneal nerve or application of radiant heat to the footpad in the acute decerebrate, low spinal cat. The results of these studies, as well as those of Pomeranz and Chiu (1976) on untreated, normal mice (see above), are compatible with the hypothesis that, at least in mice, rats, and cats, responses to potentially or actually painful stimuli are modulated by release of endogenous morphinelike substances at central sites.

However, Grevert and Goldstein (1978) found that naloxone (1, 2, and 10 mg intravenously) had no effects that could be distinguished statistically from those of saline on subjective pain ratings and responses to mood-state questionnaires after ischemic pain (inflating a sphygmomanometer cuff to 250 mm Hg and pulling a dynamometer with a 12-kg load 20 times), or on subjective pain ratings, mood-state questionnaires, and finger plethysmograph recordings after immersion of the other hand in circulating water at 10°C; an earlier report of antagonistic action of naloxone on "tension-anxiety" (Grevert & Goldstein, 1977a) could not be confirmed. Grevert and Goldstein (1978) concluded that endorphins are not released under the conditions of experimental pain in man used in their studies and that perhaps for this to occur, more painful and stressful stimuli may be needed. Nor could Goldstein and Hilgard (1975) demonstrate an antagonistic action of naloxone on hypnotic analgesia. Three easily hypnotizable subjects reported "pain" and "distress" on two separate numerical scales (0 = no pain or distress, 1 = just noticeable pain or distress, etc., to 10 = intense pain or distress, and higher ratings), while pressing a hand dynamometer with a 10-kg load 20 times (2-sec hold and 2-sec release) under ischemic conditions (sphygmomanometer cuff above the elbow inflated to 250 mm Hg). Before hypnosis, the pain and distress curves rose monotonically and in parallel in two of the subjects, and they deviated somewhat in the third.

After hypnosis, no "overt" pain was reported by any of the subjects; no "overt" distress was reported by two; and the third reported mild "overt" distress toward the end of the 6-min period of ischemia. Neither naloxone (1.2 mg) nor saline, both given subcutaneously, made any difference when these agents were given under double-blind conditions to each subject on different occasions under hypnotic analgesia and the test procedure was repeated. Similar lack of effect of naloxone or saline was observed on "covert" pain and distress elicited by suggestion during hypnosis. It appears, therefore, that release of an endogenous morphinelike substance is not involved in the mechanism of hypnotic analgesia.

Physical Dependence

Wei and Loh (1976) precipitated morphinelike abstinence syndromes in rats by administration of naloxone (10 mg/kg intraperitoneally) after continuous infusion of methionine-enkephalin or β-endorphin for 70 hr into the frontal cortex or the periaqueductal gray matter; the precipitated abstinence phenomena observed (escape attempts, increased "wet-dog" shakes, and teeth chattering) were very similar to those observed after a 70-hr infusion of morphine into the periaqueductal gray matter, followed by administration of naloxone. That these "natural" endogenous opioid peptides can produce physical dependence if they are present at opioid receptor sites continuously for a relatively long time (e.g., 70 hr) suggests that normally, their presence at opioid receptor sites is transient; indeed, it has already been noted that their activity in cerebrospinal fluid appears to be lower than normal in patients with pain (Terenius & Wahlström, 1975a; Akil et al., 1978). One intriguing possibility that may be inferred from Wei and Loh's (1976) findings is that the actions of morphine, including the generation of physical dependence, may be mediated through *release* of endogenous opioid peptides; testing this inference would require testing the actions of morphine before and after depleting the brain (including the spinal cord) of endogenous opioid peptides. Compatible with the view that morphine may act through the release of endogenous peptides (e.g., endorphins and ACTH) is the evidence adduced by Jacquet et al. (1977) of the existence of two kinds of opioid receptors in the rat: one in the periaqueductal gray matter and midbrain reticular formation, which is nonstereospecific and is strongly activated by local microinjection of (+)-morphine and transiently by (−)-morphine to produce hyperactivity and rotation, not antagonized by naloxone (such behavior was specific for morphine and heroin but did not occur after microinjection of levorphanol, methadone, etorphine, or dextrorphan); the other in the periaqueductal gray matter, which is stereospecific and is strongly activated by (−)-morphine or β-endorphin to produce pronounced analgesia and catatonia, reversible by naloxone. After microinjection of (−)-morphine into the periaqueductal gray matter, both types of receptors are activated, but the analgesic–catatonic effects predominate. Jacquet et al. (1977) equated the excitatory effects with those seen in naloxone-precipitated opioid abstinence syndromes. Further, Jacquet (1978) reported that microinjections of the naturally occurring peptide ACTH into the periaqueductal gray matter produced a dose-dependent excitatory effect similar to that produced by local microinjections of (+)-morphine, which resembles the naloxone-precipitated opioid abstinence syndrome. Jacquet (1978) concluded that when morphine is given systemically, it activates both ACTH and β-endorphin receptors, the effects of the latter predominating; that tolerance develops to the effects of morphine on the β-endorphin receptor, but not on the ACTH receptor; and that when naloxone is administered, the effects of morphine on the β-endorphin receptor only are blocked, thereby unmasking the excitatory effects of morphine on the ACTH receptor, which constitutes the naloxone-precipitated morphine-abstinence syndrome. The "dual actions" of morphine on the ACTH and β-endorphin receptors concretize the "dual action" hypothesis of morphine physical dependence as revised by Seevers and Deneau in 1961. They may also explain the fact that a narcotic antagonist, nalorphine, can precipitate what appears to be a morphine-abstinence syndrome after the administration of a single large dose of morphine in the chronic spinal dog (Wikler & Carter, 1953), and that in man, the dose of nalorphine needed to precipitate abstinence phenomena decreases progressively as the subject becomes increasingly tolerant to and physically dependent on morphine, methadone, or heroin (Wikler et al., 1953).

Snyder (1977) has reviewed evidence that enkephalin neurons block the release of excitatory neurotransmitters from the central terminal axons of sensory neurons by releasing enkephalin onto opioid receptors located presynaptically (i.e., on the same terminal axons). Administered morphine binds to unoccupied opioid receptors, and if administration of morphine is continued, release of enkephalin is inhibited through a hypothetical neuronal feedback loop, thereby making more opioid receptors available for morphine; when administration of morphine is stopped suddenly, morphine leaves the opioid receptors, which now also lack enkephalin; the morphine-abstinence syndrome is attributed to the lack or decrease in enkephalin, which, however, is only temporary, as levels of enkephalin at opioid receptors are eventually restored.

Snyder (1977, 1979) cited evidence that the presence or absence of morphine or enkephalin at opioid receptors may be reflected intraneuronally by changes in cyclic AMP and the cyclic-AMP-forming enzyme, adenylate cyclase. Thus, in neuroblastoma–glioma cell cultures, opioid agonists reduce endogenous levels of cyclic AMP and inhibit the activity of adenylate cyclase. Incubation of these cells with opioid agonists results in *increase* in the basal level of adenylate cyclase activity (possibly through an enzymatic derepression feedback mechanism), so that higher concentrations of opioid agonists are required to reduce cyclic AMP activity ("tolerance"); when a narcotic antagonist is added to or opioid agonists are withdrawn from the medium, a marked *increase* in cyclic AMP levels occurs because of the increased adenylate cyclase activity present; presumably, the "rebound" increase in cyclic AMP accounts for the opioid-abstinence syndrome *in vivo*. Snyder (1979) also suggested that the locus ceruleus in the brain stem, containing high densities of noradrenergic neurons and opioid receptors, may account for symptoms of opioid abstinence. Thus, opioid agonists slow the firing of neurons in the locus ceruleus (Bird & Kuhar, 1977), and tolerance develops to this action without cross-tolerance to clonidine, an α-noradrenergic compound that slows the firing of locus ceruleus cells presynaptically (Aghajanian, 1978); clonidine has been reported to suppress the opioid-withdrawal syndrome in animals (Aghajanian, 1978) and the symptoms of opioid withdrawal in man (Gold *et al.*, 1978a,b). However, loci other than the locus ceruleus must be involved in the genesis of tolerance to and physical dependence on morphine, since both phenomena have been shown to occur in the chronic spinal dog (Wikler & Frank, 1948; Wikler and Carter, 1953) and in a chronic spinal man (Wikler & Rayport, 1954).

Mental Disorders

Bloom *et al.* (1976) noted that while the endogenous opioid peptides (methionine-enkephalin, α-endorphin, β-endorphin, and γ-endorphin) may have varying degrees of analgesic activity, resembling that of morphine on intracerebral injection, their effects in other respects differ from those of morphine and among each other. Thus, when injected into the cerebrospinal fluid either through the cisterna magna or through ventricular cannulae, β-endorphin produced a long-lasting catatonic state (different from the immobility produced by morphine), which, according to the authors, was reminiscent of schizophrenic catatonia (catalepsy), and a marked fall in rectal temperature; these effects were promptly antagonized by naloxone. This catatonic syndrome could not be reproduced by the other endogenous opioid peptides even after high doses. In contrast to β-endorphin, γ-endorphin produced marked elevation of rectal temperature, sometimes with hyperactivity to sensory testing and handling. All endogenous opioid peptides produced wet-dog shakes when they were injected into the lateral ventricles (but not when they were injected through the cisterna magna), and such wet-dog shakes were *antagonized* by naloxone. Bloom *et al.* (1976) concluded that subtle derangements in the biochemical or physiological mechanisms normally regulating the cleavage of the postulated prohormone β-lipotropin into the several endogenous opioid peptides may lead to mental illness. They suggested that this hypothesis may be tested by therapeutic trials of opioid antagonists in patients with mental disorders (see below). A diametrically opposed interpretation of the "catatonia" induced by intracerebral injection of β-endorphin in the rat was made by Jacquet and Marks (1976), who compared it with the immobility produced by systematic administration of neuroleptics, effective in the treatment of schizophrenia and other psychotic disorders. It should be noted that in their experiments, Jacquet and Marks (1976) gave β-endorphin (also α-endorphin, methionine-enkephalin, leucine-enkephalin, and morphine) by microinjection into the periaqueductal gray matter, rather than into ventricular cerebrospinal fluid as did Bloom *et al.* (1976). All of the endogenous opioid peptides produced varying degrees of catalepsy, but that produced by β-endorphin was by far the most profound and longest lasting and was completely reversed by naloxone, given intraperitoneally. The features of this catalepsy differed from those produced by morphine. Like morphine, β-endorphin also produced analgesia, but none of the other endogenous opioid peptides showed any analgesic activity. Jacquet and Marks (1976) pointed out that neuroleptics have been reported to bind opioid receptors (Creese *et al.*, 1976). Conversely Czlonkowski *et al.* (1978) have reported that some opioids with morphinan or benzmorphan structures (but not morphine, etorphine, β-endorphin, methionine-enkephalin, and leucine-enkephalin) bind to neuroleptic receptor sites (measured by inhibition of ^{3}H-spiroperidol binding) in the corpus striatum of the rat. Jacquet and Marks (1976) concluded that a *deficiency* of β-endorphin at its receptor sites may be involved in those psychotic states that are improved by neuroleptics. However, Segal *et al.* (1977) compared the behavioral effects of β-endorphin microinjected into the periaqueductal gray matter (also into the cerebrospinal fluid through ventricular cannulae) with those produced by the neuroleptic haloperidol (0.5–12 mg/kg) given subcutaneously. They found that in rats, β-endorphin in the periaqueductal gray matter produced rigidity similar to though less intense than when injected into the lateral ventricle, impairment of ability to stay on a vertical grid, and loss of the righting reflex. In contrast, rats given haloperidol showed flaccidity, remained stationary on the vertical grid, and retained the righting reflex. The effects of β-endorphin, but not those of haloperidol, were reversible by naloxone. Segal *et al.* (1977) concluded that contrary to the view of Jacquet and Marks (1976), β-endorphin does *not* act like an endogenous neuroleptic.

If β-endorphin-produced catalepsy in the rat (reversible by naloxone) is considered analogous to the effects of a psychotogen (Bloom *et al.*, 1976), then administration of naloxone to schizophrenic patients should ameliorate, whereas if it is considered analogous to the effects of a neuroleptic (Jacquet & Marks, 1976), naloxone should intensify their psychotic behavior. However, reports on the effects of naloxone on the psychotic behavior of schizophrenic patients, particularly their hallucinations, have been inconclusive. Gunne *et al.* (1977) found that naloxone reversed hallucinations in four of six chronic schizophrenic patients, but in double-blind studies, Volavka *et al.* (1977), Janowsky *et al.* (1977), and Kurland *et al.* (1977) reported that naloxone had no effects on schizophrenic hallucinations that could be distinguished from placebo. On the other hand, in a double-blind, placebo-controlled study on nine schizophrenic patients selected on the basis of having auditory hallucinations at least twice per hour and other criteria, Watson *et al.* (1978) found a significant ($p < 0.05$) reduction of hallucinations after intravenous administration of naloxone (10 mg) lasting several hours. Of the nine patients, six reported clear-cut improvement in hallucinations, one showed borderline improvement, and two did not improve; after placebo, improvement occurred in one, while the eight others showed no or borderline improvement. When two other patients were studied single-blind after naloxone (10 mg intravenously), hallucinations were reduced in both. The 11 patients used in these studies were screened from approximately 1000 general psychiatric patients; no data are given for the effects of naloxone in schizophrenic patients with less frequent hallucinations. Watson *et al.* (1978) pointed out that the use of a longer-acting opioid antagonist like naltrexone might be useful in studying such subjective and variable phenomena as hallucinations. Noting that β-endorphin and ACTH are secreted concomitantly by the pituitary gland (Guillemin *et al.*, 1977), Lehmann *et al.* (1979) investigated the possible relationship between a favorable response to naloxone and endogenous β-endorphin levels in schizophrenic patients by measuring ratings on the Brief Psychiatric Rating Scale (BPRS) and diurnal variation in plasma ACTH levels (as an indicator of brain β-endorphin levels). In a double-blind, placebo-controlled study, the thought disturbance factor and the hallucinatory behavior item on the BPRS showed significant improvement ($p < 0.01$) when evaluated 6 hr after administration of naloxone, 10 mg intravenously, at 8:00 A.M. Plasma ACTH levels in five patients (it is not clear that all of these were the same as the five patients tested with the BPRS) showed no change, a rise or a fall, 6 hr after naloxone or placebo, but Lehmann *et al.* (1979) pointed out that the subject who showed the greatest variability of ACTH (diurnal drop) showed the greatest clinical improvement (after naloxone). Terenius *et al.* (1977) observed no improvement in five depressed patients given naloxone, 0.4–0.8 mg three times daily in six trials over 6–12 days. In cerebrospinal fluid obtained by lumbar puncture, every treatment session resulted in a lowering of "Fraction I" endorphin values, generally accompanied by an increase in 5-hydroxy-indoleacetic acid values, indicating a reciprocal relationship between endorphin "Fraction I" and brain serotonin.

In a report on the effects of synthetic β-endorphin on three depressed and three chronic schizophrenic ambulatory patients treated in a private setting (for the most part still on psychotropic medication), Kline *et al.* (1977) described improvement of mood in the depressed patients after intravenous administration of β-endorphin (1.5 mg) on one occasion and no effects after a repeat injection with a new batch of β-endorphin; in the schizophrenic patients, this (or a slightly higher) dose of β-endorphin produced worsening of schizophrenic behavior. After repeat doses of β-endorphin, one of the three schizophrenic patients appeared to become less paranoid and more energetic and hopeful, but no change occurred in the other two; the effects of naloxone were equivocal. The improvement in mood of the depressed patients is reminiscent of the effects of opium on patients with agitated depressions, a treatment not infrequently used (with warnings of the dangers of addiction) before the introduction of electroconvulsive and modern pharmacotherapy (Schmitz, 1925–1926). As β-endorphin has morphine-like analgesic activity, at least when given intracerebrally, it would be interesting to know whether it produces moisis and decrease in respiratory rate when given intravenously in man; however, no such data are included in the report of Kline *et al.* (1977).

Verhoeven *et al.* (1979) have reported transient or semipermanent improvement in 14 patients with long-lasting, relapsing schizophrenic or schizoaffective psychoses resistant to conventional neuroleptics when they were treated with intramuscular injections of β-LPH $_{62-77}$, which is γ-endorphin with the tyrosine at the N-terminal removed (DTγE). In animals, this nonopioidlike peptide showed neuroleptic activity similar to that produced by haloperidol. Verhoeven *et al.* (1979) speculated that schizophrenia may be due to reduced availability of DTγE or a closely related neuropeptide consequent to disturbances in the mechanisms regulating β-lipotropin-endorphin metabolism, and that administration of DTγE may normalize the level of this or of a closely related peptide.

After observing the disappearance of schizophrenic symptoms in a hypertensive patient treated by hemodialysis, Wagemaker and Cade (1977) began systematic studies of the effects of dialysis in patients with chronic schizophrenia. Remarkable improvement as long as dialysis was continued was noted by the time of their report, some patients relapsing after dialysis was discontinued. Wagemaker and Cade speculated that a substance is removed from the blood during dialysis and builds up again after dialysis is stopped. They pointed out the need for double-blind, sham-dialysis-controlled studies. Palmour et al. (cited by Lewis et al., 1979) reported that they found a peptide, β_H-leu^5-endorphin, identical with β-endorphin except for leucine instead of methionine in the fifth amino-acid position, in dialysates of chronic schizophrenic patients. However, Lewis et al. (1979) could not detect β_H-leu^5-endorphin in ultrafiltrates of arterial blood (which were not diluted in large volumes of outer dialysis fluid but were collected directly and replaced intravenously with sterile saline solution) from two drug-resistant schizophrenic patients and two controls.

REFERENCES

Adams, J. E., 1976, Naloxone reversal of analgesia produced by brain stimulation in the human, Pain 2:161–166.

Aghajanian, G. K., 1978, Tolerance of locus coeruleus neurones to morphine and suppression of withdrawal response by clonidine, Nature (London) 276:183–188.

Akil, H., Mayer, D. J., and Liebeskind, J. C., 1972, Comparaison chez le rat entre l'analgésie induite par stimulation de la substance grise périaqueducale et l'analgésie morphinique, C. R. Acad. Sci. (Paris) 274:3603–3605.

Akil, H., Mayer, D. J., and Liebeskind, J. C., 1976, Antagonism of stimulation-produced analgesia by naloxone, a narcotic antagonist, Science 191:961–962.

Akil, H., Richardson, D. E., Hughes, J., and Barchas, J. S., 1978, Enkephalin-like material elevated in ventricular cerebrospinal fluid of patients after analgetic focal stimulation, Science 201:463–465.

Ariëns, E. J., van Rossum, J. M., and Simonis, A. M., 1956, A theoretical basis of molecular pharmacology. Part I. Interactions of one or two compounds with one receptor system, Arzneimittelforschung 6:282–293.

Ariëns, E. J., Simonis, A. M., and van Rossum, J. M., 1964a, Drug-receptor interaction: Interaction of one or more drugs with different receptor systems, in Molecular Pharmacology: The Mode of Action of Biologically Active Compounds, Vol. 1 (E. J. Ariëns, Ed.), pp. 287–393. Academic Press, New York.

Ariëns, E. J., Simonis, A. M., and van Rossum, J. M., 1964b, Drug-receptor interaction: Interaction of one or more drugs with one receptor system, in Molecular Pharmacology: The Mode of Action of Biologically Active Compounds, Vol. 1 (E. J. Ariëns, Ed.), pp. 119–286. Academic Press, New York.

Atweh, S. F., and Kuhar, M. J., 1977, Autoradiographic localization of opiate receptors in rat brain. I. Spinal cord and lower medulla, *Brain Res. 124:53–67.*

Bell, J. A., and Martin, W. R., 1977, The effect of the narcotic antagonists naloxone, naltrexone and nalorphine on spinal cord C-fiber reflexes evoked by electrical stimulation or radiant heat, *Eur. J. Pharmacol. 42:147–154.*

Belluzzi, J. D., Grant, N., Garsky, V., Sarantakis, D., Wise, C. D., and Stein, L., 1976, Analgesia induced *in vivo* by central administration of enkephalin in rat, *Nature* (London) 260:625–626.

Bird, S. J., and Kuhar, M. J., 1977, Iontophoretic application of opiates to the locus coeruleus, *Brain Res. 122:523–533.*

Bloom, F., Segal, D., Ling, N., and Guillemin, R., 1976, Endorphins: Profound behavioral effects in rats suggest new etiological factors in mental illness, *Science* 194:630–632.

Cox, B. M., Opheim, K. E., Teschemacher, H., and Goldstein, A., 1975, A peptide-like substance from pituitary that acts like morphine. 2. Purification and properties. *Life Sci. 16:1777–1782.*

Cox, B. M., Goldstein, A., and Li, C. H., 1976, Opioid activity of a peptide, beta-lipotropin-(61-91), derived from beta-lipotropin, *Proc. Natl. Acad. Sci. USA 73:1821–1823.*

Creese, I., Feinberg, A. P., and Snyder, S. H., 1976, Butyrophenone influences on the opiate receptor, *Eur. J. Pharmacol. 36:231–235.*

Czlonkowski, A., Höllt, V., and Herz, A., 1978, Binding of opiates and endogenous opioid peptides to neuroleptic receptor sites in the corpus stratum, *Life Sci. 22:953–962.*

Ehrlich, P., 1913, Chemotherapeutics: Scientific principles, methods and results, *Lancet 185:445–451.*

Frederickson, R. C. A., and Norris, F. H., 1976, Enkephalin-induced depression of single neurons in brain areas with opiate receptors-antagonism by naloxone, *Science 194:440–442.*

Gero, A., 1971, Intimate study of drug action. III. Mechanisms of molecular drug action, in *Drill's Pharmacology in Medicine* (J. R. DiPalma, Ed.), pp. 67–98. McGraw-Hill Book Company, New York.

Gilbert, P. E., and Martin, W. R., 1976, The effects of morphine- and nalorphine-like drugs in the nondependent, morphine-dependent and cyclazocine-dependent chronic spinal dog, *J. Pharmacol. Exp. Ther. 198:66–82.*

Gold, M. S., Redmond, D. E., and Kleber, H. D., 1978a, Clonidine blocks acute opiate-withdrawal symptoms, *Lancet 2:599–602.*

Gold, M. S., Redmond, D. E., and Kleber, H. D., 1978b, Clonidine in opiate withdrawal, *Lancet 1:929–930.*

Goldstein, A., 1973, The search for the opiate receptor, in *Pharmacology and the Future of Man. Proc. 5th Congr. Pharmacology, San Francisco 1972,* Vol. 1 (J. Cochin, Ed.), pp. 140–159. Karger, Basel.

Goldstein, A., and Cox, B. M., 1977, Opioid peptides (endorphins) in pituitary and brain, *Psychoneuroendocrinology 2:11–16.*

Goldstein, A., and Hilgard, E. R., 1975, Failure of the opiate antagonist naloxone to modify hypnotic analgesia, *Proc. Nat. Acad. Sci. USA 72:2041–2043.*

Goldstein, A., Lowney, K. E., and Pal, B. K., 1971, Stereospecific and non-specific interactions of the morphine congener levorphanol in subcellular fractions of mouse brain, *Proc. Nat. Acad. Sci. USA 68:1742–1747.*

Grevert P., and Goldstein, A., 1977a, Effects of naloxone on experimentally induced ischemic pain and on mood in human subjects, *Proc. Natl. Acad. Sci. USA 74:1291–1294.*

Grevert, P., and Goldstein, A., 1977b, Some effects of naloxone on behavior in the mouse, *Psychopharmacology* 53:111–113.

Grevert, P., and Goldstein, A., 1978, Endorphins: Naloxone fails to alter experimental pain or mood in humans, *Science* 199:1093–1095.

Guillemin, R., 1978, Peptides in the brain: The new endocrinology of the neuron, *Science* 202:390–402.

Guillemin, R., Vargo, T., Rossier, J., Minick, S., Ling, N., Rivier, C., Vale, W., and Bloom, F., 1977, β-endorphin and adrenocorticotropin are secreted concomitantly by the pituitary gland, *Science* 197:1367–1369.

Gunne, L. M., Lindström, L., and Terenius, L., 1977, Naloxone-induced reversal of schizophrenic hallucinations, *J. Neural Transmission* 40:13–19.

Hosobuchi, T., Rossier, J., Bloom, F. E., and Guillemin, R., 1979, Stimulation of human periaqueductal gray for pain relief increases immunoreactive beta-endorphin in ventricular fluid, *Science* 203:279–281.

Hughes, J., 1975, Isolation of an endogenous compound in the brain with pharmacological properties similar to morphine, *Brain Res.* 88:295–308.

Hughes, J., Smith, T. W., Kosterlitz, H. W., Fothergill, L. A., Morgan, B. A., and Morris, H. R., 1975a, Identification of two related pentapeptides from the brain with potent opiate agonist activity, *Nature* (London) 258:577–579.

Hughes, J., Smith, T., Morgan, B., and Fothergill, L., 1975b, Purification and properties of enkephalin—The possible endogenous ligand for the morphine receptor, *Life Sci.* 16:1753–1758.

Hutchison, M., Kosterlitz, H. W., Leslie, F. M., Waterfield, A. A., and Terenius, L., 1975, Assessment in the guinea-pig ileum and mouse vas deferens of benzomorphans which have strong antinociceptive activity but do not substitute for morphine in the dependent monkey, *Brit. J. Pharmacol.* 55:541–546.

Jacob, J. J., Tremblay, E. C., and Colombel, M. C., 1974, Facilitation de réactions nociceptives par la naloxone chez la souris et chez le rat, *Psychopharmacologia* 37:217–223.

Jacquet, Y. F., 1978, Opiate effects after adrenocorticotropin or beta-endorphin injection in the periaqueductal gray matter of rats, *Science* 201:1032–1034.

Jacquet, Y. F., and Marks, N., 1976, The C-fragment of beta-lipotropin: An endogenous neuroleptic or antipsychotogen? *Science* 194:632–634.

Jacquet, Y. F., Klee, W. A., Rice, K. C., Ijima, I., and Minamikawa, J., 1977, Stereospecific and nonstereospecific effects of (+)- and (−)-morphine: Evidence for a new class of receptors? *Science* 198:842–845.

Janowsky, D. C., Segal, D. S., Abrams, A., Bloom, F., and Guillemin, R., 1977, Negative naloxone effects in schizophrenic patients, *Psychopharmacology* 53:295–297.

Kline, N. S., Li, C. H., Lehmann, H. E., Lajtha, A., Laski, E., and Cooper, T., 1977, Beta-endorphin-induced changes in schizophrenic and depressed patients, *Arch. Gen. Psychiat.* 34:1111–1113.

Kurland, A. A., McCabe, O. L., and Hanlon, T. E., 1977, The treatment of perceptual disturbances in schizophrenia with naloxone hydrochloride, *Amer. J. Psychiat.* 134:1408–1410.

Lehmann, H., Nair, V., and Kline, N. S., 1979, Beta-endorphin and naloxone in psychiatric patients: Clinical and biological effects, *Amer. J. Psychiat.* 136:762–766.

Lewis, R. V., Gerber, L. D., Stein, S., Stephen, R. L., Grosser, B. I., Velick, S. F., and Udenfriend, S., 1979, On β_H-leu^5-endorphin and schizophrenia, *Arch. Gen. Psychiat.* 36:237–239.

Li, C. H., 1964, Lipotropin, a new active peptide from pituitary glands, *Nature* (London), 201:924.

Li, C. H., and Chung, D., 1976, Isolation and structure of an untriakontapeptide with opiate activity from camel pituitary glands, *Proc. Natl. Acad. Sci. USA 73*:1145–1148.

Ling, N., Burgus, R., and Guillemin, R., 1976, Isolation, primary structure, and synthesis of alpha-endorphin and gamma-endorphin, two peptides of hypothalamic-hypophysial origin with morphinomimetic activity, *Proc. Natl. Acad. Sci. USA 73*:3942–3946.

Loh, H. H., Tseng, L. F., Wei, E., and Li, C. H., 1976, β-endorphin is a potent analgesic agent, *Proc. Natl. Acad. Sci. USA 73*:2895–2898.

Lord, J. A. H., Waterfield, A. A., Hughes, J., and Kosterlitz, H. W., 1976, Multiple opiate receptors, in *Opiates and Endogenous Opioid Peptides* (H. W. Kosterlitz, Ed.), pp. 275–280. Elsevier/North-Holland Biomedical Press, Amsterdam.

Lord, J. A. H., Waterfield, A. A., Hughes, J., and Kosterlitz, H. W., 1977, Endogenous opioid peptides: Multiple agonists and receptors, *Nature* (London) 267:495–499.

Mains, R. E., Eipper, A. B., and Ling, N., 1977, Common precursor to corticotropins and endorphins, *Proc. Nat. Acad. Sci. USA* 74:3014–3018.

Martin, W. R., 1967, Opioid antagonists, *Pharmacol. Rev. 19*:463–521.

Martin, W. R., Eades, C. G., Thompson, J. A., Huppler, R. E., and Gilbert, P. E., 1976, The effects of morphine- and nalorphine-like drugs in the nondependent and morphine-dependent chronic spinal dog, *J. Pharmacol. Exp. Ther. 197*:517–532.

Mayer, D. J., Price, D. D., and Rafii, A., 1977, Antagonism of acupuncture analgesia in man by the narcotic antagonist naloxone, *Brain Res. 121*:368–372.

Meglio, M., Hosobuchi, Y., Loh, H. H., Adams, J. E., and Li, C. H., 1977, β-endorphin: Behavioral and analgesic activity in cats, *Proc. Natl. Acad. Sci. USA* 74:774–776.

Michaelis, L., and Menten, M., 1913, Kinetik der Invertinwirkung, *Biochem. Ztschr. 49*:333–369.

Palmour, R. M., Ervin, F. R., Wagemaker, H., and Cade, R., 1977, Characterization of a peptide derived from the serum of psychiatric patients, *Abstr. Soc. Neurosi. 7*:320 (cited in Lewis *et al.*, 1979).

Pasternak, G. W., Goodman, R., and Snyder, S. H., 1975, An endogenous morphine-like factor in mammalian brain, *Life Sci. 16*:1765–1769.

Pert, C. B., and Snyder, S. H., 1973, Opiate receptor: Demonstration in nervous tissue, *Science 179*:1011–1014.

Pert, C. B., Pasternak, G., and Snyder, S. H., 1973, Opiate agonists and antagonists discriminated by receptor binding in the brain, *Science 182*:1359–1361.

Pert, A., Simantov, R., and Snyder, S. H., 1977, A morphine-like factor in mammalian brain: Analgesic activity in rats, *Brain Res. 136*:523–533.

Pomeranz, B., and Chiu, D., 1976, Naloxone blockade of acupuncture analgesia: Endorphin implicated, *Life Sci. 19*:1757–1762.

Pomeranz, B., Cheng, R., and Law, P., 1977, Acupuncture reduces electrophysiological and behavioral responses to noxious stimuli: pituitary is implicated, *Exp. Neurol. 54*:172–178.

Schmitz, H., 1925–1926, Die Opiumbehandlung bei Geisteskrankheiten insbesondere bei Melancholie, ihre Geschichte, ihr heutiger Stand und eigene Erfahrungen, *Allg. Ztschr. Psychiat. 83*:92–113.

Seevers, M. H., and Deneau, G. A., 1961, A critique of the "dual action" hypothesis of morphine physical dependence, *Arch. Int. Pharmacodyn. Thér. 140*:514–520.

Segal, D. S., Browne, R. G., Bloom, F., Ling, N., and Guillemin, R., 1977, β-endorphin: Endogenous opiate or neuroleptic? *Science 198*:411–413.

Simon, E. J., Hiller, J. M., and Edelman, I., 1973, Stereospecific binding of the potent narcotic analgesic (³H)etorphine to rat-brain homogenate, *Proc. Nat. Acad. Sci.* (Washington) 70:1947–1949.

Snyder, S. H., 1977, Opiate receptors and internal opiates, *Sci. American 236*(3): 44–56.

Snyder, S. H., 1979, Receptors, neurotransmitters and drug responses, *New Engl. J. Med.* 300:465–472.

Suda, T., Liotta, A. S., and Krieger, D. T., 1978, β-endorphin is not detectable in plasma from normal human subjects, *Science* 202:221–223.

Takagi, H., Satoh, M., Akaike, A., Shibata, T., and Kuraishi, Y., 1977, The nucleus reticularis gigantocellularis of the medulla oblongata is a highly sensitive site in the production of morphine analgesia in the rat, *Eur. J. Pharmacol.* 45:91–92.

Takagi, H., Satoh, M., Akaike, A., Shibata, T., Yajima, H., and Ogawa, H., 1978, Analgesia by enkephalins injected into the nucelus reticularis gigantocellularis of rat medulla oblongata, *Eur. J. Pharmacol.* 49:113–116.

Terenius, L., 1973, Characteristics of the "receptor" for narcotic analgesics in synaptic plasma membrane fraction from rat brain, *Acta Pharmacol. Toxicol.* 33:377–384.

Terenius, L., and Wahlström, A., 1974, Inhibitors of narcotic receptor binding in brain extracts and cerebrospinal fluid, *Acta Pharmacol. Toxicol.* 35 (Suppl. 1):55.

Terenius, L., and Wahlström, A., 1975a, Morphine-like ligand for opiate receptors in human CSF, *Life Sci.* 16:1759–1764.

Terenius, L., and Wahlström, A., 1975b, Search for an endogenous ligand for the opiate receptor, *Acta Physiol. Scand.* 94:74–81.

Terenius, L., Wahlström, A., and Ågren, H., 1977, Naloxone (Narcan) treatment in depression: Clinical observations and effects on CSF endorphins and monoamine metabolites, *Psychopharmacology* 54:31–33.

Teschemacher, H., Opheim, K. E., Cox, B. M., and Goldstein, A., 1975, A peptide-like substance from pituitary that acts like morphine. 1. Isolation, *Life Sci.* 16:1771–1776.

Verhoeven, W. M. A., van Praag, H. M., van Ree, J. M., and de Wied, D., 1979, Improvement of schizophrenic patients treated with (des-tyr¹)-γ-endorphin (DTγE), *Arch. Gen. Psychiat.* 36:294–298.

Volavka, J., Mallya, A., Baig, S., and Perez-Cruet, J., 1977, Naloxone in chronic schizophrenia, *Science* 196:1227–1228.

Wagemaker, H., and Cade, R., 1977, The use of hemodialysis in chronic schizophrenia, *Amer. J. Psychiat.* 134:684–685.

Watson, S. J., Berger, P. A., Akil, H., Mills, M. J., and Barchas, J. S., 1978, Effects of naloxone on schizophrenia: Reduction in hallucinations in a subpopulation of subjects, *Science* 201:73–76.

Wei, E., and Loh, H., 1976, Physical dependence on opiate-like peptides, *Science* 193:1262–1263.

Wikler, A., and Carter, R. L., 1953, Effects of single doses of N-allylnormorphine on hindlimb reflexes of chronic spinal dogs during cycles of morphine addiction, *J. Pharmacol. Exp. Ther.* 109:92–101.

Wikler, A., and Frank, K., 1948, Hindlimb reflexes in chronic spinal dogs during cycles of addiction to morphine and methadone, *J. Pharmacol. Exp. Ther.* 94:382–400.

Wikler, A., and Rayport, M., 1954, Lower limb reflexes of a chronic "spinal" man in cycles of morphine and methadone addiction, *Arch. Neurol. Psychiat.* (Chicago) 71:160–174.

Wikler, A., Fraser, H. F., and Isbell, H., 1953, N-allylnormorphine; Effects of single doses and precipitation of acute "abstinence syndromes" during addiction to morphine, methadone or heroin in man (post-addicts), *J. Pharmacol. Exp. Ther.* 109:8–20.

CHAPTER 5

Mechanisms of Opioid Analgesia

THE NATURE OF PAIN AND ITS RELIEF BY MORPHINE

In man, the presence of pain is inferred by the observer from the verbal reports of the subject and/or certain behavioral characteristics expressing his or her emotional state, and from evidence, actual or presumed, of tissue injury. Given the same or equivalent degrees of tissue injury, the severity of pain and demands for its relief vary widely. For example, Beecher (1956, 1968) noted that at the Anzio Beachhead in World War II, 150 soldiers with severe war wounds (trauma to bones, intrathoracic and intra-abdominal trauma) complained far less of pain, and only 32% wanted a narcotic within 7.2–12.5 hr after the trauma, compared with 150 males who had sustained comparable injuries in civilian disasters, 83% of whom wanted a narcotic within 3.0–4.4 hr after the trauma. In animals, pain is inferred by the observer from certain "nociceptive" reflexes and behaviors (attempts to escape, struggling, attacking, vocalizing). Yet here, too, the manifestations of pain, given the same or equivalent degrees of injury, are not invariable. Thus, Pavlov (1927) reported an experiment by Eroféeva in which she used strong electric (faradic) stimulation of the skin (which normally evokes vigorous unconditioned defense reflexes) as the conditioned stimulus for the formation of an alimentary conditioned reflex, by repeatedly pairing the former with presentation of food to the food-deprived dog. In response to this ("noxious") conditioned stimulus applied to the same skin area or a new area, the dog salivated, smacked its lips, and turned to the place where the food was about to be presented; there was no evidence of any motor defense reflex, nor was there any appreciable change in pulse or respiration. Similar results were obtained from dogs in which cauterization or pricking of the skin deep enough to draw blood was made to acquire the properties of an alimentary conditioned reflex. Pavlov (1927) noted that dogs frequently join in a scuffle for food in which they sustain skin wounds, which, however, play no dominant role as stimuli for any defense reflex, being entirely subordinated to the reflex for food. However, there were limits to the possibility of transforming an unconditioned defense reflex into a conditioned alimentary reflex; for example, when the stimulus for the unconditioned defense reflex was a strong electric current applied to the skin overlying bone with no muscular layer intervening, it was found impossible to replace the unconditioned defense reflex by a conditioned alimentary reflex, presumably because the electrical stimulus signalized far greater danger to the life of the animal than injury to the skin.

Observations such as these suggest strongly that pain is not merely a graded response (subjective, behavioral, or reflex) to the number of afferent impulses set up in "pain fibers" of peripheral nerve by tissue injury.

Hardy *et al.* (1952) conceptualized pain as an experience composed of "sensations" and "reactions" (to tissue injury). To measure pain sensations in man experimentally, they advised a "dolorimeter," consisting of the light from an incandescent lamp, which was focused by a biconvex condensing lens through an aperture in a non-heat-conducting screen for exactly 3 sec (exposure time controlled by an electronic shutter fixed just behind the aperture) onto an area of about 1.5 cm^2 in the center of the subject's forehead, which was previously blackened with India ink. The intensity of the thermal stimulus could be decreased or increased by a variac transformer in series with the lamp. The intensity of the thermal stimulus delivered was measured in mc/sec/cm^2 by a calibrated radiometer, the thermopile of which was placed in exactly the same position as the stimulated skin. *Pain sensation* was defined as the "pain threshold," namely, the thermal stimulus at which the subject (in accordance with instructions) perceived that the sensation of warmth and heat seemed to change into a more localized pricking pain at the very end of the 3-sec exposure time. In Hardy *et al.*'s hands, this pain threshold was remarkably constant in one individual and among different individuals, the mean being 232 mc/sec/cm^2 and the range, 202–252 mc/sec/cm^2 (Hardy *et al.*, 1952, p. 89), and morphine produced dose-related elevations of such pain thresholds (Hardy *et al.*, 1952, pp. 340–345). Nevertheless, they felt that pain reactions were more important in the total pain experience. To measure pain reactions, they recorded the excursions of the needle of a galvanometer connected through a Wheatstone bridge with the forearm and palmar surface of the middle finger, in response to graded thermal stimuli applied for 3 sec to the forehead, as in their pain threshold measurements. The minimal intensity of the thermal stimulus that caused the galvanometer needle to swing sharply across the scale immediately following the application of the stimulus (drop in skin resistance) was taken as the threshold of the "alarm reaction." Unlike the pain threshold, the threshold for the alarm reaction varied widely from test to test in the same individual and among different individuals. Ingestion of 40 ml of 95% ethyl alcohol markedly elevated the thresholds for the alarm reaction in the three subjects tested (Hardy *et al.*, 1952, pp. 264–267). Curiously, Hardy *et al.* furnished no data on the effects of morphine on the alarm reaction, possibly because of its variability and nonspecificity.

However, in the hands of investigators other than Hardy *et al.*, even the "pain threshold" proved to be variable and/or unpredictable with regard to the effects of morphine or saline (Beecher, 1957). Thus, Andrews (1943a) found that the pain threshold of postaddicts (former narcotic addicts) was within the range reported by Wolff *et al.* (1940) for nonaddicts, but that single analgesic doses of morphine had no significant effects on this threshold; yet, clinical experience showed that the same doses of morphine relieved pain in postaddicts. On the other hand, Andrews (1943b) found that morphine reduces changes in skin resistance following exposure to radiant heat in both postaddicts and nonaddicts; he concluded, therefore, that the reduction in the alarm reaction is more important in morphine analgesia than elevation of the pain threshold. Even greater discrepancies with the Wolff *et al.* (1940) pain threshold were found by Denton and Beecher (1949); they reported that not uncommonly, saline elevated while morphine lowered pain thresholds in well-trained college students. Other experimental methods for measuring pain and morphine analgesia in man have been reviewed in detail by Wikler (1950) and Beecher (1957). Like the Wolff *et al.* pain threshold, these measures are, for the most part, measures of sensory-discrimination functions, and the effects of morphine thereon have been inconsistent.

Noting that uncontrolled emotional factors could account, at least in part, for the divergent effects of morphine on the pain threshold reported by different investigators (see above), Hill *et al.* (1952a,b) hypothesized that morphine analgesia is due not to any effect it may have on sensory discriminative functions like the pain threshold, but to its effect on the alarm reaction, which they equated with *pain-anticipatory anxiety.* In a preliminary study, Hill *et al.* (1952a) correlated subjects' (postaddicts') judgments of the relative pain *intensity* of electric shocks of exactly 0.1-sec duration delivered to the skin of one had through bipolar saline-paste electrodes, with the actual wattage, amperage, and voltage of such electric shocks; they found that the subjects' estimation of relative pain intensity correlated best with the delivered wattage. In the next study (Hill *et al.*, 1952b), two groups of subjects were used, designated "informal" and "formal." The experiments on the informal group were carried out in a well-lighted room from which all unnecessary apparatus had been removed and the door to which was left open; the subjects (one at a time) were greeted by the experimenter in a friendly manner, the apparatus and procedure were discussed in a casual manner, and questions were answered reassuringly; when the subject was ready, the electrodes were applied and he was invited to deliver the shocks himself, the experimenter varying the wattage randomly over a preselected range, ending with four successive shocks of constant intermediate wattage (judged painful by the experimenters in tests on themselves), the perceived intensity of which the subject was asked to remember as the "standard." Then, half the subjects were given morphine (15 mg) and the other half, placebo, both intramuscularly, and each subject was sent back to the ward. One hour later, each subject was recalled to the experimental room and was given (or if he so preferred, delivered to himself) six series (separated by rest periods) of nine shocks each, the wattage of which was varied randomly in either direction from the "standard" by the experimenter; after each shock, the subject was asked to judge whether the shock was "stronger" or "weaker" than the remembered standard. The experiments in the formal group were carried out in the same manner *except* that the room was dimly lighted and cluttered with unnecessary electronic instruments, the door was closed, each subject was greeted in a polite but impersonal manner, discussion of the apparatus and procedure was limited to what was necessary, all electric shocks were delivered by the experimenter, and the subject was admonished to "be accurate and, above all, calm."

For each of the four groups (informal, morphine and placebo; formal, morphine and placebo), ogive curves were plotted, showing on the abscissa the known mean delivered wattage and, on the ordinate, the percentage of shocks (at each wattage) judged "stronger" than the remembered standard by the subjects. A perpendicular dropped onto the abscissa from the point on the ogive curve corresponding to 50% judged "stronger" (equivalent to 50% judged "weaker"), indicated the wattage of the subjects' judgment of the standard under each of the four particular conditions of the study. In the informal group, the wattage of the standard after placebo or after morphine was not significantly different from the wattage of the pretreatment standard. In other words, under conditions designed to *minimize* pain-anticipatory anxiety, the subjects' judgment of the pain intensity of the electric shocks after placebo was the same as before treatment, and morphine made no difference. On the other hand, in the formal group, the wattage of the standard after placebo was significantly *less* than before treatment, but the wattage of the standard after morphine was not significantly different from the wattage of the pretreatment standard. In other words, under conditions designed to *maximize* pain-anticipatory anxiety, the subjects *overestimated* the pain intensity of shocks at the wattage perceived as standard after placebo (compared with the pretreatment standard), and morphine *corrected this error*. Another way of stating this interpretation of the data is to say that morphine reduced pain-anticipatory anxiety and its effects on pain estimation (i.e., overestimation) of standard electric shocks; in the absence of pain-anticipatory anxiety, pain estimation of standard electric shocks was correct, and the same dose of morphine had no effect on such judgments.

Similar conclusions were reached by Kornetsky (1954) in a study employing radiant heat stimuli instead of electric shocks, but retaining the formal–informal experimental design, likewise carried out on postaddicts. In addition to measurements of "stronger or weaker than standard" judgments, several measures of "anticipation" were included, as well as measures of galvanic response to the radiant heat stimuli (changes in skin conductance). It was found that although control (no-drug) measures under formal and informal conditions did not differ significantly (probably because radiant heat stimuli were perceived as less threatening than electric shocks), morphine decreased significantly the number of "stronger" judgments and anticipatory galvanic responses, and it increased latencies to motor and galvanic responses measured from the onset of the heat stimuli, *only under formal conditions*.

Further evidence that morphine reduces pain-anticipatory anxiety was obtained by Hill *et al.* (1952c, 1955) in another series of investigations. In these studies, visual–manual reaction times were measured in a large group of postaddicts under "no-penalty" and "shock-penalty" conditions. In each condition, six series (separated by brief rest periods) of 18 light-flash stimuli were presented, to each of which the subjects were required to respond by moving a key as quickly as possible. In the no-penalty condition, responses had no consequences for the subject, and mean reaction times in each of the six series differed little from each other; morphine (15 mg intramuscularly) significantly slowed reaction times compared with the condition in which no drug was given. In the shock-penalty condition, however, the subject was informed (and soon experienced) that if any given reaction time was "slow" (the criterion for "slow" was not explained to the subject), another light would flash, and when he responded to it, he would deliver a brief, strong, but physically harmless faradic shock to his hand through saline-paste electrodes attached thereto. For the first series of 18 light-flash stimuli, the criterion for slow reaction times was a mean obtained in "practice" sessions (without shock penalties); for subsequent series, the criterion was revised downward if the mean reaction time on the last previous series was faster than the criterion used for the series preceding it, but no upward revision was made if the mean on the last previous series was slower. When no medication was given, marked slowing and increased variability of reaction times developed by the end of the second or third series, and such disruption of performance increased progressively through the fifth series, subsiding somewhat in the sixth (final) series. Inasmuch as reaction times were measured from the onset of the light not followed by shock penalty and from the onset of the other light signifying that reaction to it would be followed by shock penalty, slowing of reaction times in the shock-penalty condition relative to the no-penalty condition was *anticipatory* of shock to be self-inflicted. When testing was begun 50 min after intramuscular injection of morphine (15 mg), such disruption of performance did not develop, or it was long delayed; in fact, for some subjects, mean reaction times were slightly faster than after the same dose of morphine in the no-penalty condition. In contrast, pentobarbital (250 mg intramuscularly) did not ameliorate the disruption of reaction time performance in the shock-penalty condition, indicating the specificity of morphine in reducing pain-anticipatory anxiety.

The specificity of morphine and some other opioids in reducing pain-anticipatory anxiety was more fully explored by Hill *et al.* (1954, 1957a, 1966, 1967) in investigations on the rat, utilizing a modified form of the "conditioned emotional response" originally devised by Estes and Skinner (1941). Partially food-deprived rats were trained to press a bar at a steady rate for delivery of a food pellet (0.1 gm) at aperiodic intervals with a 2-min mean. When steady food-conditioned bar-pressing had been established, a tone was sounded at an intensity that just failed to affect the bar-pressing rate. Then the tone was presented for 4 min and terminated with a strong electric shock delivered to the feet through the grid floor, care being exercised to make sure that the rat had no contact with the bar when the shock was delivered (i.e., that the rat's bar-pressing behavior was not punished). After several such tone–shock pairings, the rats "froze" at the onset of the tone, and bar pressing was completely suppressed or nearly so for the 4 min of the tone's duration, but it was resumed at a somewhat faster rate immediately after cessation of the tone accompanied by delivery of electric shock to the feet. Measurement of the effects of drug on suppression of responding during the 4 min of the tone before delivery of the electric shock was made at the time of peak action of the drug as determined in experiments on food-conditioned bar-pressing before commencing tone–shock pairings. Dose-related decreases in suppression of responding during the 4 min of the tone relative to the immediately preceding 4-min pretone rate were found for morphine, methadone, and meperidine, the last-mentioned analgesic being tested as an "unknown." In contrast, no effects nor dose-related effects were found with amphetamine, pentobarbital, nalorphine, chlorpromazine, and cocaine. The ineffectiveness of nalorphine was rather surprising, since it had been reported (Lasagna & Beecher, 1954; Keats & Telford, 1956) that despite its psychotomimetic "side effects," it has analgesic properties in man. However, unlike morphine nalorphine has no effect on animal nociceptive reflexes, such as the tail flick in the rat (Woods, 1956). The diethylamide of D-lysergic acid (LSD-25) produced dose-related decreases in suppression when predrug suppression was incomplete (the tone frequency was irregular, predominantly 50–60 Hz with higher frequency harmonics, presented 2 db above an ambient noise level of 42 db), but it had no effects when predrug suppression was almost complete (the tone frequency was 523 Hz with no harmonics, of slightly squared sine waves, presented at 32 db above an ambient level of 42 db). The partial analgesic action of LSD-25 revealed by this "screening technique" is in accordance with the report by Kast and Collins (1964) of pain relief from LSD-25 in human patients with terminal cancer. It is important to note that in this animal "screening technique," the 4-min tone terminated concomitantly with electric shock to the feet was presented only *once* for a given dose of a given drug on a given day (to minimize the effect of repeated shocks on aversive learning in the morphine state), and care was exercised *not* to shock the rat while it is in contact with the bar (i.e., not to punish the rat for bar-press responding). Presenting tone–shock stimuli repeatedly in a single session, Lauener (1963) found that morphine did not decrease tone-produced suppression of responding, whereas chlordiazepoxide did. Kelleher and Morse (1964) found that in the pigeon, morphine did not reduce suppression of peck responding produced by repeated punishment. On the other hand, when they used methods very similar to those of Hill *et al.* (1954, 1957a, 1966, 1967), results in agreement with these investigators were reported by Maxwell *et al.* (1961) on the effects of morphine, 5 mg/kg, and by Black and Grosz (1974) on morphine, 9 mg/kg. Basing their investigations on Chorazyna's (1962) finding that stimuli that inhibit fear or anxiety retard the extinction of that fear, Morris and Gebhart (1978) reported that in doses greater than 0.75 mg/kg, morphine did indeed block extinction of suppression of food-reinforced bar-pressing in the presence of a flashing light, which, prior to the extinction sessions, had been accompanied by electric shocks to the rat through the grid floor; morphine was administered only in the extinction sessions (repeated presentation of flashing light without electric shock), and testing was carried out in the nondrug state. From these data, Morris and Gebhart (1978) concluded, in agreement with Hill *et al.* (1954, 1957a, 1966, 1967), that morphine has antianxiety properties (i.e., morphine reduces pain-anticipatory anxiety).

The concept that morphine relieves pain through reduction of the pain-anticipatory anxiety component without affecting the sensory-discriminative component of pain implies, besides a preferential action of morphine, that pain-anticipatory anxiety is acquired through a conditioning process. Thus, Wikler (1958) has hypothesized that early in life, only intense, noxious stimuli evoke an unconditioned emotional response; however, such intense noxious stimuli often begin as mild ones that evoke only specific, discriminable sensations such as "pricking" and "distending," without an unconditioned emotional response, and they gradually or rapidly increase in intensity to a degree evoking an unconditioned emotional response; hence, after many such "pairings," even mild noxious stimuli come to evoke an emotional response as a conditioned phenomenon (pain-anticipatory anxiety), and the sensory experiences evoked by mild noxious stimuli are transformed into "pricking pain," "distending pain," etc.

The effects of morphine so far described have been exerted primarily on the consequences of pain-anticipatory anxiety on pain-intensity judgments (Hill *et al.*, 1952a,b) and visual–manual reaction times (Hill *et al.*, 1952c, 1955) in man, and on inhibition of bar pressing in the presence of a tone heralding electric shock in rats (Hill *et al.*, 1954, 1957a, 1966, 1967). The effects of morphine on autonomic functions are more complex. Kornetsky (1954) reported that morphine reduced the number of anticipatory electrodermal responses and increased electrodermal response latencies measured from the onset of thermal stimuli in man, *but only under anxiety-promoting (so-called formal) conditions.* On the other hand, comparing unconditioned and tone-conditioned "phasic" (electrodermal) and "tonic" (basal) changes in skin conductance during intermittent, presumably mild electric shocks delivered to the calf in man, Jones *et al.* (1965) found that during *acquisition,* morphine (16 mg) attenuated the increase in tonic (basal) conductance and tended to reduce the degree of conditioning of the phasic (electrodermal) response, but that it had no effect on the responsivity of the latter. In another study, comparing unconditioned and tone-conditioned tonic and phasic responses to intermittent electric shocks delivered to one hand during *retention*, Jones and Ayres (1968) found that again, morphine reduced the unconditioned increase in basal skin conductance that developed during continued testing, but that it had no effect on conditioned tonic or phasic responses. Whether or not morphine would have reduced the amplitude (responsivity) of the conditioned tonic and/or phasic responses if pain-anticipitory anxiety had been deliberately induced as part of the experimental design cannot be determined from the report of Jones and Ayres. However, it is known that conditioned autonomic responses are more resistant to morphine than are conditioned motor responses. Thus, Stephens and Gantt (1956) observed that in dogs, morphine (0.5–5.0 mg/kg) reduced or abolished classically conditioned motor reflexes but left the concomitant cardiac conditioned reflexes unaffected—a phenomenon illustrative of what they termed, "schizokinesis."

Inspection of the data obtained by Hill *et al.* (1952a,b,c; 1955) on pain-anticipatory anxiety in man indicates that unlike pentobarbital, morphine "stabilizes" performance; that is, after morphine, pain-estimations and visual–manual reaction times are relatively uninfluenced by the procedures designed to induce pain-anticipatory anxiety and are more like those obtained in the no-drug, no-anxiety control condition. These data, together with observations of the "euphoric" general behavior of postaddicts after morphine on the ward, suggested that "stabilization" of performance may be a specific action of morphine extending beyond pain-anticipatory anxiety to include rewarding motivational determinants of behavior. To test this hypothesis, 182 postaddict volunteers were used as subjects of another study (Hill *et al.*, 1957a). All subjects were prisoners with long histories of narcotic addiction and repeated relapses and were serving sentences for violation of the federal narcotic laws, were considered to have very poor prognoses for continued abstention from narcotics after discharge, and had sentences sufficiently long to ensure at least six months in a drug-free state prior to the earliest prospective date of discharge. In this study, visual–manual reaction times were measured under four incentive conditions, defined in terms of different schedules of morphine rewards for participation in the experiments. In nonmedicated subjects, group-mean reaction times were slowest when a fixed morphine reward was given at least a week *before* the reaction time tests ("low incentive"), intermediate when the same fixed morphine reward was given *after* completion of the reaction time tests ("standard incentive"), faster when the amount of morphine given *after* completion of the reaction time tests varied directly with the mean speed of reaction ("high incentive"), and slightly faster when some of the subjects in the "high-incentive" condition volunteered for another experiment in which the same fixed morphine reward as in the standard-incentive condition was given *after* completion of the reaction time tests (standard II incentive). In subjects given morphine (15 mg intramuscularly) 50 min before the reaction time tests in each incentive condition, the differences in group-mean reaction times in the four incentive conditions were significantly *smaller* than in the corresponding no-drug control condition; that is, with reference to the no-drug condition, morphine acted as a "stimulant" under low incentive, as a "depressant" under standard II incentive, and as a placebo under standard I incentive and high incentive, thus *narrowing* the "range of change" in group-mean reaction times as a function of varying incentives, compared with the no-drug condition. In contrast, when the subjects were given pentobarbital (250 mg intramuscularly) 50 min before the reaction time tests in each incentive condition, the differences in group-mean reaction times in the four incentive conditions were significantly *greater* than in the no-drug control condition; that is, with reference to the no-drug condition, pentobarbital acted as a depressant under low incentive, as a stimulant under high incentive, and as a placebo in standard I and standard II incentives, thus *expanding* the range of change in group-mean reaction times as a function of varying incentives, compared with the no-drug condition (and the morphine condition).

These data indicate that the "analgesic" action of morphine in man is part of a more general action of this drug, namely, to "stabilize" performance, or to produce relative "indifference" to punishing or rewarding stimuli. This conclusion is in accordance with Wikler's (1952) opinion that morphine reduces all "primary" drives, and Schaumann's (1954) concept that morphine's analgesic action is part of a more general "antiprotective" action. In persons beset with punitive expectancies, even in the absence of pain, such morphine-produced indifference may be interpreted by the subject as a feeling of unusual well-being, and by the observer as euphoria. On the other hand, in persons whose expectancies are, on the whole, rewarding, morphine-produced indifference may be interpreted by the subject as unpleasant, and by the observer as dysphoric. The outcome of studies of Lasagna *et al.* (1955) may be viewed in this light. Thus, these investigators found that in 30 male postaddict prisoners at the Lexington, Kentucky, hospital, morphine (15 and 22.3 mg) produced euphoria in 22 and dysphoria in only three, while heroin (4 and 6 mg) produced euphoria in 15 and dysphoria in only 4; on the other hand, in 20 male students at Harvard Medical School, morphine (8 and 15 mg) produced "euphoria" in 8 and dysphoria in 10, while heroin (2 and 4 mg) produced euphoria in 9 and dysphoria in 10. In the remaining subjects—both prisoner postaddicts and Harvard Medical School students—clear-cut ratings of euphoria or dysphoria could not be made. Other interpretations of the data of Lasagna *et al.* (1955) are possible, but these and the interpretation based on the assumed difference in expectancies (punitive in the case of the prisoner postaddicts, rewarding in the case of the Harvard Medical School students) are not mutually exclusive.

In contrast to the indifference-producing action of morphine, so-called sedative doses of the shorter-acting barbiturates (e.g., pentobarbital) render the subject more responsive to punishing or rewarding stimuli. In doses that do not produce unconsciousness, thiopental and pentobarbital are not only devoid of analgesic properties but lower pain threshold in man (verbal report of pain and/or withdrawal of the leg, on graded pressure applied to the surface of the tibia) and antagonize the analgesic effects of meperidine or nitrous oxide (Dundee, 1960; Clutton-Brock, 1961). The "disinhibiting" effects of the shorter-acting barbiturates on behavior in the absence of pain are dramatically illustrated by the use of these drugs in "narcoanalysis" and "narcosynthesis" (Wikler, 1957). Taken orally in smaller amounts, the shorter-acting barbiturates like pentobarbital, amobarbital, or secobarbital have milder disinhibiting actions much like one or two alcoholic drinks. In a social-interaction setting, such disinhibiting effects may be reported as "relaxing" by the subject, though to a (nonintoxicated) observer, the behavior of the subject may appear to be quite the opposite. It would be interesting to compare euphoric–dysphoric reactions to "sedative" doses of pentobarbital in prisoner postaddicts (presumed punitive expectancies) and Harvard Medical School students (presumed rewarding expectancies). One would expect results opposite to those of morphine or heroin, but the data available are not quite appropriate because they were obtained by two groups of investigators using different methods. Thus, Lasagna *et al.* (1955) reported nine euphoric and eight dysphoric reactions to pentobarbital (0.05 and 0.1 g intravenously) in Harvard Medical School students, but they did not administer pentobarbital to prisoner postaddicts. Hill *et al.* (1963) used a 550-item true–false questionnaire (the Addiction Research Center Inventory, or ARCI) to characterize the subjective effects of pentobarbital, 200 or 250 mg intramuscularly (as well as other drugs), in prisoner postaddicts at the Lexington, Kentucky, hospital. The most common reactions to pentobarbital were similar to those of alcohol and consisted of affirmation of such dysphoric items as tiredness, weakness, general slowing, and drowsiness, accompanied by affirmation of some euphoric items; on the other hand, fewer dysphoric items and many more euphoric items were affirmed after morphine, 10 or 20 mg intramuscularly. To the extent that the findings of Lasagna *et al.* (1955) and of Hill *et al.* (1963) may be compared, it appears probable that in contrast to morphine, pentobarbital produces euphoria more commonly in Harvard Medical School students (rewarding expectancies) than in prisoner postaddicts (punitive expectancies), and the reverse for dysphoria.

From this survey of the nature of pain and its relief by morphine, it is evident that a neurophysiological model of these phenomena must describe not only transmission of neural activity evoked by noxious peripheral stimuli in the spinal cord, but also inhibitory and facilitatory circuits at "higher" levels, including those (presumably limbic–cortical) that are activated in pain-anticipatory anxiety. One such model has been proposed by Melzack and Wall (1965) and by Casey and Melzack (1967), involving three interconnected processes, each with its own neural substrate: sensory–discriminative, motivational–affective, and central control. The sensory–discriminative and motivational–affective dimensions of pain are subject to "gate control" through inhibitory influences of the substantia gelatinosa on "transmission cells" (T) in the spinal cord, the substantia gelatinosa being itself inhibited by small-fiber ("pain" fiber) input, with resultant increase in firing of T cells, and excited by large-fiber ("nonpain" fiber) input, with resultant decrease in firing of T cells. The large-fiber input is derived not only from the dorsal roots but also from supraspinal levels (rhombencephalic, mesencephalic, diencephalic, and limbic–cortical "central control" circuits). When the resultant output from the T cells exceeds a critical value, the organism is triggered into action (fight, flight, vocalization, and/or other overt responses, in part based on past experiences and cognitive appraisal of the present situation). The neural substrate of the sensory–discriminative dimension is the classical neospinothalamic tract, which transmits the output from the dorsal horn T cells in the anterolateral spinal cord to the ventrobasal nuclei of the thalamus and the somatosensory cortex. The neural substrates of the motivational–affective dimension are the "paramedial ascending system" (spinoreticular, spinomesencephalic, and paleospinothalamic components of the anterolateral somatosensory pathway), which transmits the output from dorsal horn T cells into the reticular core of the brain stem and the medial thalamus; the fibers of the paramedial ascending system also penetrate the midbrain central gray matter, which is part of the limbic midbrain area that, among other projections, connects reciprocally with the hypothalamic area and receives connections from the frontal granular cortex. The neural basis of the central control dimension is mainly the frontal cortex with its reciprocal connections with intracortical fiber systems from virtually all sensory and associational areas, and with reticular and limbic structures. Not included in this brief digest of Melzack and Wall's (1965) and Casey and Melzack's (1967) neurophysiological model of pain are numerous citations of evocation of pain and of relief of pain by stimulation or lesioning of many of the specific structures in the neural substrates of the three interconnected dimensions of pain.

SITES OF MORPHINE'S ANTINOCICEPTIVE ACTIONS IN THE CENTRAL NERVOUS SYSTEM

Spinal Cord

Although it is profoundly influenced by supraspinal mechanisms, the sensory–discriminative dimension of pain is primarily integrated at the spinal cord level (including the descending spinal trigeminal sensory tract). Some of the most widely used analgesia-screening methods in animals, like the tail-flick response to radiant heat in the rat (D'Amour & Smith, 1941) and the skin-twitch response to radiant heat or skin pinches in the dog (Andrews & Workman, 1941) can be demonstrated after spinal cord transection at appropriate levels, and these nociceptive reflexes are depressed by morphine, though to a lesser degree than in the intact animal (Irwin et al., 1951; House & Wikler, 1951). Herr et al. (1952) reported that the threshold of the tail-flick response in the rat was lowered about 30% by decortication and about 50% by spinal transection; to achieve equal degrees of depression of the tail-flick response, the dose of morphine had to be twice as large in decorticated rats and five times as large in spinal rats than in the intact animal. Similarly, Houde and Wikler (1951) found that in dogs with spinal cords hemisected at the C-6 or C-7 level, the amplitude of the skin-twitch response to radiant heat was slightly but significantly greater on the spinal than on the intact side, and morphine (5 mg/kg subcutaneously) depressed the amplitude of the response on both sides, but to a greater degree on the intact side (thresholds, or latencies to skin-twitch responses, were difficult to evaluate because of concomitant changes in amplitude). These data suggest that in the intact organism, the depressive effect of morphine on nociceptive segmental reflexes in the spinal cord is augmented by tonic supraspinal inhibitory influences on their thresholds and amplitudes, and perhaps by supraspinal actions of morphine that increase such inhibition (see below).

Morphine depresses nociceptive spinal reflexes predilectively. Wikler and Frank (1948) investigated the effects of morphine and other drugs on hind-limb reflexes of the chronic spinal dog, after full recovery from initial "spinal shock," several weeks following complete transection or removal of a transverse segment of the spinal cord in the midthoracic or lower thoracic region. Morphine (e.g., 5 mg/kg subcutaneously or intramuscularly) markedly depressed the ipsilateral flexor and crossed extensor reflexes (responses to nociceptive stimulation), enhanced the ipsilateral extensor thrust (a response to stretch of the toe pads or displacement of the hairs between the toes), and had little or no effect on the knee jerk (a response to sudden stretch of the quadriceps muscle). These findings were confirmed by Martin and Eades (1964). Analogous effects of morphine and methadone were found by Wikler and Rayport (1954) in a chronic "spinal" man, namely, depression of ipsilateral flexion and crossed extension of the lower limbs in response to "pinwheel" stimuli applied to the skin of a lower limb, and no effect or enhancement of the knee and ankle jerks. Likewise, Berlin et al. (1954) reported that in three paraplegic patients, morphine (15–20 mg intramuscularly) markedly elevated the reflex movement threshold of the lower extremities in response to radiant heat applied to a blackened area on the thigh, and that it reduced or abolished spontaneous reflex movements, if present.

Another reflex response to noxious stimulation, which has been used extensively in the analysis of morphine's antinociceptive action, is the flexor reflex in the spinal cat. Blume (1927) reported that morphine depressed the flexor reflex in the decapitated cat. In an analysis of the effects of morphine on the patterns of behavior and reflex activity in the cat, Wikler (1944) found that in the spinal preparation, morphine depressed the ipsilateral flexor and cross-extensor reflex responses to noxious stimulation, but that it had little or no effect on the knee jerk, a tendon reflex response to phasic stretch. Using electrographic techniques in cats with spinal cords transected through the atlanto occipital membrane (Lloyd preparation), Wikler (1945) found that morphine (5–15 mg/kg intravenously) depressed polysynaptic (multineuronal) discharges evoked by single electric shocks to the sural or deep peroneal nerves and recorded from L-7 or S-1 ventral roots; in doses of 5 mg/kg, morphine enhanced, and in doses of 15 mg/kg, morphine depressed the monosynaptic discharges evoked by single electrical shocks to the ipsilateral gastrocnemius or deep peroneal nerves and recorded from L-7 or S-1 ventral roots. Takagi et al. (1955) reported that morphine (7 mg/kg) depressed sciatic nerve to S-1 ventral root polysynaptic discharges markedly for 10–30 min in curarized intact cats and for 5–10 min in "high" spinal cats (spinal cords transected between C-1 and C-2 segments) but not at all in "low" spinal cats (spinal cords transected between T-1 and T-2 or L-2 and L-3 segments) even after 14 mg/kg of morphine; in addition, these investigators reported that in intact cats, the depressant action of morphine (7 mg/kg) on this reflex discharge was augmented by electrolytic destruction of the "facilitatory" area in the brain-stem reticular formation, and that the same dose of morphine augmented the reflex discharge when the "inhibitory" area of the brain-stem reticular formation was destroyed. Takagi *et al.* (1955) concluded that the depressive action of morphine on the polysynaptic reflex discharge (in the intact cat) is due not to a direct depressive action on the spinal segmental reflex, but to stimulation of the inhibitory and facilitatory regions in the brain-stem and cervical reticular formations, the former usually predominating. However, contradictory to the findings of Takagi *et al.* (1955) on low spinal cats are the observations of Krivoy *et al.* (1973) on last lumbar dorsal root to ventral root reflex electrical discharges in cats decerebrated and made spinal by transection of the spinal cord at the L-2 level. These investigators found that in such low spinal cats, polysynaptic reflex discharges were depressed by morphine (0.5- 12.5 mg/kg intravenously) in a dose-dependent manner, and that they were restored to control values by naloxone. Krivoy *et al.* (1973) suggested that one of the reasons Takagi *et al.* (1955) failed to observe the depressive action of morphine on polysynaptic reflex discharges in the low spinal cat was that the latter investigators observed their preparations for only 5–7 min (after injection of morphine); Krivoy *et al.* (1973) also pointed out that in one of the figures in the paper of Takagi *et al.* (1955), the major polysynaptic potential was depressed after morphine.

Interestingly, Krivoy *et al.* (1973) also found that morphine depressed the monosynaptic reflex discharge, but this depressant action of morphine was dependent on the frequency of afferent stimulation, being greatest at 12.5 Hz and least at 0.5 Hz, the depression at 0.5 Hz not reaching statistical significance. The selective depressant action of morphine on *repetitive* activity, whether polysynaptic or monosynaptic, at the spinal segmental reflex level is further illustrated by the investigations of Jurna *et al.* (1973), who reported that in cats decerebrated and made spinal by transection of the spinal cord at the lower thoracic level, morphine (2 mg/kg) depressed polysynaptic excitatory postsynaptic potentials (EPSPs), the repetitive discharge from interneurons in the vicinity of the motoneurons (but not in the dorsal gray matter), and the temporal facilitation of EPSPs produced in motoneurons by *repetitive* stimulation of afferents from the gastrocnemius–soleus muscles; all of these depressant effects of morphine were reversed by levallorphan. In contrast, morphine did not affect monosynaptic EPSPs in motoneurons evoked by *single* dorsal root stimuli, antidromic potentials in the motoneuron evoked by ventral root stimulation, or the inhibitory post-synaptic potentials (IPSPs) evoked in gastrocnemius–soleus moto-neurons by sural nerve stimulation. Jurna *et al.* (1973) concluded that in the spinal cord, the depressive action of morphine is due not to a selective effect on interneurons, but to interference with special pro-cesses built up by *repetitive* stimulation in the terminals of afferent fibers converging on interneurons or motoneurons. To some extent, the ob-servations of Krivoy *et al.* (1973) and of Jurna *et al.* (1973) may explain discordant reports on the effects of morphine on the knee jerk, perhaps dependent on the frequencies of the stimuli (muscle stretch) by which this reflex was elicited: marked depression (Luckhardt & Johnson, 1928); slight depression (DeBodo & Brooks, 1937); and no effect or enhance-ment (Wikler, 1944; Cook & Bonnycastle, 1953).

The effects of morphine on inhibitory processes in the spinal cord were investigated by Kruglov (1964). Polysynaptically mediated (indi-rect) inhibition of a dorsal root to ventral root segmental reflex discharge was plotted as a function of the interval between conditioning and test stimuli. Subthreshold conditioning stimuli were delivered to one part of a dorsal root at increasing intervals before test stimuli (maximal for Group 1 afferent fibers) were delivered to the other part of the dorsal root. Prior to drug treatment, the inhibitory effect of such conditioning appeared as a sharp decrease in the percentage of facilitation of the monosynaptic arc; such inhibition first became evident at a stimulus in-terval of about 1.5–2.0 msec and passed over into absolute inhibition at about 3.0 msec, continuing to 12 msec. Morphine markedly diminished or, in doses of 5–10 mg/kg, completely eliminated such inhibitory de-viations of the facilitatory curve. Likewise, antidromic inhibition was depressed by morphine. A maximal test stimulus was applied to L-6 dorsal root, severed intradurally, and the monosynaptic spike-response was recorded from the severed nerve to one head of the quadriceps muscle; the preceding inhibitory volley was delivered antidromically to the nerve severed from the other head of the quadriceps muscle. The inhibitory action of the antidromic volley (maximal at intervals of about 2.5 msec and continuing up to 40–50 msec) was significantly reduced by morphine or codeine (5–10 mg/kg). On the other hand, morphine, in doses of less than 5 mg/kg, had no effect on direct inhibition and, in doses of 5–10 mg/kg, markedly increased direct inhibition as measured by the inhibitory effect of a preceding conditioning stimulus to the severed deep peroneal nerve on the monosynaptic discharge elicited by a maximal test stimulus delivered to the severed gastrocnemius nerve and recorded from severed S-1 ventral root. Kruglov (1964) concluded that morphine blocks neither excitatory nor inhibitory synapses of primary afferent fibers on motoneurons, but that it does block polysynaptic and antidromic inhibition. Noting that in previous research, analgesics of the morphine group were found to prolong the central conduction time of the flexor reflex and to depress polysynaptic afterdischarges, he pointed out that acetylcholine is the neurotransmitter not only at interneuronal synapses in the spinal cord but also in the motoneuron collateral synapses to the somas of the Renshaw cells, which are activated by antidromic stimulation. Thus, the loci of the depressant actions of morphine in the spinal cord (flexor reflex, polysynaptic afterdischarge, polysynaptic inhibition, antidromic inhibition) appear to coincide with the loci at which acetylcholine is the neurotransmitter.

Though, except for Takagi et al. (1955), there is general agreement that even in low spinal cats, relatively small doses of morphine regularly depress electrical polysynaptic reflex discharges, the relationship of such discharges to "pain" has not been clear. Koll et al. (1961, 1963) have adduced evidence that included in such polysynaptic discharges are reflex responses to nonnoxious as well as to noxious stimulation of peripheral nerve. The polysynaptic reflex discharges to nociceptive stimulation appear after a longer latency and they persist for a longer time. In order of their temporal appearance, Koll et al. (1961, 1963) designated these polysynaptic discharges as "postdelta" and "C" reflexes (presumably correlated with subjective reports of "first" and "second" pain, respectively). In cats decerebrated and made spinal at L-7, morphine, in doses of 0.3–0.4 mg/kg intravenously, regularly and markedly depressed the postdelta and C reflexes, while exerting less constant depressive effects on the polysynaptic reflex discharge with shorter latency. Koll et al. (1963) concluded that morphine has a predilective action on certain interneurons belonging to the postdelta and C nociceptive reflex arcs.

In addition to depressing nociceptive polysynaptic segmental spinal cord reflexes, morphine and other opioids have been shown to exert depressant actions on unit activity of neurons in the laminae of the dorsal gray matter specifically responding to noxious stimulation of peripheral nerve, and in the transmission of impulses from such neurons in the anterolateral spinothalamic tract. Thus, recording from glass pipette microelectrodes filled with 1 M K-acetate inserted into the lumbar gray matter in cats with spinal cords transected at T-5, Iwata and Sakai (1971) found that in doses of 40 μg/kg intravenously, the potent opioid fentanyl depressed firing of spinal interneurons activated by A-delta but not by A-alpha fibers of cutaneous ipsilateral saphenous nerve. With extracellular microelectrode recording, Kitahata *et al.* (1973, 1974) reported that in cats decerebrated and made spinal by transection of the spinal cord between L-1 and L-2, morphine sulfate (0.5, 1, and 2 mg/kg intravenously) suppressed in a dose-related manner single-unit activities in Rexed (1952) laminae I and V, known to respond principally to noxious stimuli, but not in laminae IV and VI, known to respond to nonnoxious stimuli; also, morphine sulfate (1 mg/kg intravenously) reduced unit activities in laminae I and V evoked by noxious cutaneous stimuli. Similarly, LeBars *et al.* (1975) observed that with extracellular microelectrode recording in the dorsal gray matter of L-6 and L-7 lumbar segments in C-1 spinal cats, morphine (2 mg/kg intravenously) depressed firing rates in responses in Rexed lamina V cells, elicited by natural nociceptive stimulation, identified by graded responses to increasing intensities of pinches and broad receptive fields; these depressive actions of morphine were reversed by nalorphine (1 mg/kg) or naloxone (0.05–0.2 mg/kg) intravenously. Calvillo *et al.* (1974) applied morphine iontophoretically to dorsal horn neurons in segments L-5 to L-7 in chloralose-anesthetized, decerebrated, or spinal cords transected at T-13. Morphine depressed ongoing activity, glutamate-evoked excitation, and responses to noxious stimulation in most neurons, but it had little effect on ongoing activity and glutamate-evoked excitation of neurons responding to nonnoxious stimuli; naloxone, intravenously and iontophoretically, reversed the morphine-produced depression. Likewise, Zieglgänsberger and Bayerl (1976) found that microelectrophoretically applied morphine and levorphanol depressed spontaneous as well as stimulus-induced activity in lamina V dorsal horn neurons (L-6,7 segments) in cats made spinal at T-9,10 or anesthetized with pentobarbital and anemically decerebrated. These depressant effects were antagonized by naloxone applied microelectrophoretically at the same sites. Morphine and levorphanol applied electrophoretically to motoneurons slowed the rate of rise of mono- and polysynaptic EPSPs by a naloxone-antagonizable mechanism at doses that had almost no effect on spike shape. Higher doses of morphine and levorphanol produced "nonspecific" effects (not antagonizable by naloxone), which are summarized as reduction in the amplitude of IPSPs and reduction in the amplitude or complete abolition of spikes evoked both directly and antidromically. Zieglgänsberger and Bayerl (1976) noted that their findings complement those of Jurna *et al.* (1973), reviewed above, and concluded that especially their additional finding that microelectrophoretically applied naloxone antagonizes the depressant effects of systemically administered morphine on dorsal horn firing in spinal cats indicates that the spinal cord is a major site of opioid analgesic action.

That in the cat, the neospinothalamic (anterolateral or ventrolateral) tract does indeed transmit pain was demonstrated by Pomeranz (1973), who recorded extracellular action potentials from axons in the ventrolateral tract at C-2 in cats made spinal at C-1 and found that 30% of the axons sampled responded exclusively to painful cutaneous stimuli (noxious heat, noxious cold, sharp probe with heavy pressure) or electrical stimulation of the radial or sural nerve and received inputs only from small-diameter fibers. These responses in the ventrolateral tract apparently were not subject to the "gating" mechanism postulated by Melzack and Wall (1965) and Casey and Melzack (1967), since they were not inhibited by concomitant stimulation of large-diameter afferent fibers or facilitated by concomitant stimulation of small-diameter afferent fibers. Pomeranz (1973) pointed out that in addition to these "monomodal" axons in the ventrolateral tract responding exclusively to noxious stimulation of the skin, there are many "multimodal" axons responding to nonnoxious as well as to noxious stimulation, constituting the dorsolateral tract and 70% of the ventrolateral tract, which are subject to a gating mechanism; he suggested that perhaps the two pathways operate in parallel to transmit "painful" information from the spinal cord to the brain. Perhaps the existence of ungated and gated mechanisms in the spinal cord could explain the apparently discordant reports of Fujita *et al.* (1953, 1954) and Satoh and Takagi (1971) on the effects of morphine on potentials in the neospinothalamic tract evoked by splanchnic nerve stimulation in spinal cats. Fujita *et al.* (1953, 1954) reported that low doses of morphine or meperidine abolished such potentials for "a long time." On the other hand, Satoh and Takagi (1971) found that in intact cats or in cats decerebrated by intercollicular section, anesthetized with pentobarbital, or prepared under ether and immobilized with *d*-tubocurarine or gallamine triethiodide with artificial respiration, 2–4 mg/kg of morphine intravenously inhibited the ventrolateral (neospinothalamic) tract responses to afferent splanchnic nerve stimulation, but this effect was reversed by acute transection of the spinal cord at C-1; in spinal cats, a dose of 10 mg/kg of morphine caused a slight depression of the response. Satoh and Takagi (1971) concluded that the depressive effect of small doses of morphine on pain-afferent pathways in the spinal cord from splanchnic (and sciatic) nerve stimulation is mediated chiefly by its facilitatory action on descending inhibitory sensory-regulating (gating) bulbar structures; after large doses of morphine, a direct suppressive effect on spinal sensory transmission is also involved, but, according to Satoh and Takagi (1971), this effect seems to be related to morphine's "side effect," since large doses of morphine (8–10 mg/kg) "produce abnormal behavior in cats." The failure of Satoh and Takagi (1971) to find depressive actions of small doses of morphine on spinal cord nociceptive transmission in C-1 spinal cats is difficult to reconcile with the work of the numerous investigators (see above) who observed depressive effects of even smaller doses of morphine on nociceptive polysynaptic reflex discharges and nociceptive lamina-specific unit activities in the dorsal gray matter in low spinal cats.

All of these data (except those of Takagi *et al.*, 1955, and Satoh and Takagi, 1971) on spinal preparations indicate strongly that in the *intact* organism, the spinal cord may be one of the important sites of morphine's analgesic action. Supporting this conclusion are the findings of Yaksh and Rudy (1976), who introduced morphine, fentanyl, codeine, and ethylmorphine in microgram quantities into the lumbar subarachnoid space in the intact rat, and tested analgesia by the tail-flick, hot-plate, squeak–escape response to forceps pinch and the operant shock-titration methods. All the opioid analgesics elevated the thresholds or depressed the test response in a dose-related manner, and these effects were reversed by naloxone, 0.5–2.0 mg/kg intravenously or 0.1–3.0 μg introduced through the spinal catheter. Diffusion of the opioid analgesic from the lumbar subarachnoid space to supraspinal regions was ruled out by the following evidence: 5% bromphenol blue introduced into the lumbar subarachnoid space stained spinal segments no more than 1.0–1.5 cm distant in either direction; 15 μg of morphine (sufficient to produce analgesia by introduction into the lumbar subarachnoid space) did not produce analgesia when injected intravenously; and radioactivity in forebrain and brain stem never exceeded 0.15% of radioactivity from spinal cord after introduction of ^{14}C-morphine into the lumbar subarachnoid space through the catheter.

Brain Stem

Recent research (see below) indicates that modulation of the sensory–discriminative dimension of pain at the spinal cord level is strongly influenced by descending pathways from the caudal brain stem, including the medullary raphe nuclei (e.g., nucleus raphe magnus), the nuclei gigantocellularis and paragigantocellularis, and possibly other structures lying close to the floor of the fourth ventricle; also, descending pathways from the periaqueductal gray matter (especially the dorsal raphe nucleus located therein) are thought to activate the medullary raphe nuclei. Modulation of the motivational-affective dimension of pain at the levels of the hypothalamus, the limbic system, the medial thalamus, and the frontal cortex is strongly influenced by ascending pathways from the rostral brain stem, including the periventricular gray matter surrounding the posterior part of the third ventricle and the periaqueductal gray matter (especially the dorsal and median raphe nuclei). The evidence for the involvement of these loci in the integration of pain is derived, in part, from studies on the effects on chronic pain or responses to noxious stimuli of local application of morphine or other opioids, of focal electrical stimulation or destruction, and of more distant anatomical lesions on these phenomena.

That structures in the brain stem lying close to the floor of the fourth ventricle are highly putative sites for the analgesic action of morphine is indicated by the findings of Herz and his collaborators (see below). In these studies, conducted on rabbits, opioids and opioid antagonists were injected through a cannula into a selected part of the ventricular system, spread of the drug solutions to a communicating part being prevented by prior plugging of the latter with eucerine (Nivea Creme). Spread of the applied drug was checked by autoradiography after injection of ^{14}C-morphine into the same selected part of the ventricular system, and also after microinjection of ^{14}C-morphine into various diencephalic and mesencephalic structures, to assess the spread of unlabeled morphine microinjected into these areas. Depression of the licking reaction to electrical stimulation of the tooth pulp of the upper incisors or depression of the flexor reflex elicited by heat was used as an index of analgesia. In brief, it was found that morphine (or fentanyl), confined in its actions to the floor of the fourth ventricle (especially its rostral part, including the aqueduct), consistently produced marked analgesia (Herz et al., 1970; Vigouret et al., 1973; Teschemacher et al., 1973). No analgesia was observed after injection of morphine into the lateral ventricles or the cisterna cerebellomedullaris, and slight analgesia was observed after injection of morphine into the third ventricle. Marked analgesia was also observed after microinjection of morphine into the hypothalamus, the subthalamus, and the mesencephalon, especially in the medial parts of the structures, but spread of the drug into the ventricular system from these areas could not be excluded with certainty. Herz et al. (1970) noted that microinjection of morphine into the periaqueductal gray matter often produced motor excitation together with depression of the licking reaction to tooth-pulp stimulation. In keeping with the localization of the analgesic action of morphine to the floor of the fourth ventricle, it was shown (Albus et al., 1970; Herz & Teschemacher, 1971) that the analgesic and respiratory-depressant effects of morphine (10 mg/kg given intramuscularly) could be reversed by injection of the morphine antagonist levallorphan into the aqueduct after plugging the third ventricle, thus permitting the antagonist to spread into the fourth ventricle but not rostrally. On the other hand, when levallorphan was injected into the lateral ventricle after plugging the aqueduct (thus confining the action of the antagonist to the lateral and third ventricles), no antagonism of the analgesic effect of systemically administered morphine was observed, and the respiratory-depressant effects were reduced only partially and temporarily. When higher doses of the morphine antagonists were allowed to spread throughout the whole ventricular system after previous systemic administration of morphine, a long-lasting excitatory state developed.

According to Taber *et al.* (1960), eight groups of cells can be distinguished in the midsagittal region (raphe) of the brain stem in the cat. Proceeding roughly in a caudal–rostral direction, these "raphe nuclei" are the raphe obscurus, the raphe pallidus, the raphe magnus, the raphe pontis, the centralis superior, the raphe dorsalis, the linearis intermedius, and the linearis rostralis. Their efferent and afferent connections have been described by Brodal *et al.* (1960a,b). Histochemical investigations by Dahlström and Fuxe (1964, 1965) and by Ungerstedt (1971) have shown that in the rat, most (if not all) the raphe nuclei contain serotonin and that serotoninergic pathways from the caudal raphe nuclei (e.g., the raphe magnus) descend to the dorsal and ventral horns and sympathetic lateral column of the spinal cord, while serotoninergic pathways from the rostral raphe nuclei (e.g., raphe dorsalis) ascend to the hypothalamus, septum, cingulum, amygdala, and cerebral cortex. Apart from the raphe-serotoninergic pathways, the brain stem of the rat also contains noradrenergic and dopaminergic pathways. The most caudal noradrenergic group of cells in the medulla oblongata gives rise to one system of axons that descends in the anterior funiculus and ventral part of the lateral funiculus and terminates in the ventral horn, and another system of axons that descends in the dorsal part of the lateral funiculus and terminates in the dorsal horn and sympathetic lateral column. Caudal and more rostral cell groups in the medulla and pons give rise to a "ventral" ascending noradrenergic system that terminates on cells in the lower brain stem, the mesencephalon, and the diencephalon (including the whole hypothalamus). Cells in the locus ceruleus give rise to a "dorsal" noradrenergic system that overlaps with the "ventral" noradrenergic system in the medulla and pons; descending axons in both adrenergic systems terminate in lower brain stem nuclei, while ascending axons in the "dorsal" adrenergic system terminate in the hypothalamus, the cingulum, the bulbus olfactorius, the cerebral cortex, and the cerebellar cortex. Dopaminergic cell bodies are located mainly in the substantia nigra, and their axons terminate in the nucleus caudatus, the tuberculum olfactorium (anterior perforated space in man), and the nucleus accumbens; dopaminergic cells in the median eminence give rise to axons that terminate within the hypothalamus.

That monoamines are involved, at least in part, in the analgesic action of morphine is indicated by the finding of Schneider (1954) that reserpine (which depletes the brain of both serotonin and the catecholamines) antagonizes morphine analgesia in mice. Lee and Fennessy (1970) reported that in the mouse, doses of morphine that were sufficient to depress the phenylquinone-writhing response (ED_{50} 0.85 mg/kg) reduced brain levels of serotonin only, whereas larger doses, sufficient to elevate the threshold for the hot-plate paw-licking response (ED_{50} 8.5 mg/kg) reduced brain levels of both serotonin and norepinephrine (both monoamines were determined fluorometrically). In rats, Tenen (1968) found that administration of p-chloraphenylalanine (pCPA, an inhibitor of tryptophan hydroxylase that blocks the synthesis of serotonin) partially antagonized the threshold-elevating actions of morphine, dl-methadone, and d-propoxyphene on the flinch–jump threshold to foot shock; the antagonism of pCPA to the analgesic effect of codeine was only suggestive, and pCPA did not antagonize the analgesic effect of meperidine. Vogt (1974) demonstrated that intraperitoneal administration of pCPA markedly lowered the serotonin concentration in the pons, medulla, and spinal cord of rats, while injection of 5,6-dihydroxytryptamine (5,6-DHT) into one lateral ventricle markedly lowered the serotonin concentration in the spinal cord but hardly affected that of the pons and medulla; the analgesic potency of morphine given systemically (as measured by depression of leg withdrawal in response to graded pressure on the foot) was markedly reduced by pCPA and to a lesser extent by 5,6-DHT. Vogt (1974) pointed out that these data do not imply a spinal site for the analgesic action of morphine, but only that the raphe–serotoninergic system is involved in morphine analgesia, as well as noradrenergic and dopaminergic systems, the exact roles of which are as yet unclear.

Proudfit and Anderson (1973) reported that the serotonin antagonists cinanserin and methysergide shifted in a facilitatory direction the time course of the curve representing facilitation and inhibition of the segmentally evoked monosynaptic reflex produced by conditioning stimuli applied to the caudal raphe nuclei (e.g., raphe magnus) in the unanesthetized decerebrate cat. These results were obtained by close intra-arterial injection of low doses of cinanserin (1.0–1.6 mg/kg) or methysergide (200 μg/kg) in the spinal cord, but not by intravenous injection of these low doses (much higher doses of the serotonin antagonists intravenously did produce the same results). Caudal raphe stimulation also evoked short-latency dorsal and ventral root potentials; the serotonin antagonists increased the dorsal root potential but depressed the segmentally evoked dorsal root potential. In a subsequent report, Proudfit and Anderson (1974b) described second, longer-latency dorsal and ventral root potentials evoked by electrical stimulation of the nucleus raphe magnus that were depressed by cinanserin, 4 mg/kg intravenously, while the first, short-latency dorsal root potential was increased. From measurements of length constants for the short- and long-latency dorsal root potentials, it appeared that the short-latency potential is generated in smaller fibers (Groups II and III) than the long-latency potential (Group I fibers). From these and other data, the authors tentatively proposed that the descending serotoninergic system consists of two basic divisions, one that terminates presynaptically on primary afferent terminals (inhibitory) and another that terminates on motoneurons or on an intercalated neuron (excitatory). The activation of these descending serotoninergic systems would be to inhibit peripheral input while increasing motoneuronal responsiveness to central activation. Noting that small-diameter dorsal root fibers carry pain impulses (Burgess & Perl, 1967), Proudfit and Anderson (1974a, 1975) hypothesized that morphine might activate the caudal raphe-descending serotoninergic pathways that depolarize primary afferent terminals and presynaptically inhibit pain impulses, thereby producing analgesia. To test his hypothesis, they compared the analgesic effects (latency of the tail flick to radiant heat) of morphine (5 mg/kg intraperitoneally) in rats with partial or complete destruction of the raphe magnus and in controls (unoperated rats or rats with extraraphe lesions). Compared with that in the controls, the analgesia produced by morphine was reduced in rats with raphe magnus lesions, the degree of analgesia reduction being proportional to the extent of raphe magnus destruction (Spearman rank correlation coefficient between analgesic index and percentage of destruction of nucleus raphe magnus was -0.91, $p < 0.001$). Prior to testing with morphine, the tail-flick latency was significantly shortened in rats with raphe magnus lesions ("hyperalgesia"), while it remained unaltered after extraraphe lesions. In 9 of 11 other rats, electrical stimulation of the raphe magnus resulted in analgesia; in the remaining 2, neither electrical stimulation of the raphe magnus nor morphine produced analgesia, and it was found that the stimulating electrodes had produced lesions in the nucleus raphe magnus. These results are in accord with those of Oliveras et al. (1975), who found that electrical stimulation of the inferior centralis of the raphe (equivalent to the raphe obscurus and raphe magnus) produced analgesia in the cat; such analgesia was antagonized by naloxone, 0.15 mg/kg given intramuscularly. These data indicate that the nucleus raphe magnus exerts a tonic inhibition of pain perception (presumably through a descending serotoninergic system that presynaptically depolarizes small-diameter primary afferent terminals), and that morphine activates this descending raphe magnus system.

Evidence that morphine analgesia is produced by activation of another descending bulbospinal inhibitory system (catecholaminergic) has been reported by Takagi and his collaborators (see below). In intact rabbits, bradykinin injected intra-arterially (through the deep femoral artery) close to the spinal cord evoked discharges in lamina V cells of the L-6,7 dorsal horns. These discharges were depressed by morphine (0.3–2.0 mg/kg) given systemically (reversible by nalorphine) or by electrical stimulation of the bulbar reticular formation (including the nucleus reticularis gigantocellularis, or NRGC); the effect of electrical stimulation was blocked by prior administration of tetrabenazine (40 mg/kg), and this effect was reversed by L-dopa (20 mg/kg) but not by L-5-hydroxytryptophan (20 mg/kg); given without electrical stimulation, tetrabenazine (40 mg/kg) increased bradykinin-evoked discharges (antagonizable by L-dopa, 20 mg/kg), while L-dopa (20 mg/kg) depressed such discharges (Takagi et al., 1975). Microinjection of morphine 40 μg into the NRGC of intact rabbits decreased bradykinin-evoked discharges in lamina V cells of the L-6,7 dorsal horns in 6 of 10 experiments (Takagi et al., 1976). In rabbits made spinal by transection of the cord at L-2, morphine (2 mg/kg given systemically) did not decrease bradykinin-evoked lamina V cell discharges, but 5 mg/kg did have depressant effects, which were reversed by nalorphine; L-dopa (20 mg/kg) likewise had depressant effects on bradykinin-evoked lamina V cell discharges (Takagi et al., 1975). Analagous results on the effects of morphine on the flexor reflex and bradykinin-evoked discharges in lamina V cells of the L-6,7 dorsal horns in intact and spinal rabbits were obtained by Takagi and Satoh (1978).

In intact rats, microinjection of 0.5–2.0 μg (Takagi et al., 1976) or 0.015–0.38 μg (Takagi et al., 1977) of morphine into the NRGC (including the closely adjacent nucleus reticularis paragigantocellularis or NRPG) produced a dose-dependent analgesia (measured by the response to tail pinches), reversible by naloxone (2 mg/kg subcutaneously). The differential sensitivity of the NRPG and the NRGC to morphine was investigated by Akaike et al. (1978). Microinjection of 0.15–15.0 ng of morphine into the NRPG produced a dose-dependent analgesia, prevented by pretreatment with naloxone (1 mg/kg subcutaneously). Microinjection of 15 ng of morphine into the NRPG produced analgesia in 9 of 12 rats, but only in 5 of 22 rats when microinjected into the NRGC. Electrical stimulation of the NRPG produced analgesia in 11 of 13 rats, but in only 1 of 11 rats in which the NRGC was electrically stimulated, while electrical stimulation of the nucleus raphe magnus (NRM) produced analgesia in 2 of 8 rats (stronger stimulation produced aversive responses). Takagi *et al.* (1976, 1977) had reported that no analgesia was produced in rats by microinjection of morphine (0.5 μg) into the NRM, or of 0.38–1.52 μg into the nucleus reticularis lateralis, the nucleus reticularis ventralis, or the nucleus reticularis pontis; microinjection of 0.5–2.0 μg of morphine into the periaqueductal gray matter (PAG) did not produce analgesia, but 10–20 μg did. Thus, from their data, Takagi *et al.* (1976, 1977), Takagi and Satoh (1978), and Akaike *et al.* (1978) concluded that the NRPG is the most sensitive site in the brain stem to the analgesic action of morphine and that such analgesia is probably mediated by activation of a descending pathway that inhibits the transmission of nociceptive impulses in the dorsal horns of the spinal cord; after larger doses of morphine, such transmission is directly depressed. In support of this concept, these authors adduced the reports of Casey (1969), which indicated that the medial reticular formation (including the NRGC and NRPG) subserves responses to noxious stimuli, and of Basbaum *et al.* (1978), which showed that the nucleus reticularis magnocellularis in the cat (which corresponds to the NRPG in the rat) projects to spinal structures with known nociceptive input. That this descending inhibitory pathway may be catecholaminergic is supported by the data on the effects of tetrabenazine and L-dopa on bradykinin-evoked discharges in lamina V cells of the spinal cord (Takagi *et al.*, 1975) and by the finding of Shimoi and Takagi (1974) that morphine increases the concentration of normetanephrine in the rat spinal cord.

In the decerebrate cat, LeBars *et al.* (1976) found that close intraarterial injection of bradykinin had little effect on discharges in lamina V cells of lumbar dorsal horns, and these were likewise but little affected by morphine (2 mg/kg) or by naloxone (0.1 mg/kg intravenously); however, when the decerebrate preparation was reversibly spinalized by cooling the spinal cord at T-11,12, bradykinin greatly increased the firing of lumbar lamina V cells in the dorsal horns, morphine (2 mg/kg intravenously) markedly depressed such firing, and naloxone (0.1 mg/kg intravenously) reversed the depressant effects of morphine. Also, in the decerebrate cat, LeBars *et al.* (1976) were unable to demonstrate after morphine administration an increase in the descending inhibition of firing of lamina V cells (evoked by transcutaneous electrical stimulation) produced by increasing intensities of electrical stimulation of the central inferior raphe nucleus (raphe obscurus and raphe magnus). LeBars *et al.*

(1976) concluded that in the decerebrate cat, descending inhibitory influences are so strong that they mask any inhibition-augmenting effect that morphine may have. On the other hand, Sinclair (1973) reported that in decerebrate, unanesthetized cats, morphine or meperidine (0.5–16.0 mg/kg intravenously) progressively *blocked* ventromedial bulbospinal inhibition of a *monosynaptic* spinal segmental reflex; meperidine was more potent in blocking such inhibition when given close to the spinal cord by intra-arterial injection than when given intravenously, suggesting that the spinal cord is the major site of this blocking action on descending bulbospinal inhibition. Apparently, the depressant effects of morphine on descending bulbospinal inhibition of the monosynaptic reflex are exerted predominantly at the spinal cord level, but the depressant effects of morphine on lamina V cell discharges at the spinal cord level may be coupled with an excitatory effect on descending bulbospinal inhibition of the same lamina V cells in the intact organism.

Though the evidence reviewed thus far indicates that the sites of morphine's analgesic actions in the brain stem are located in its caudal portion, more rostral sites—notably the periaqueductal and periventricular gray matter—also appear to be involved. Tsou and Jang (1964) reported that in rabbits, analgesia (depression of a motor response to a heat stimulus) was produced by injection of morphine (20–100 μg) into a lateral ventricle, or by microinjection of morphine (10–20 μg) into the periventricular gray matter (PVG) of the third ventricle; bilateral microinjection of nalorphine (10-50 μg) into the PVG antagonized the analgesic effects of morphine (8 mg/kg) given intravenously 15–20 min later. Analgesic responses to microinjection of morphine into the periaqueductal gray matter (PAG) were equivocal. No analgesic response followed lumbar subarachnoid injection of morphine, or microinjection of morphine into the midbrain reticular formation, the nucleus dorsomedialis of the thalamus, the caudate nucleus, the septum, the tectum, or the dorsomedial region of the medial geniculate body. Tsou and Jang (1964) noted that the PVG is connected with the frontal lobe and that prefrontal lobotomy can relieve pain; they concluded that by its action on the PVG, morphine affects frontal lobe function, implying that the relief of pain by morphine is similar to the relief of pain by prefrontal lobotomy. Likewise, analgesic effects of microinjection of morphine into the PVG were reported by Foster *et al.* (1967), Jacquet and Lajtha (1973), and Yaksh *et al.* (1976) in rats, and by Pert and Yaksh (1974) in monkeys; in the studies of Pert and Yaksh (1974) and of Yaksh *et al.* (1976), the analgesic effects of morphine were reversed by naloxone, given systemically. The effects of microinjection of morphine into the PAG are more complex. Jacquet and Lajtha (1973) reported that microinjection of morphine, 10 µg into the PAG of rats, produced *hyperalgesic* responses on the flinch–jump test; similar hyperalgesic responses were observed after microinjection of morphine into the medial septal nucleus or the caudate nucleus. In a subsequent study, Jacquet and Lajtha (1974) abandoned the flinch–jump test, using reactivity to hemostat pinches of the limbs and tail as an index of analgesia, and responses to air puffs or sudden movements within the rat's visual field as measures of hyperreactivity. Following bilateral microinjection of morphine (5, 10, and 20 µg) into the PAG, hyperreactivity to the auditory and visual stimuli were observed, together with hyporeactivity (analgesia) to the noxious stimuli. Hyperreactivity was not observed after morphine given intraperitoneally or after etorphine, levorphanol, or methadone microinjected into the PAG or given intraperitoneally. Naloxone microinjected into the PAG antagonized both the hyperreactivity and the hyporeactivity produced by morphine microinjected into the PAG, and the hyporeactivity following microinjection of etorphine into the PAG or intraperitoneal injection of etorphine or levorphanol. Jacquet and Lajtha (1974) noted that marked tolerance to morphine given intraperitoneally developed after one or two doses of morphine microinjected into the PAG, but only weak cross-tolerance to intraperitoneal doses of levorphanol or methadone, and that the analgesic potencies of morphine, etorphine, levorphanol, and methadone microinjected into the PAG do not parallel their potencies after systemic administration. Sharpe *et al.* (1974) likewise reported analgesia and hyperreactivity in the rat following microinjections of morphine into the PAG, encompassing the dorsal raphe nucleus and bordering tissue. The analgesic effects (decreased responses to limb pinching) were observed after smaller doses of morphine (3–6 µg); higher doses (10–50 µg) eliminated the pain response but produced hyperreactivity to nonnoxious stimuli. Yaksh *et al.* (1976) found that within the PAG of rats, the predominant concentration of sites at which microinjection of morphine produced analgesia (minimum estimated ED_{50}, 1.5 µg) lay within the ventrolateral aspect of its posterior segment. At more rostral sites within the PAG, blockade of squealing or escape responses occurred only in response to pinching of the face and forepaws, while at more caudal sites within the PAG the whole body was involved in the analgesic effect. Some analgesic rats retained all basic reflexes measured (blink to touching the cornea; pinna twitch to insertion of a probe into the ear; righting and placing responses) and showed no hyperreactivity to loud clicks or air puffs, while others lost all basic reflexes and showed exaggerated motor startle responses. Using the shock-titration technique to assess analgesia in monkeys confined to restraining chairs, Pert and Yaksh (1974) delineated two active sites in the brain stem at which microinjection of morphine sulfate (20 μg) produced analgesia (reversible by naloxone, 1 mg/kg intravenously): one in the PAG–PVG region, extending from the lower portion of the third ventricle along the aqueduct and possibly into the floor of the fourth ventricle, and also near the midline in the subthalamic nucleus and in the vicinity of the ventromedial borders of the centromedian and parafascicular nuclei; the other more laterally, passing in the vicinity of the lateral reticular nucleus up through the substantia nigra dorsolateral to the red nucleus and into the most lateral borders of the centromedian and parafascicular nuclei of the thalamus. Pert and Yaksh (1974) suggested that morphine blocks the affective–motivational dimension of pain primarily by its action on the PAG–PVG region and by a secondary action on the collaterals of the neospinothalamic tract. Microinjection of morphine base (10 μg) bilaterally into the mesencephalic reticular formation (MRF) of rats was reported by Haigler and Mittleman (1978) to produce elevation of the tail-flick threshold. About 30% of the analgesic rats were hyperreactive to "mild stimuli." Naloxone injected into the MRF (15 μg bilaterally) or given subcutaneously (10 mg/kg) reversed the effects of morphine microinjected into the MRF. Haigler and Mittleman concluded that the MRF is a site where morphine may act to produce analgesia by a specific narcotic mechanism of action.

Microinjection of morphine sulfate (0.1–0.2 μg) into the anterior thalamic nuclei in the rat was reported to produce dose-dependent analgesic effects similar to 2–16 mg/kg of morphine sulfate given intramuscularly (Buxbaum et al., 1970); analgesia was also observed after microinjection of morphine into other thalamic and hypothalamic areas, but not after microinjection into the caudate nucleus, the olfactory bulb or the reticular formation.

Classically, electrical stimulation of many of these morphine-sensitive sites in the brain stem of cats, particularly the PAG–PVG region, has elicited flight–fight responses, together with their autonomic concomitants; therefore, it would be surmised that the analgesic effects of morphine microinjected into the PAG–PVG areas are depressant ones, though it should be noted that in the cat, morphine produces analgesia accompanied by dilated pupils and, at doses of 5 mg/kg or higher, by motor excitement and flight reactions (Wikler, 1944). Thus, in unanesthetized, freely moving cats, localized electrical stimulation has delineated an unbroken field in the diencephalon and mesencephalon from which effective defense reactions, including rage, can be elicited. This field lies mainly in the perifornical area of the hypothalamus (ventrolaterally below the massa intermedia, extending caudally and laterally into the posterior hypothalamus dorsal to the mammillary bodies) and in the PAG, but it includes also the preoptic and ventral septal regions (Hess, 1954, 1969; Hess & Akert, 1955; Hunsperger, 1956; Skultety, 1963; see also Crosby et al., 1962; Grossman, 1967, pp. 518–524). Bilateral electrocoagulation of the PAG temporarily abolishes affective defense reactions elicited by electrical stimulation of the affectively active zones in the hypothalamus, but bilateral lesions of the posterior hypothalamus or pretectal region do not affect defense reactions elicited by electrical stimulation of the PAG, caudal to the lesions (Hunsperger, 1956; Skultety, 1958, 1963). These data indicate that the PAG is not merely an area traversed by pathways for affective reactions from the hypothalamus but represents a "station" (relay station) in the brainstem substrate for affective reactions (Hunsperger, 1956). Complex reciprocal connections exist between these hypothalamic-periaqueductal areas and the limbic system, broadly conceived. Ablation or stimulation of the amygdala, hippocampus, septum, cingulate gyrus, or orbitofrontal cortex has resulted in enhancement or reduction of affective reactions (Grossman, 1967, p. 552).

In line with the affective reactions elicited in cats by electrical stimulation of the PAG is the observation of Schmidek et al. (1971) that in unanesthetized squirrel monkeys with stereotoxically implanted electrodes and access to a lever that could turn off electric shocks delivered in increments to the tail, electric stimulation of the PAG lowered the tail-shock threshold; however, electrical stimulation of the septal–preoptic region (where Hess, 1954, 1969, and Hess and Akert, 1955, found that electrical stimulation elicited affective defense reactions in the cat) elevated the tail-shock threshold. Nashold et al. (1969) reported that in a patient with intractable pain, electrical stimulation of the PAG (and the tegmentum surrounding it) through bipolar stereotoxically implanted electrodes produced feelings that the patient described as "fearful," "frightful," or "terrible," as well as pain always localized in the central portion of the body, deep within the head, neck, and abdomen. Complementing such reports on the effects of electrical stimulation of the PAG is the finding of Liebman et al. (1970) that lesions in the ventrolateral mesencephalic gray matter impaired the performance of rats in a passive-avoidance task and abolished defecation in an open-field test; they concluded that the ventrolateral portion of the mesencephalic gray matter is critical for the normal expression of fear in rats.

On the other hand, Reynolds (1969) reported that in rats, electrical stimulation of the dorsolateral perimeter of the PAG (much the same area electrically stimulated by Nashold et al., 1969, in man) produced analgesia (no response to hemostat pressure applied to the paws or the tail) sufficient to permit abdominal laparotomy and wound closure without aversive reactions, and without impairing responses to nonnoxious stimuli such as loud noises or quick visual movements in the rat's visual field. Mayer *et al.* (1971) observed analgesic effects in rats on electrical stimulation not only of the central gray matter (ventral posterior region) but also of the ventral tegmentum, the medial thalamus, and the junctural region between the ventral tegmentum and the posterior hypothalamus. In most rats, the stimulation-produced analgesia was limited to one-half or one quadrant of the body, with normal reactions to noxious stimuli elsewhere and to visual, auditory, or tactile stimuli (some rats were hyperreactive to such nonnoxious stimuli). Akil *et al.* (1972) reported that electrical stimulation of the dorsal raphe nucleus in the PAG of the rat produced analgesia of the hind limbs, which was partially antagonized by naloxone (1 mg/kg, given systemically). In cats also, electrical stimulation in the vicinity of the dorsal raphe nucleus of the PAG was found by Liebeskind *et al.* (1973) and Oliveras *et al.* (1974) to produce decreased escape and defense reactions to pinches of the four limbs or the tail with hemostat or toothed forceps; mixed analgesic and motor and/or emotional reactions were obtained from electrical stimulation of broader areas of the PAG and adjacent reticular formation. In man, chronic intractable pain has been relieved by electrical stimulation of the PAG–PVG region. Thus, Adams (1976) reported that in a patient with diabetic neuropathy, self-stimulation of the PVG in the coronal and sagittal plane of the posterior commissure through a sterotaxically implanted electrode produced relief of his pain, outlasting PVG stimulation by 22–23 hr. Likewise, Hosobuchi *et al.* (1977) found that in six patients with chronic intractable pain from various sources, electrical stimulation of the PAG–PVG region through sterotaxically implanted electrodes relieved the pain, usually without altering pin–prick perception or Hardy *et al.* (1952) pain thresholds. Effective control of chronic pain in patients by low-amplitude and low-frequency electrical stimulation of the PVG in the area between the nucleus parafascicularis and the third ventricle at the level of the posterior commissure was reported by Richardson and Akil (1977a,b). In some of these patients, such relief of chronic pain was accompanied by analgesia, increase tolerance to ischemic pain, and/or increased latency to withdrawal of a limb from radiant heat (Richardson and Akil, 1977b). Electrical stimulation of the PAG also relieved chronic pain but produced dizziness, shortness of breath, nystagmus, eye movement, contralateral tingling paresthesias, and other unpleasant effects (Richardson & Akil, 1977a). Adams (1976), Hosobuchi (1977), and Richardson and Akil (1977b) also reported that naloxone antagonized the relief of chronic pain by intracerebral electrical stimulation, indicating that the latter caused release of an endogenous opioid substance.

The reasons for the differences reported on the effects of electrical stimulation of the PAG–PVG region are not at all clear; Richardson and Akil (1977a) suggested that they may be due to differences in the parameters of electrical stimulation, but no consistency can be found in the descriptions of waveform, duration, frequency, voltage, or amperage used by investigators who have reported affective defense reactions or unpleasant feelings, including pain, and those who have reported analgesia. That stimulation-produced analgesia (SPA) is due to *activation* of a neural system concentrated in the PAG–PVG region that inhibits transmission of nociceptive impulses at the spinal cord level (Mayer *et al.*, 1973) is indicated by the findings of Liebeskind *et al.* (1973) and Oliveras *et al.* (1974). In cats under light chloralose anesthesia, paralyzed by Flaxedil and maintained under artificial ventilation, recordings were made of spontaneous activity and of activity evoked by noxious (strong pinches to the limbs, tail, and ears) and nonnoxious (light touch and movement of hairs) stimuli in interneurons of the L-7 dorsal horn. Electrical stimulation of the dorsal raphe nucleus in the PAG through chronically implanted electrodes markedly inhibited spontaneous activity and activity evoked by noxious stimuli in most of the lamina V cells (known to respond preferentially to noxious stimuli) but only in a few of the lamina IV cells (known to respond preferentially to nonnoxious stimuli) in the dorsal horn. Inhibition of lamina V cells was also obtained by electrical stimulation of adjacent regions in the PAG and the reticular formation. Using much the same technique, Duggan and Griersmith (1979) found that in the cat, electrical stimulation near the dorsal raphe nucleus *nonselectively* inhibited dorsal horn responses to both noxious and nonnoxious stimuli, while electrical stimulation in the vicinity of the medullary raphe nuclei selectively inhibited responses to noxious stimuli; in neither case was the inhibition reversed by naloxone, contrary to the finding of Oliveras *et al.* (1975). Further evidence that SPA is not due to postseizure depression or to some nonspecific "rewarding" effect of brain stimulation was reported by Mayer and Liebeskind (1974). In rats, they compared the effects of SPA and morphine (10–60 mg/kg intraperitoneally) on three tests for analgesia (pinch, jump, and tail flick), recorded electrographic seizure activity from areas where SPA was tested (PVG, mesencephalic central gray, ventral tegmentum, dorsomedial thalamic nucleus, ventrobasal thalamic complex, lateral hypothalamus, septum), and measured rates of self-stimulation through the electrodes used to test for SPA. Morphine produced analgesia by all three analgesic tests and so did electrical stimulation in the mesencephalic gray matter and the PVG, without electrographic seizure activity; in the other areas, SPA ranged from 0% (septum, lateral hypothalamus) to 33% (ventral tegmentum), and seizure activity ranged from 0% (ventral tegmentum) to 80–100% (ventrobasal thalamic complex, dorsomedial thalamic nucleus, septum). Self-stimulation rates and analgesia as measured by any of the three tests were not positively correlated; highest rates of self-stimulation were supported by electrodes in the course of the medial forebrain bundle running through the ventral tegmentum (SPA, 33%) and the lateral hypothalamus (SPA, 0%). Mayer and Liebeskind (1974) also noted that lesions of the mesencephalic gray matter do not alter thresholds of an operant turning off electric shocks delivered subcutaneously to the flanks in cats (Kelly and Glusman, 1968), indicating that SPA is unlikely to be due to functional depression of the mesencephalic gray matter.

Mayer *et al.* (1973) pointed out that both SPA and morphine-produced analgesia are antagonized by naloxone, and both have been shown to inhibit lamina V cell interneurons in the dorsal horn of the spinal cord; these and other similarities suggest that like SPA, morphine produces its analgesic effects, at least in part, through *activation* of the PAG–PVG regions. Thus, Mayer and Hayes (1975) found that rats made tolerant to morphine (given subcutaneously in increasing doses over a period of 21 days to a level of 600 mg/kg/day) were cross-tolerant to SPA; loss of tolerance to SPA was gradual after withdrawal of morphine (75% SPA by the 44th abstinence day). On the other hand, no difference was found in the analgesic effects of morphine (4 mg/kg) given systemically in unstimulated, nontolerant rats and rats made tolerant to SPA by continuous electrical stimulation of the mesencephalic central gray for 24 hr, repeated twice at intervals of 48 hr; this finding was explained on the grounds that tolerance to SPA develops locally in the area electrically stimulated, whereas morphine (administered systemically) acts on various structures in the PVG, the PAG, and the floor of the fourth ventricle. Tolerance to the pain-relieving effects of electrical stimulation of the PVG on prolonged self-stimulation by patients with chronic pain was noted by Richardson and Akil (1977b). Tolerance to the pain-relieving effects of electrical stimulation of the PAG-PVG regions and cross-tolerance to narcotics was reported by Hosobuchi *et al.* (1977); such tolerance disappeared after stopping electrical stimulation temporarily. Also, biogenic monoamines appear to be involved in similar ways both in morphine analgesia (Schneider, 1954; Lee & Fennesy, 1970; Tenen, 1968; Proudfit & Anderson, 1973, 1974b; Vogt, 1974; Takagi *et al.*, 1975) and in SPA elicited from the vicinity of the dorsal raphe nucleus in the PAG. Akil *et al.* (1972) and Akil and Mayer (1972) reported that in unstimulated rats, tail-flick latencies to radiant heat did not change 72 hr after injection of pCPA, 300 mg/kg intraperitoneally, but pCPA reduced latencies if they had been prolonged by electrical stimulation of ventral mesencephalic central gray matter in the vicinity of the dorsal raphe nucleus. pCPA did not alter or enhance SPA if the stimulating electrodes were in the dorsal mesencephalic central gray matter or outside it; interestingly, in the cat, the antiserotonin drug LSD (100 μg/kg intravenously) blocked inhibition of lamina V cells in the dorsal horn of the spinal cord if such inhibition was elicited by electrical stimulation of the dorsal raphe nucleus but not by electrical stimulation elsewhere (Liebeskind et al., 1973; Guilbaud et al., 1973). Further studies by Akil and Liebeskind (1975) indicated that, in general, serotonin and dopamine facilitate SPA elicited from the PAG, while norepinephrine appears to inhibit it. Depletion of all three monoamines by tetrabenazine markedly reduced such SPA, which was restored to original levels by injection of either 5-hydroxytryptophan or L-dopa. Elevation of serotonin levels by injection of 5-hydroxytryptophan enhanced SPA, while selective depletion of serotonin by pCPA reduced SPA. Dopamine receptor blockade by pimozide decreased SPA, whereas administration of the dopamine precursor L-dopa or the dopamine receptor stimulant apomorphine increased SPA. On the other hand, selective depletion of norepinephrine by disulfiram increased SPA. Combined lowering of norepinephrine levels by injection of alpha-methyl-paratyrosine and elevation of dopamine levels by injection of L-dopa resulted in marked enhancement of SPA. The dopaminergic link in SPA has been elucidated by the studies of Barnes et al. (1979). In cats made decerebrate precollicularly, paralyzed by gallamine triethiodide (Flaxedil) and artificially ventilated, extracellular recordings were made of unit activity in lamina V cells of the L-6,7 dorsal horns evoked by noxious stimuli (pinches and sural nerve stimulation of the ipsilateral limb) and by nonnoxious stimuli (touch). Inhibition of responses to noxious (but not to nonnoxious stimuli) was obtained by electrical stimulation of the substantia nigra, the PAG, and the dorsal raphe nucleus. Nigral inhibition was abolished by tetrabenazine (40 mg/kg) and reestablished by L-dopa (20 mg/kg) or apomorphine (20 mg/kg), all drugs given intravenously. Inhibition from electrical stimulation of all three brain sites was reduced by methysergide (1 mg/kg) and partially restored by 5-hydroxytryptophan (70 mg/kg), both drugs given intravenously. According to the scheme proposed by Barnes et al. (1979), the common descending inhibitory pathway from the raphe nucleus is serotoninergic; the raphe nucleus is activated by a dopaminergic pathway from the substantia nigra and by activation of the PAG (transmitter unspecified).

That morphine analgesia is produced, in part, by activation of mesencephalic raphe nuclei is further indicated by studies on the effects of lesions in these nuclei and their descending connections in morphine-treated animals. Samanin *et al.* (1970) reported that electrolytic lesions of the midbrain raphe nuclei decreased morphine analgesia in rats (measured by the hot-plate test, pressure on the tail required for vocalization, and voltage required for first escape response and vocalization to electrical stimulation through the skin at the base of the tail); such lesions resulted in marked and long-lasting decrease in forebrain serotonin levels without affecting levels of norepinephrine. Basbaum *et al.* (1977) found that unilateral lesions in the dorsal part of the lateral funiculus (DLF) but not elsewhere in the white matter of the mid-thoracic spinal cord reduced or abolished the analgesic response (predominantly or exclusively ipsilateral) below the level of the lesion to electrical stimulation of the dorsal raphe nucleus in the PAG, or to morphine (3–5 mg/kg intraperitoneally); despite the presence of DLF lesions, larger doses of morphine (20–25 mg/kg) did produce analgesia below the level of the lesions. Basbaum *et al.* (1977) cited Dahlström and Fuxe's (1964) demonstration of a serotoninergic pathway from the nucleus raphe magnus in the medulla, coursing in part in the DLF, and terminating in the dorsal and ventral gray horns of the spinal cord; Oleson and Liebeskind's (1975) findings that central gray stimulation and morphine increased spontaneous activity in the raphe nuclei of rats; and Proudfit and Anderson's (1975) finding that lesions of the nucleus raphe magnus reduced or abolished morphine analgesia in rats, as well as other data indicating that the descending (serotoninergic) pathway from the raphe magnus nucleus is pain-inhibitory. Basbaum *et al.* (1977) concluded that although no direct connection between the dorsal raphe nucleus and the nucleus raphe magnus has been demonstrated, the latter must be activated indirectly by activation of the dorsal raphe nucleus either by electrical stimulation (SPA) or by morphine; large doses of morphine (e.g., 20–25 mg/kg) are presumed also to exert direct depressant effects on the spinal cord. In keeping with the concept that morphine's analgesic action is mediated by activation of the dorsal raphe nucleus is the report of Sasa *et al.* (1977) that in rats, lesions of the dorsal raphe nucleus, which reduced the serotonin content of the forebrain, lowered the threshold of paw pulling in response to progressively increasing pressure applied to the hind paw and almost completely inhibited morphine analgesia. Puzzling, however, is their finding that lesions of the locus ceruleus, which selectively reduced the norepinephine content of the forebrain, elevated the paw-pulling threshold and inhibited morphine analgesia; perhaps the analgesic effect of morphine was masked by the already elevated paw-pulling threshold produced by the lesion of the locus ceruleus.

More direct data on morphine's excitant or depressant actions in the brain stem are less conclusive. Oleson and Liebeskind (1975) reported that in awake, restrained rats, either electrical stimulation of the mesencephalic central gray matter or systemic administration of morphine increased spontaneous activity and inhibited evoked potentials and unit activity recorded from the dorsal raphe nucleus, the median raphe nucleus, and the nucleus raphe magnus in response to noxious (but not to nonnoxious) stimulation of the limbs. These findings suggest that like SPA, morphine activates the raphe nuclei and blocks nociceptive input into them (perhaps through descending serotoninergic inhibition of transmission of nociceptive impulses at the level of the dorsal horns of the spinal cord). On the other hand, Buxbaum and Pamplin (1975) found that in rats anesthetized with chloral hydrate, morphine given systemically caused a marked decrease or cessation of firing of single neurons in the dorsal raphe nucleus, which could be prevented by pretreatment with naloxone. These divergent observations on the effects of morphine given systemically on spontaneous firing in the raphe nuclei can perhaps be reconciled by Buxbaum and Pamplin's (1975) hypothesis that the decreased firing observed by them may have been due to negative feedback on the serotonin-containing cells of the dorsal raphe nucleus, consequent to enhanced serotonin-receptor interactions in the forebrain produced by the increase in serotonin turnover after administration of large doses of morphine. Mayer and Price (1976) cited Bennet and Mayer's (1976) finding that microinjection of morphine into the PAG of rats inhibits the responses of spinal cord dorsal horn neurons to noxious stimulation. Investigating acceleration of neuronal firing in the mesencephalic reticular formation (MRF) and adjacent areas (e.g., the longitudinal fasciculus) and the dorsal raphe nucleus evoked by graduated pressure on a foot in rats anesthetized with chloral hydrate, Haigler (1976) found that the dorsal raphe nucleus was relatively unresponsive to noxious stimulation, only 4 of 50 cells being accelerated; in one of these 4 responding cells, morphine was applied iontophoretically, and it blocked the response to nociceptive stimulation. In 24 nonresponding cells, iontophoretically applied morphine slowed spontaneous firing in only 1. In contrast, cells in the MRF responded readily to noxious stimulation; such acceleration of neuronal firing was blocked by iontophoretically applied morphine, oxymorphone, or methadone and was antagonized by prior administration of naloxone applied iontophoretically or given intravenously; iontophoretically applied chlorpromazine or sodium pentobarbital did not affect firing in the MRF. Haigler (1976) concluded that at least under the limits imposed by chloral hydrate anesthesia, his data support the MRF rather than the dorsal raphe nucleus as a possible site for morphine analgesia in the brain stem. However, in unanesthetized cats decerebrated at the supracollicular level, Henry (1975) found that morphine or meperidine applied iontophoretically to the mesencephalic central gray matter or the dorsal raphe nucleus depressed ongoing neuronal activity and gluta- mate excitation and reduced spike size. In an attempt to reconcile such conflicting data on morphine's pharmacological receptor action, Yaksh et al. (1976) suggested that within the PAG, morphine depresses an *inhibitory* neuron, thus releasing PAG excitation (effected directly by electrical stimulation) of both the ascending (raphe dorsalis, raphe medianus) and descending (raphe magnus, raphe pallidus) serotoniner- gic systems, the former related to perception and the latter to spinal cord nociceptive reflexes.

Cerebral Cortex

In man, chronic intractable pain may be relieved by prefrontal lobotomy (Koskoff et al., 1948; Watts & Freeman, 1948; Dynes & Pop- pen, 1949; Hamilton & Hayes, 1949; King et al., 1950) or by more re- stricted surgical interventions such as rostral cingulumotomy (Foltz & White, 1966), which interrupt thalamoorbitofrontal or limbic–orbito- frontal connections, respectively. In some ways, the relief of chronic intractable pain by such surgical procedures resembles that produced by morphine. Thus, what is relieved is "suffering," or the motivational– affective dimensions of pain. Like morphine (Denton & Beecher, 1949), unilateral frontal lobotomy (King et al., 1950) relieves chronic pain without altering the cutaneous pain perception threshold. Also like morphine, which reduces anticipatory responses to radiant heat stimuli (Kornetsky, 1954), prefrontal lobotomy reduces anticipatory responses to radiant heat (Malmo and Shagass, 1950) or to electric shock stimuli (Elithorn et al., 1955). On the other hand, whereas morphine elevates the threshold for wincing or head withdrawal in intact man (Jones & Chapman, 1944), such thresholds are lowered by prefrontal lobotomy (Chapman et al., 1948).

Kuhar et al. (1973) reported that opioid receptor binding in both monkey and human brain was greater in the frontal pole than in the amygdala, the medial thalamus, the hypothalamus, and the PAG. Direct data on the actions of morphine in the orbitofrontal cortex of man are lacking. However, Pert and Snyder (1973) having demonstrated a rela- tively high density of opioid receptor binding in the sensorimotor cortex of the rat, Satoh *et al.* (1976) investigated the actions of morphine in rats' sensorimotor cortex by iontophoretic techniques. They found that at low doses, the iontophoretic application of morphine depressed spontaneous discharge activity; higher doses and repeated iontophoretic application of morphine often converted this effect into excitation. Only the depressant effect was antagonized by naloxone applied iontophoretically. Morphine, applied iontophoretically, depressed the excitatory actions of L-glutamate and of acetylcholine by a naloxone-antagonizable mechanism. The late response to transcallosal stimulation was depressed by iontophoretically applied morphine and by fentanyl given systemically, and such depression was antagonized by iontophoretically applied naloxone. In contrast, the primary (or early) response to transcallosal stimulation was little affected by morphine, fentanyl, or naloxone.

The evidence of opioid receptor binding sites in the frontal pole of the human brain and of the depressant actions of low doses of morphine in the sensorimotor cortex of the rat suggests that in addition to its well-demonstrated actions at the levels of the spinal cord and the brain stem, morphine may exert its analgesic effects through actions in the orbitofrontal cortex. Though one-to-one anatomical–functional correlations are open to question, the data reviewed in this chapter do indicate that the mechanisms of morphine analgesia involve all three dimensions of pain: the sensory–discriminative (integrated mainly at the spinal cord level), the motivational–affective (integrated mainly at the brain-stem level), and the central control (integrated mainly at the thalamoorbitofrontal and limbic–orbitofrontal levels).

REFERENCES

Adams, J. E., 1976, Naloxone reversal of analgesia produced by brain stimulation in the human, *Pain* 2:161–166.

Akaike, A., Shibata, T., Satoh, M., and Takagi, H., 1978, Analgesia induced by microinjection of morphine into, and electrical stimulation of, the nucleus reticularis paragigantocellularis of rat medulla oblongata, *Neuropharmacol.* 17:775–778.

Akil, H., and Liebeskind, J. C., 1975, Monoaminergic mechanisms of stimulation-produced analgesia, *Brain Res.* 94:279–296.

Akil, H., and Mayer, D. J., 1972, Antagonism of stimulation-produced analgesia by p-CPA, a serotonin synthesis inhibitor, *Brain Res.* 44:692–697.

Akil, H., Mayer, D. J., and Liebeskind, J. C., 1972, Comparaison chez le rat entre l'analgésie induite par stimulation de la substance grise périaqueducal et l'analgésie morphinique, *C. R. Acad. Sci.* (Paris) 274:3603–3605.

Albus, K., Schott, M., and Herz, A., 1970, Interaction between morphine and morphine antagonists after systemic and intraventricular application, *Eur. J. Pharmacol.* 12:53–64.

Andrews, H. L., 1943a, The effects of opiates on the pain thresholds in post-addicts, *J. Clin. Invest.* 22:511-516.

Andrews, H. L., 1943b, Skin resistance changes and measurements of pain threshold, *J. Clin. Invest.* 22:517-520.

Andrews, H. L., and Workman, W., 1941, Pain threshold measurements in the dog, *J. Pharmacol. Exp. Ther.* 73:99-103.

Barnes, C. D., Fung, S. J. and Adams, W. L., 1979, Inhibitory effects of substantia nigra on impulse transmission from nociceptors, *Pain* 6:207-215.

Basbaum, A. I., Marley, N. J. E., O'Keefe, J., and Clanton, C. H., 1977, Reversal of morphine and stimulus-produced analgesia by subtotal spinal cord lesions, *Pain* 3:43-56.

Basbaum, A. I., Clanton, C. H., and Fields, H. I., 1978, Three bulbospinal pathways from the rostral medulla of the cat: An autoradiographic study of pain modulating systems, *J. Comp. Neurol.* 178:209-224.

Beecher, H. K., 1956, Relationship of significance of wound to pain experienced, *J. Amer. Med. Ass.* 161:1609-1613.

Beecher, H. K., 1957, The measurement of pain, *Pharmacol. Rev.* 9:59-209.

Beecher, H. K., 1968, Some complexities of the pain experience as seen in comparative studies of pathological and experimental pain, in *The Addictive States: Research Publications of the Association for Research in Nervous and Mental Disease*, Vol. 46 (A. Wikler, Ed.), pp. 157-164. Williams & Wilkins, Baltimore, Maryland.

Bennett, G. J., and Mayer, D. J., 1976, Effects of microinjected narcotic analgesics into the periaqueductal gray (PAG) on the response of rat spinal cord dorsal horn interneurons, *Soc. Neurosci. Abstr.* 2:928.

Berlin, L., Guthrie, T. C., Goodell, H., and Wolff, H. G., 1954, Studies on central excitatory state; factors responsible for variability of motor response to cutaneous stimulation in human subjects with isolated spinal cords, *Arch Neurol. Psychiat* (Chicago) 72: 764-779.

Black, W. C., and Grosz, H. J., 1974, Propranolol antagonism of morphine-influenced behavior, *Brain Res.* 65:362-367.

Blume, W., 1927, Über die Wirkung des Morphins auf das Rückenmark der dekapitierten Katze, *Arch. Exper. Path. Pharmakol.* 119:24-30.

Brodal, A., Taber, E., and Walberg, F., 1960a, The raphe nuclei of the brain stem in the cat. II. Efferent connections, *J. Comp. Neurol.* 114:239-259.

Brodal, A., Walberg, G., and Taber, E., 1960b, The raphe nuclei of the brain stem in the cat. III. Afferent connections, *J. Comp. Neurol.* 114:261-281.

Burgess, P. R., and Perl, E. R., 1967, Myelinated afferent fibres responding specifically to noxious stimulation of the skin, *J. Physiol.* 190:541-562.

Buxbaum, D. M., and Pamplin, W., 1975, Effects of morphine on single unit activity of neurons in the nucleus raphe dorsalis, *The Pharmacologist* 17:187.

Buxbaum, D. M., Yarbrough, G. G., and Carter, M. E., 1970, Dose-dependent behavioral and analgesic effects produced by microinjections of morphine sulfate into the anterior thalamic nuclei, *The Pharmacologist* 12:211.

Calvillo, O., Henry, J. L., and Neuman, R. S., 1974, Effects of morphine and naloxone on dorsal horn neurons in the cat, *Canad. J. Physiol. Pharmacol.* 52:1207-1211.

Casey, K. L., 1969, Somatic stimuli, spinal pathways, and size of cutaneous fibers influencing unit activity in the medial medullary reticular formation, *Exp. Neurol.* 25:35-56.

Casey, K. L., and Melzack, R., 1967, Neural mechanisms of pain: A conceptual model, in *New Concepts in Pain and Its Clinical Management* (E. L. Way, Ed.), pp. 13-31. F. A. Davis Company, Philadelphia, Pennsylvania.

Chapman, W. P., Rose, A. S., and Solomon, H. C., 1948, Measurements of heat stimulus producing motor withdrawal reaction in patients following frontal lobotomy, in "The Frontal Lobes: Research Publication of the Association for Research in Nervous and Mental Disease, Vol. 27 (J. F. Fulton, C. D. Aring, and S. B. Wortis, Eds.), pp. 754–768. Williams & Wilkins, Baltimore, Maryland.

Chorazyna, H., 1962, Some properties of conditioned inhibition, *Acta Biol. Exp.* 22:5.

Clutton-Brock, J., 1961, Pain and the barbiturates, *Anaesthesia* 16:80–88.

Cook, L., and Bonnycastle, D. D., 1953, An examination of some spinal and ganglionic actions of analgetic materials, *J. Pharmacol. Exp. Ther.* 109:35–44.

Crosby, E. C., Humphrey, T., and Lauer, E. W., 1962, *Correlative Anatomy of the Nervous System*, p. 338. Macmillan, New York.

Dahlström, A., and Fuxe, K., 1964, Evidence for the existence of monoamine-containing neurons in the central nervous system. I. Demonstration of monoamines in the cell bodies of brain stem neurons, *Acta Physiol. Scand.* 62 (Suppl. 232):1–78.

Dahlström, A., and Fuxe, K., 1965, Evidence for the existence of monoamine neurons in the central nervous system. II. Experimentally induced changes in the intraneuronal amine levels of bulbospinal neuron systems, *Acta Physiol. Scand.* 64 (Suppl. 247):1–85.

D'Amour, F. E., and Smith, D. L., 1941, A method for determining loss of pain sensation, *J. Pharmacol. Exp. Ther.* 72:74–79.

DeBodo, R. E., and Brooks, C. McC., 1937, The effects of morphine on blood sugar and reflex activity in the chronic spinal cat, *J. Pharmacol. Exp. Ther.* 61:82–88.

Denton, J. E., and Beecher, H. K., 1949, New analgesics. I. Methods in the clinical evaluation of new analgesics, *J. Amer. Med. Ass.* 141:1051–1057.

Duggan, A. W., and Griersmith, B. T., 1979, Inhibition of the spinal transmission of nociceptive information by supraspinal stimulation in the cat, *Pain* 6:149–161.

Dundee, J. W., 1960, Alterations in response to somatic pain associated with anaesthesia. II. The effect of thiopentone and pentobarbitone, *Brit. J. Anaesthesia* 32:407–414.

Dynes, J. B., and Poppen, J. L., 1949, Lobotomy for intractable pain, *J. Amer. Med. Ass.* 140:15–19.

Elithorn, A., Piercy, M. F., and Crosskey, M. A., 1955, Prefrontal leucotomy and the anticipation of pain, *J. Neurol. Neurosurg. Psychiat.* 18:34–43.

Estes, W. M., and Skinner, B. F., 1941, Some quantitative properties of anxiety, *J. Exper. Psychol.* 29:390–400.

Foltz, E. L., and White, L. E., 1966, Rostral cingulumotomy and pain "relief," in *Pain: Henry Ford Hospital International Symposium* (R. S. Knighton and P. R. Dumke, Eds.), pp. 469–491. Little, Brown and Co., Boston, Massachusetts.

Foster, R. S., Jenden, D. J., and Lomax, P., 1967, A comparison of the pharmacologic effects of morphine and N-methyl morphine, *J. Pharmacol. Exp. Ther.* 157:185–195.

Fujita, S., Yasuhara, M., and Ogiu, K., 1953, Studies on sites of action of analgesics. I. The effect of analgesics on afferent pathways of several nerves, *Jap. J. Pharmacol.* 3:27–38.

Fujita, S., Yasuhara, M., Tamamoto, S., and Ogiu, K., 1954, Studies on the sites of action of analgesics. 2. The effect of analgesics on afferent pathways of pain, *Jap. J. Pharmacol.* 4:41–51.

Grossman, S. P., 1967, *A Textbook of Physiological Psychology*, pp. 518–524. John Wiley & Sons, New York.

Guilbaud, G., Besson, J. M., Oliveras, J. L., and Liebeskind, J. C., 1973, Suppression by LSD of the inhibitory effect exerted by dorsal raphe stimulation on certain spinal cord interneurons in the cat, *Brain Res.* 61:417–422.

Haigler, H. J., 1976, Morphine: Ability to block neuronal activity evoked by a nociceptive stimulus, *Life Sci.* 19:841–858.

Haigler, H. J., and Mittleman, R. S., 1978, Analgesia produced by direct injection of morphine into the mesencephalic reticular formation, *Brain Res. Bull.* 3:655–662.

Hamilton, F. E., and Hayes, G. J., 1949, Prefrontal lobotomy in the management of intractable pain, *Arch. Surg.* 58:731–738.

Hardy, J. D., Wolff, H. G., and Goodell, H., 1952, *Pain Sensations and Reactions*, Williams & Wilkins, Baltimore, Maryland.

Henry, J. L., 1975, Effects of morphine and meperidine on neurones in cat midbrain, *Fed. Proc.* 34:757.

Herr, F., Nyiri, M., and Venulet, J., 1952, Studies on the mode of analgesic action of morphine and morphine derivatives, *Acta Physiol. Acad. Scient. Hungaricae* 3:199–208.

Herz, A., and Teschemacher, H. J., 1971, Activities and sites of antinociceptive action of morphine-like analgesic substances and kinetics of distribution following intravenous, intracerebral intraventricular application, *Adv. Drug Res.* 6:79–118.

Herz, A., Albus, K., Metys, J., Schubert, P., and Teschemacher, H. J., 1970, On the central sites for the antinociceptive action of morphine and fentanyl, *Neuropharmacol.* 9:539–551.

Hess, W. R., 1954, *Das Zwischenirn: Syndrome, Lokalisationen, Funktionen* (2nd, expanded ed.), pp. 102–103. Benno Schwabe Verlag, Basel, Switzerland.

Hess, W. R., 1969, *Hypothalamus and Thalamus: Experimental Documentation* (2nd, enlarged ed.), pp. 66–67. Georg Thieme Verlag, Stuttgart, Germany.

Hess, W. R., and Akert, K., 1955, Experimental data on role of hypothalamus in mechanism of emotional behavior, *Arch. Neurol. Psychiat.* (Chicago) 73:127–129.

Hill, H. E., Flanary, H. G., Kornetsky, C. H., and Wikler, A., 1952a, Relationship of electrically induced pain to the amperage and the wattage of shock stimuli, *J. Clin. Invest.* 31:464–472.

Hill, H. E., Kornetsky, C. H., Flanary, H. G., and Wikler, A., 1952b, Effects of anxiety and morphine on discrimination of intensities of painful stimuli, *J. Clin. Invest.* 31:473–480.

Hill, H. E., Kornetsky, C. H., Flanary, H. G., and Wikler, A., 1952c, Studies on anxiety associated with anticipation of pain. I. Effects of morphine, *Arch. Neurol. Psychiat.* (Chicago) 67:612–619.

Hill, H. E., Belleville, R. E., and Wikler, A., 1954, Reduction of pain-conditioned anxiety by analgesic doses of morphine in rats, *Proc. Soc. Exper. Biol. & Med. (N.Y.)* 86:881–884.

Hill, H. E., Belleville, R. E., and Wikler, A., 1955, Studies on anxiety associated with anticipation of pain. II. Comparative effects of pentobarbital and morphine, *Arch. Neurol. Psychiat.* (Chicago) 73:602–608.

Hill, H. E., Belleville, R. E., and Wikler, A., 1957a, Motivational determinants in the modification of behavior by morphine and pentobarbital, *Arch. Neurol. Psychiat.* (Chicago) 77:28–35.

Hill, H. E., Pescor, F. T., Belleville, R. E., and Wikler, A., 1957b, Use of differential bar-pressing rates of rats for screening analgesic drugs. I. Techniques and effects of morphine, *J. Pharmacol. Exp. Ther.* 120:388–397.

Hill, H. E., Haertzen, C. A., Wolbach, A. B., and Miner, E. J., 1963, The Addiction Research Center Inventory: Standardization of scales which evaluate subjective effects of morphine, amphetamine, pentobarbital, alcohol, LSD-25, pyrahexyl and chlorpromazine, *Psychopharmacologia* 4:167–183.

Hill, H. E., Belleville, R. E., Pescor, F. T., and Wikler, A., 1966, Comparative effects of methadone, meperidine and morphine on conditioned suppression, *Arch. Int. Pharmacodyn. Thér.* 163: 341–352.

Hill, H. E., Bell, E. C., and Wikler, A., 1967, Reduction of conditioned suppression:

Actions of morphine compared with those of amphetamine, pentobarbital, nalorphine, cocaine, LSD-25 and chlorpromazine, *Arch. Int. Pharmacodyn. Thér.* 165:212–
226.

Hosobuchi, Y., Adams, J. E., and Linchiz, R., 1977, Pain relief by electrical stimulation of
the central gray matter in humans and its reversal by naloxone, *Science* 197:183–
185.

Houde, R. W., and Wikler, A., 1951, Delineation of the skin-twitch response in dogs and
the effects thereon of morphine, thiopental and mephenesin, *J. Pharmacol. Exp. Ther.*
103:236–242.

Hunsperger, R. W., 1956, Affektreaktionen auf elektrische Reizung im Hirnstamm der
Katze, *Helv. Physiol. Acta* 14:70–92.

Irwin, S., Houde, R. W., Bennet, D. R., Hendershot, L. C., and Seevers, M. H., 1951, The
effects of morphine, methadone and meperidine on some reflex responses of spinal
animals to nociceptive stimulation, *J. Pharmacol. Exp. Ther.* 101:132–143.

Iwata, N., and Sakai, Y., 1971, Effects of fentanyl upon spinal interneurons activated by
A-delta afferent fibers of the cutaneous nerve of the cat, *Jap. J. Pharmacol.* 21:413–416.

Jacquet, Y., and Lajtha, A., 1973, Morphine action at central nervous system sites in rat:
Analgesia or hyperalgesia depending on site and dose, *Science* 182:490–492.

Jacquet, Y. F., and Lajtha, A., 1974, Paradoxical effects after microinjection of morphine in
the periaqueductal gray matter of rats, *Science* 185:1055–1057.

Jones, B. E., and Ayres, J. J. B., 1968, Effects of morphine on differentially conditioned
electrodermal responses, in *The Addictive States: Research Publications of the Association
for Research in Nervous and Mental Disease*, Vol. 46 (A. Wikler, Ed.), pp. 166–175.
Williams & Wilkins, Baltimore, Maryland.

Jones, B. E., Ayres, J. J. B., Flanary, H. G., and Clements, T. H., 1965, Effects of morphine
and pentobarbital on conditioned electrodermal responses and basal conductance in
man, *Psychopharmacologia* 7:159–174.

Jones, C. M., and Chapman, W. P., 1944, Comparative study of analgesic effect of
morphine sulfate and monoacetyl-morphine, *Arch. Int. Med.* 73:322–328.

Jurna, I., Grossmann, W., and Theres, C., 1973, Inhibition by morphine of repetitive
activation of cat spinal motoneurones, *Neuropharmacol.* 12:983–993.

Kast, E. C., and Collins, V. J., 1964, Lysergic acid diethylamide as an analgesic agent,
Anesthes. Analg. 43:285–291.

Keats, A. S., and Telford, J., 1956, Nalorphine, a potent analgesic in man, *J. Pharmacol.
Exp. Ther.* 117:190–196.

Kelleher, R. T., and Morse, W. H., 1964, Escape behavior and punished behavior, *Fed.
Proc.* 23:808–817.

Kelly, D. D., and Glusman, M., 1968, Aversive thresholds following midbrain lesions, *J.
Comp. Physiol. Psychol.* 66:25–34.

King, H. E., Clausen, H., and Scarff, J. E., 1950, Cutaneous thresholds for pain before and
after unilateral frontal lobotomy: A preliminary report, *J. Nerv. Ment. Dis.* 112:93–96.

Kitahata, L. M., Kosaka, Y., Taub, A., and Collins, W. F., 1973, Lamina-specific suppression of dorsal horn unit activity by morphine sulphate, *Fed. Proc.* 32(1):693.

Kitahata, L. M., Kosaka, Y., Taub, A., Bonnikos, K., and Hoffert, M., 1974, Lamina
specific suppression of dorsal-horn unit activity by morphine, *Anesthesiology* 41:39–48.

Koll, W., Haase, J., Schütz, R. M., and Mühlberg, B., 1961, Reflexentladungen der
tiefspinalen Katze durch afferente Impulse aus hochschwelligen nociceptiven
A-Fasern (post delta-Fasern) und aus nociceptiven C-Fasern cutaner Nerven, *Pflügers
Archiv.* 272:270–289.

Koll, W., Haase, J., Block, G., and Mühlberg, B., 1963, The predilective action of small
doses of morphine on nociceptive spinal reflexes of low spinal cats, *Int. J. Neuropharmacol.* 2:57–65.

Kornetsky, C., 1954, Effects of anxiety and morphine on the anticipation and perception of painful radiant thermal stimuli, *J. Comp. Physiol.* 47:130–132.

Koskoff, Y. D., Dennis, W., Lazovik, D., and Wheeler, E. T., 1948, The physiological effects of frontal lobotomy performed for the alleviation of pain, in *The Frontal Lobes: Research Publications of the Association for Research in Nervous and Mental Disease*, Vol. 27 (J. F. Fulton, C. D. Aring, and S. B. Wortis, Eds.), pp. 723–753. Williams & Wilkins, Baltimore, Maryland.

Krivoy, W., Kroeger, D., and Zimmerman, E., 1973, Actions of morphine on the segmental reflex of the decerebrate-spinal cat, *Brit. J. Pharmacol.* 47:457–464.

Kruglov, N. A., 1964, Effect of the morphine-group analgesics on the central inhibitory mechanisms, *Int. J. Neuropharmacol.* 3:197–203.

Kuhar, M. J., Pert, C. B., and Snyder, S. H., 1973, Regional distribution of opiate receptor binding in monkey and human brain, *Nature* (London) 245:447–450.

Lasagna, L., and Beecher, H. K., 1954, The analgesic effectiveness of nalorphine and nalorphine–morphine combinations in man, *J. Pharmacol. Exp. Ther.* 112:356–363.

Lasagna, L., von Felsinger, J. M., and Beecher, H. K., 1955, Drug induced chanes in man. I. Observations on healthy subjects, chronically ill patients and "post-addicts." *J. Amer. Med. Ass.* 157:1006–1020.

Lauener, H., 1963, Conditioned suppression in rats and the effect of pharmacological agents thereon, *Psychopharmacologia* 4:311–325.

LeBars, D., Menetrey, D., Conseiller, C., and Besson, J. M., 1975, Depressive effect of morphine upon lamina V cells activities in the dorsal horn of the spinal cat, *Brain Res.* 98:261–277.

LeBars, D., Menetrey, D., and Besson, J. M., 1976, Effects of morphine upon the lamina V type cells activities in the decerebrate cat, *Brain Res.* 113:293–310.

Lee, J. R., and Fennessy, M. R., 1970, The relationship between morphine analgesia and the levels of biogenic amines in the mouse brain, *Eur. J. Pharmacol.* 12:65–70.

Liebeskind, J. C., Guilbaud, G., Besson, J. M., and Oliveras, J. L., 1973, Analgesia from electrical stimulation of the periaqueductal gray matter in the cat: Behavioral observations and inhibitory effects on spinal cord interneurons, *Brain Res.* 50:441–446.

Liebman, J. M., Mayer, D. J., and Liebeskind, J. C., 1970, Mesencephalic central gray lesions and fear-motivated behavior in rats, *Brain Res.* 23:353–370.

Luckhardt, A. B., and Johnson, C. A., 1928, Studies on the kneejerk. IV. The effect of moderate doses of morphine sulfate on the kneejerk of the cat, *Am. J. Physiol.* 83:653–657.

Malmo, R. B., and Shagass, C., 1950, Behavioral and physiologic changes under stress after operation on the frontal lobes, *Arch. Neurol. Psychiat.* (Chicago) 63:1–12.

Martin, W. R., and Eades, C. G., 1964, A comparison between acute and chronic physical dependence in the chronic spinal dog, *J. Pharmacol. Exp. Ther.* 146:385–394.

Mayer, D. J., and Hayes, R. L., 1975, Stimulation-produced analgesia: Development of tolerance and cross-tolerance to morphine, *Science* 188:941–943.

Mayer, D. J., and Liebeskind, J. C., 1974, Pain reduction by focal electrical stimulation of the brain: An anatomical and behavioral analysis, *Brain Res.* 68:73–93.

Mayer, D. J., and Price, D. D., 1976, Central nervous system mechanisms of analgesia, *Pain* 2:379–404.

Mayer, D., Akil, H., and Liebeskind, J., 1973, Pain reduction: A comparison of stimulation-produced and narcotic analgesia, *Fed. Proc.* 32(1):693.

Mayer, D. J., Wolfle, T. L., Akil, H., Carder, B., and Liebeskind, J. C., 1971, Analgesia from electrical stimulation in the brainstem of the rat, *Science* 174:1351–1354.

Maxwell, D. R., Palmer, H. T., and Ryall, R. W., 1961, A comparison of the analgesic and some other central properties of methotrimeprazine and morphine, *Arch. Int. Pharmacodyn. Thér.* 132:60–73.

Melzack, R., and Wall, P. D., 1965, Pain mechanisms: A new theory, *Science* 150:971–978.

Morris, M. D., and Gebhart, G. F., 1978, The effect of morphine on fear extinction in rats, *Psychopharmacology* 57:267–271.

Nashold, B. S., Wilson, W. P., and Slaughter, D. G., 1969, Sensations evoked by stimulation in the midbrain of man, *J. Neurosurg.* 30:14–24.

Oleson, T. D., and Leibeskind, J. C., 1975, Relationship of neural activity in the raphe nuclei of the rat to brain stimulation-produced analgesia, *The Physiologist* 18:338.

Oliveras, J. L., Besson, J. M., Guilbaud, G., and Liebeskind, J. C., 1974, Behavioral and electrophysiological evidence of pain inhibition from midbrain stimulation in the cat, *Exp. Brain Res.* 20:32–44.

Oliveras, J. L., Redjemi, F., Guilbaud, G., and Besson, J. M., 1975, Analgesia induced by electrical stimulation of the inferior centralis of the raphe in the cat, *Pain* 1:139–145.

Pavlov, I. P., 1927, *Conditioned Reflexes: An Investigation of the Physiological Activity of the Cerebral Cortex* (G. V. Anrep, Trans. and Ed.), Oxford University Press, London. Reprinted by Dover Publications, Inc., New York, 1960, pp. 29–32.

Pert, C. B., and Snyder, S. H., 1973, Opiate receptor, demonstration in nervous tissue, *Science* 179:1011–1014.

Pert, A., and Yaksh, T., 1974, Sites of morphine induced analgesia in the primate brain: Relation to pain pathways, *Brain Res.* 80:135–140.

Pomeranz, B., 1973, Specific nociceptive fibers projecting from spinal cord neurons to the brain: A possible pathway for pain, *Brain Res.* 50:447–451.

Proudfit, H. K., and Anderson, E. G., 1973, Influence of serotonin antagonists on bulbospinal systems, *Brain Res.* 61:331–341.

Proudfit, H. K., and Anderson, E. G., 1974a, Blockade of morphine analgesia by destruction of a bulbo-spinal serotonergic pathway, *The Pharmacologist* 16:203.

Proudfit, H. K., and Anderson, E. G., 1974b, New long latency bulbospinal evoked potentials blocked by serotonin antagonists, *Brain Res.* 65:542–546.

Proudfit, H. K., and Anderson, E. G., 1975, Morphine analgesia: Blockade by raphe magnus lesions, *Brain Res.* 98:612–618.

Rexed, B., 1952, The cytoarchitectonic organisation of the spinal cord of the cat, *J. Cell. Comp. Neurol.* 96:415–495.

Reynolds, D. V., 1969, Surgery in the rat during electrical analgesia induced by focal brain stimulation, *Science* 164:444–445.

Richardson, D., and Akil, H., 1977a, Pain reduction by electrical brain stimulation in man. Part I. Acute administration in periaqueductal and periventricular sites, *J. Neurosurg.* 47:178–183.

Richardson, D. E., and Akil, H., 1977b, Pain reduction by electrical brain stimulation in man. Part 2. Chronic self-administration in the periventricular gray matter, *J. Neurosurg.* 47:184–194.

Samanin, R., Gumulka, W., and Valzelli, L., 1970, Reduced effect of morphine in midbrain raphe lesioned rats, *Eur. J. Pharmacol.* 10:339–343.

Sasa, M., Munekiyo, K., Osumi, Y., and Takaori, S., 1977, Attenuation of morphine analgesia in rats with lesions of the locus coeruleus and dorsal raphe nucleus, *Eur. J. Pharmacol.* 42:53–62.

Satoh, M., and Takagi, H., 1971, Enhancement by morphine of the central descending inhibitory influence on spinal sensory transmission, *Eur. J. Pharmacol.* 14:60–65.

Satoh, M., Zieglgänsberger, W., and Herz, A., 1976, Actions of opiates upon single unit activity in the cortex of naive and tolerant rats, *Brain Res.* 115:99–110.

Schaumann, O., 1954, Analgetika und protektives System, *Dtsch. med. Wchnschr.* 79:1571–1573.

Schmidek, H. H., Fohanno, D., Ervin, F. R., and Sweet, W. H., 1971, Pain threshold alterations by brain stimulation in the monkey, *J. Neurosurg.* 35:717–722.

Schneider, J. A., 1954, Reserpine antagonism of morphine analgesia in mice, *Proc. Soc. Exp. Biol. Med.* (N.Y.) 87:614–615.

Sharpe, L. J., Garnett, J., and Cicero, T., 1974, Analgesia and hyper-reactivity produced by intracranial microinjections of morphine into the periaqueductal grey matter of the cat, *Behav. Biol.* 11:303–313.

Shiomi, H., and Takagi, H., 1974, Morphine analgesia and the bulbospinal noradrenergic system: Increase in the concentration of normetanephrine in the spinal cord of the rat caused by analgesics, *Brit. J. Pharmacol.* 52:519–526.

Sinclair, J. G., 1973, Morphine and meperidine on bulbospinal inhibition of the monosynaptic reflex, *Eur. J. Pharmacol.* 21:111–114.

Skultety, F. M., 1958, The behavioral effects of destructive lesions of the periaqueductal gray matter in adult cats, *J. Comp. Neurol.* 110:337–365.

Skultety, F. M., 1963, Stimulation of periaqueductal gray and hypothalamus, *Arch. Neurol.* (Chicago) 8:608–620.

Stephens, J. H., and Gantt, W. H., 1956, The differential effect of morphine on cardiac and motor conditional reflexes—Schizokinesis, *Johns Hopkins Hosp. Bull.* 98:245–254.

Taber, E., Brodal, A., and Walberg, F., 1960, The raphe nuclei of the brain stem in the cat. I. Normal topography and cytoarchitecture and general discussion, *J. Comp. Neurol.* 114:161–182.

Takagi, H., and Satoh, M., 1978, Neurological models for the study of narcotics: Bradykinin-induced nociceptive responses and site of anti-nociceptive action of morphine, in *Factors Affecting the Action of Narcotics* (M. L. Adler, L. Manara, and R. Samanin, Eds.), pp. 39–62. Raven Press, New York.

Takagi, H., Matsumura, M., Yanai, A., and Ogiu, K., 1955, The effect of analgesics on the spinal reflex activity of the cat, *Jap. J. Pharmacol.* 4:176–187.

Takagi, H., Doi, T., and Kawasaki, K., 1975, Effects of morphine, *l*-dopa and tetrebenazine on the lamina V cells of spinal dorsal horn, *Life Sci.* 17:67–72.

Takagi, H., Doi, T., and Akaike, A., 1976, Microinjection of morphine into the medial part of the bulbar reticular formation in rabbit and rat: Inhibitory effect on lamina V cells of spinal dorsal horn and behavioral analgesia, in *Opiates and Endogenous Opioid Peptides* (H. W. Kosterlitz, Ed.), pp. 191–198. Elsevier/North Holland Biomedical Press, Amsterdam, The Netherlands.

Takagi, H., Satoh, M., Akaike, A., Shibata, T., and Kuraishi, Y., 1977, The nucleus reticularis gigantocellularis of the medulla oblongata is a highly sensitive site in the production of morphine analgesia in the rat, *Eur. J. Pharmacol.* 45:91–92.

Tenen, S. S., 1968, Antagonism of the analgesic effect of morphine and other drugs by *p*-chloropheylalanine, a serotonin depletor, *Psychopharmacologia* 2:278–285.

Teschemacher, H. J., Schubert, P., and Herz, A., 1973, Autoradiographic studies concerning the supraspinal site of the antinociceptive action of morphine when inhibiting the hindleg flexor reflex in rabbits, *Neuropharmacol.* 12:123–131.

Tsou, K., and Jang, C. S., 1964, Studies on the site of analgesic action of morphine by intracerebral micro-injection, *Scientia Sinica* 13:1099–1109.

Ungerstedt, U., 1971, Sterotaxic mapping of the monoamine pathways in the rat brain, *Acta Physiol. Scand.* Suppl. 367:1–48.

Vigouret, J., Teschemacher, H., Albus, K., and Herz, A., 1973, Differentiation between spinal and supraspinal sites of action of morphine when inhibiting the hindleg withdrawal reflex, *Neuropharmacol.* 12:111–121.

Vogt, M., 1974, The effect of lowering of the 5-hydroxytryptamine content of the rat spinal cord on analgesia produced by morphine. *J. Physiol.* (London) 236:483–498.

Watts, J. W., and Freeman, W., 1948, Frontal lobotomy in the treatment of intractable pain, in *The Frontal Lobes: Research Publications of the Association for Research in Nervous and Mental Disease*, Vol. 27 (J. F. Fulton, C. D. Aring, and S. B. Wortis, Eds.), pp. 715–722. Williams & Wilkins, Baltimore, Maryland.

Wikler, A., 1944, Studies on the action of morphine on central nervous system of cat, *J. Pharmacol. Exp. Ther.* 80:176–187.

Wikler, A., 1945, Effects of morphine, nembutal, ether and eserine on two-neuron and multineuron reflexes in the cat, *Proc. Soc. Exper. Biol. & Med.* (N.Y.) 58:193–196.

Wikler, A., 1950, Sites and mechanisms of action of morphine and related drugs in the central nervous system, *Pharmacol. Rev.* 2:435–506.

Wikler, A., 1952, A psychodynamic study of a patient during experimental self-regulated re-addiction to morphine, *Psychiat. Quart.* 26:270–293.

Wikler, A., 1957, *The Relation of Psychiatry to Pharmacology*, Williams & Wilkins, Baltimore, Maryland.

Wikler, A., 1958, *Mechanisms of Action of Opiates and Opiate Antagonists*, Public Health Monograph No. 52, Department of Health, Education and Welfare, Public Health Service Publication No. 589. p. 20. U.S. Government Printing Office, Washington, D.C.

Wikler, A., and Frank, K., 1948, Hindlimb reflexes of chronic spinal dogs during addiction to morphine and methadone, *J. Pharmacol. Exp. Ther.* 94:382–440.

Wikler, A., and Rayport, M., 1954, Lower limb reflexes of a chronic "spinal" man in cycles of morphine and methadone addiction, *Arch. Neurol. Psychiat.* (Chicago) 71:160–170.

Wolff, H. G., Hardy, J. D., and Goodell, H., 1940, Studies on pain: Measurement of the effects of morphine, codeine and other opiates on the pain threshold and an analysis of their relation to the pain experience, *J. Clin. Invest.* 19:659–680.

Woods, L. A., 1956, The pharmacology of nalorphine (N-allylnormorphine), *Pharmacol. Rev.* 8:175–198.

Yaksh, T. L., and Rudy, T. A., 1976, Analgesia mediated by a direct spinal action of narcotics, *Science* 192:1357–1358.

Yaksh, T. L., Yeung, J. C., and Rudy, T. A., 1976, Systematic examination in the rat of brain sites sensitive to the direct application of morphine: Observation of differential effects within the periaqueductal gray, *Brain Res.* 114:83–103.

Zieglgänsberger, W., and Bayerl, H., 1976, The mechanism of inhibition of neuronal activity by opiates in the spinal cord of cat, *Brain Res.* 115:111–128.

CHAPTER 6

Theories of Tolerance to and Physical Dependence on Opioids

Though under certain conditions (see below), tolerance to opioids can develop without concomitant physical dependence, the two phenomena will be considered together inasmuch as most explanatory theories postulate common mechanisms and assume that one sort or another of "counteradaptation" to the agonistic actions of opioids develops during repeated drug administration (accounting for tolerance); this results in "latent hyperexcitability" of the central nervous system, which is suppressed as long as opioids are administered; when opioids are abruptly withdrawn, or when a narcotic antagonist is administered, the latent hyperexcitability becomes manifest as the opioid-abstinence syndrome (indicative of physical dependence).

Thus, in nontolerant human subjects, morphine produces miosis, bradypnea, bradycardia, slight hypothermia; after repeated administration of morphine, miosis persists, but partial tolerance develops to the respiratory-depressant effect, while cardiac rate and rectal temperature are elevated (Martin & Jasinski, 1969); during the "primary" (or "early") morphine-abstinence syndrome, the pupils are dilated, while respiratory and cardiac rates as well as rectal temperature are increased far above preaddiction control values. In the nontolerant chronic spinal dog (Wikler & Frank, 1948), single doses of morphine have little or no effect on the knee jerk but depress the ipsilateral flexor and crossed extensor reflexes, while enhancing the ipsilateral extensor thrust. When the same dose of morphine is administered four times daily, tolerance develops to the depressant effects on the ipsilateral flexor and crossed extensor reflexes, as well as to the excitant effect on the ipsilateral extensor thrust (Martin, 1968). About 17 hr after abrupt withdrawal of morphine, the ipsilateral flexor and crossed extensor reflexes become hyperactive, while the ipsilateral extensor thrust becomes depressed; at about 41 hr of morphine abstinence, spontaneous "stepping" or "running" movements appear (with the chronic spinal dog in the lateral recumbent position, in which such spontaneous movements do not occur normally) and may persist for as long as 96 hr. Analogous changes in the (paralyzed) lower limbs of a chronic "spinal" man have been observed after single doses of morphine, and after abrupt withdrawal of morphine (Wikler & Rayport, 1954). In both the chronic spinal dog (Wikler & Carter, 1953) and chronic spinal man (Wikler & Rayport, 1954), similar but much more rapidly developing morphine-abstinence syndromes can be precipitated within a few minutes by the subcutaneous injection of nalorphine.

GENERAL THEORIES OF TOLERANCE TO AND PHYSICAL DEPENDENCE ON MORPHINE

Homeostatic Counteradaption

In 1943, Himmelsbach proposed, as an explanation of the autonomic changes that occur during morphine tolerance and morphine abstinence, that through its actions on hypothalamic centers in the nontolerant subject, morphine disturbs homeostasis. In response to such repeated "stresses," autonomic adjustments take place that partly restore homeostasis. With continued administration of morphine, such adjustments gain strength "disproportionately," so that a new level of homeostasis is reached, requiring the presence of morphine to maintain equilibrium. When morphine is abruptly withdrawn, the equilibrium is upset, and the autonomic adjustments that had developed now become manifest as the morphine-abstinence syndrome. That the counteradaptive autonomic adjustments represent latent hyperexcitability is indicated by Himmelsbach's (1941) observation that vasopressor responses to a standard cold stimulus were greater and recovery after removal of the stimulus was slower in morphine-tolerant than in nontolerant subjects.

Cellular Counteradaptation

The changes in hind-limb reflexes of the chronic spinal dog (Wikler & Frank, 1948; Wikler & Carter, 1953) and in lower-limb reflexes of a chronic spinal man (Wikler & Rayport, 1954) during cycles of addiction to morphine, which have already been described, can be explained as counteradaptations to the initial effects of morphine, but it is difficult to postulate a homeostatic mechanism to account for such somatic changes. Wikler (1953, p. 44) suggested that on repeated administration of morphine, cellular adaptation to the depressant actions of morphine takes place in the spinal cord, thus accounting for tolerance; when morphine is withdrawn abruptly or a narcotic antagonist is administered, the cellular adaptations (counteradaptations) are unmasked, thus accounting for the morphine abstinence syndrome.

Dual Action

In 1929, Tatum *et al.*, on the basis of observation of effects of single and repeated doses of morphine in the dog, proposed that morphine simultaneously exerts direct depressant and stimulant actions on the central nervous system, the stimulant effect outlasting the depressant one, and the net effect at any given time being the resultant of the two; with continuing morphine administration and increase in dosage, tolerance develops to the depressant effects but not to the stimultant ones, so that in general, the level of irritability increases, and if morphine is withheld, the stimulant actions continue to increase in intensity (unopposed by the depressant actions, already attenuated by tolerance), giving rise to the morphine-withdrawal or -abstinence syndrome. One problem with this theory is identifying the "stimulant" actions. In dogs, convulsions may be regarded as a stimulant action of morphine, but convulsions are not characteristic of the canine morphine-abstinence syndrome. In the nontolerant chronic spinal dog, morphine enhances the extensor thrust (Wikler & Frank, 1948), yet tolerance develops to this stimulant effect (Martin, 1968) and on abrupt withdrawal of morphine in morphine-tolerant chronic spinal dogs, the extensor thrust becomes markedly depressed (Wikler & Frank, 1948). Furthermore, in chronic spinal dogs given morphine (2.5 mg/kg every 6 hr) and nalorphine (5 mg/kg every 3 hr) for 28 days, no morphine effects were observed, and on abrupt withdrawal of both drugs, the morphine-abstinence syndrome was found to be greatly attenuated (Wikler, 1952, unpublished, cited by Martin, 1967, p. 492). Likewise, Seevers and Deneau (1961) found that in the monkey, the morphine-abstinence syndrome is attenuated or abolished in proportion to the dose of levallorphan (0.25–5.0 mg/kg) administered concomitantly with morphine, 5 mg/kg every 4 hr for 35 days. If it is assumed that only the depressant actions of morphine are antagonized by narcotic antagonists, then these observations are incompatible with the Tatum *et al.* hypothesis as originally proposed, since the postulated stimulant actions of morphine should have remained unopposed and should have given rise to marked morphine-abstinence syndromes. For this and for other reasons, Seevers and Deneau (1961) revised the Tatum *et al.* hypothesis extensively. They postulated that morphine does indeed have "dual actions," but that the specific signs and symptoms of the morphine-abstinence syndrome are due to adaptive changes to the prolonged occupation of sites of action involved in the depressive phases of morphine action, while the stimulant actions of morphine increase the intensity of the first portion of the specific morphine-abstinence syndrome through heightening of the potential excitability of synapses throughout the central nervous system, until the stimulant actions are dissipated following morphine withdrawal. According to this revised hypothesis, the stimulant effects of morphine play little, if any, role in the genesis of the later portion of the morphine-withdrawal syndrome, but they do contribute to the rapidly peaking abstinence syndrome precipitated by the administration of a specific opioid-antagonist, which displaces morphine from the sites of its depressive actions.

Seevers and Deneau (1961) explained certain observations of Wikler and Carter (1953) in terms of this revision of the original Tatum *et al.* hypothesis. Wikler and Carter (1953) reported that in the chronic spinal dog, the morphine-abstinence syndrome could be precipitated by nalorphine even before there was any evidence of tolerance to morphine. Furthermore, in the morphine-tolerant chronic spinal dog, morphine *enhanced* the running movements (characteristic of morphine abstinence) that were precipitated by nalorphine, but it promptly *suppressed* the running movements that emerged following the abrupt withdrawal of morphine. Wikler and Carter (1953) suggested that

> ... the processes responsibile for physical dependence begin very early during morphine addiction, possibly after a single dose, that they are distinct from those which subserve tolerance, and that they are "masked" by the narcotic actions of morphine. N-allylnormorphine appears to antagonize the narcotic effects of morphine, thereby "unmasking" such physical dependence as has developed. (p. 101)

According to Seevers and Deneau (1961), the enhancement of running movements by morphine in the nalorphine-precipitated abstinence syndrome is due to the direct stimulant actions of morphine, unopposed by morphine's depressant effects, which are antagonized by nalorphine; in contrast, when morphine is given during the morphine-withdrawal abstinence syndrome, running movements are suppressed because the stimulant actions of morphine are opposed by its depressant actions. This view is in accord with the dual-action hypothesis as revised by Seevers and Deneau (1961), which, as already noted, holds that the direct stimulant properties of morphine play only a minor role in the morphine-withdrawal abstinence syndrome, but a more significant one in the abstinence syndrome precipitated by narcotic antagonists in both acutely and chronically morphine-tolerant subjects; in such subjects, narcotic antagonists not only unmask the counteradaptive responses that have developed to the depressant abstinence actions of morphine but also intensify the precipitated syndrome as a whole by unmasking the direct stimulant actions of morphine.

THEORIES OF THE MECHANISMS OF COUNTERADAPTATION TO THE AGONISTIC EFFECTS OF DRUGS

These theories address themselves to the problem of how counteradaptation may develop to the continued agonistic actions of opioids or other drugs in the central nervous system. Though, in some cases, the data on which they are based were obtained with nonopioid drugs, these theories may serve as models for future research on the mechanisms of counteradaptations that are presumed to underly tolerance to opioids and the opioid-abstinence syndrome.

Disuse Supersensitivity (Pharmacological Denervation Supersensitivity)

The nictitating membrane of the cat develops supersensitivity to epinephrine after denervation or decentralization (Hampel, 1935) or, with innervation anatomically intact, to norepinephrine after brain stores of norepinephrine have been depleted by reserpine (Fleming & Trendelenburg, 1961). The latter phenomenon may properly be called *pharmacological denervation supersensitivity*. However, in peripheral tissues with dual innervation, supersensitivity to one neurotransmitter may develop when another transmitter is prevented from acting either by denervation or by protracted administration of a specific pharmacological blocking agent. Thus, in the cat, the submaxillary glands have both parasympathetic and sympathetic innervation. Emmelin and Murén

(1952) reported that removal of the parasympathetic innervation by section of the chorda tympani resulted in the development of supersensitivity to the sialagogic effects of the sympathomimetic agents epinephrine and norepinephrine, given by intracardiac injection. Similarly, supersensitivity to the sialagogic effects of epinephrine developed when the cat, with chorda tympani intact, was treated daily with the parasympathetic blocking agent atropine. Such supersensitivity to sympathomimetic agents declined rapidly when the cats with chorda tympani cut were treated daily with the parasympathomimetic agent pilocarpine, or when atropine was discontinued in cats with chorda tympani intact.

By analogy with such supersensitivity phenomena in peripheral tissues, Jaffe and Sharpless (1968) hypothesized that in the central nervous system, "latent hyperexcitability" can develop in postsynaptic neurons as a consequence of prolonged "disuse" of such synapses either through continuous pharmacological blockade or through continuous reduction of neural activities converging on such synapses as a result of the agonistic actions of a drug elsewhere in the brain. Supporting this hypothesis is the demonstration by Jaffe and Sharpless (1965) that in the cat, pentylenetetrazol-induced seizure thresholds, measured 22–24 hr after the last dose of pentobarbital, were significantly below control values even after only 26 hr of pentobarbital anesthesia, and that they continued to fall as chronic pentobarbital intoxication was maintained. Maximal "supersensitivity" to pentylenetetrazol was achieved in 2–3 weeks. After abrupt withdrawal of pentobarbital, such seizure thresholds rose gradually toward control values over time courses that were the more prolonged, the longer the period of chronic barbiturate intoxication had been. Also supporting the disuse hypothesis are the demonstrations by Friedman and Jaffe (1969) and Friedman *et al.* (1969) that in the mouse, the muscarinic cholinergic agent, pilocarpine, produces a dose-dependent fall in rectal temperature, presumably through a central (hypothalamic) action, as it is blocked by the tertiary muscarinic blocking agent, scopolamine, but not by its quaternary analogue, methscopolamine. Testing hypothermic responses to pilocarpine intraperitoneally 24 hr after withdrawal of scopolamine from the drinking water, these authors found that the pilocarpine dose–response curve was shifted to the left (increased hypothermic responsivity) after continuous ingestion of scopolamine for 5 days to 4 weeks, and that the hyperresponsiveness (supersensitivity) to pilocarpine lasted longer after 4 weeks of chronic scopolamine intoxication than after 5 days. The development of tolerance to scopolamine was indicated by decreased effectiveness in blocking pilocarpine-induced hypothermia as chronic scopolamine intoxication continued; on abrupt withdrawal of scopolamine, rectal temperature fell spontaneously, indicative of a scopolamine-abstinence syndrome.

Pharmacological Redundancy

To explain *chronic* tolerance and physical dependence (e.g., on morphine), Martin and his associates (Martin, 1968, 1970; Martin & Eades, 1967; Martin et al., 1968) have proposed a theory, the essential features of which are as follows. The central neural pathways to the final common pathway innervating a given effector tissue are of two kinds: a "primary" multisynaptic pathway (with a specific neurotransmitter) that normally maintains the function of the effector tissue; and one or more "redundant" multisynaptic pathways (with other neurotransmitters) that normally are inactive or minimally active in maintaining the function of the effector tissue. Both the primary and the redundant pathways are normally inhibited by negative feedback loops originating from post-synaptic fibers in the final common pathway acting on synapses proximal in the multisynaptic pathways. It is assumed that morphine activates an inhibitory neuron in the multisynaptic primary pathway located between the neuron inhibited by the negative feedback loop and the final common pathway, but that it has no action whatever on the multisynaptic redundant pathway. In consequence, the activity of the effector tissue will be decreased (morphine-agonistic action) though such decrease in activity will be tempered somewhat by decrease in the inhibitory effects of the negative feedback loops on the primary (and redundant) multisynaptic pathways. As morphine continues to be administered, its inhibitory actions in the multisynaptic primary pathway continue unchanged, but the multisynaptic redundant pathways became increasingly active (they "hypertrophy") through decrease in negative feedback inhibition, and in consequence, the function of the effector tissue is partially or wholly restored (tolerance). When morphine is abruptly withdrawn, activity in the previously inhibited primary multisynaptic pathway is rapidly restored and this restoration summates with the increased activity in the redundant multisynaptic pathways to excite the effector tissue far above control values (morphine-abstinence syndrome) until negative feedback inhibition has been restored in both the primary and the redundant multisynaptic pathways. The slow regression of hypertrophied redundant multisynaptic pathways may account for the phenomenon of "protracted abstinence" (Martin & Jasinski, 1969). Variations in the degrees of tolerance and physical dependence that develop for different agonistic actions of morphine are explained on the basis of at least two factors: "(1) the importance of the morphine sensitive pathway in mediating the physiological response and (2) the capacity of the redundant pathway to hypertrophy" (Martin, 1968, p. 219).

It should be noted that mere occupation by a drug of a receptor in the primary pathway is not sufficient to initiate the chain of events that leads to hypertrophy of the redundant pathways; rather, the drug-receptor interaction must exert agonistic effects. Thus, no tolerance to the opioid-antagonistic actions of naloxone or physical dependence on this drug develops on repeated administration; naloxone presumably occupies the same receptor sites as morphine but exerts virtually no agonistic actions (Jasinski et al., 1967). Also, in the case of drugs that do produce agonistic effects, such agonistic actions in the primary multisynaptic pathway continue unchanged despite the development of tolerance and physical dependence. Thus, Martin et al. (1968) employed the "rebreathing" technique for measuring the responsiveness of the respiratory center to carbon dioxide inhalation in man. For respiratory minute volumes of 10 liters/min, the mean pCO_2 value in the nontolerant state was 51.7 before morphine, 60.1 after 15 mg/70 kg, and 62.8 after 30 mg/70 kg of morphine (difference between pCO_2 values after the two doses of morphine were nonsignificant). In subjects receiving 60 mg/70 kg four times daily for periods up to 8 months, predrug pCO_2 values (4–5 hr after the last previous dose) ranged from 61.0 to 62.1, indicating no attenuation of the depressant effects of morphine on the respiratory center. Yet, there was definite evidence of partial tolerance to this effect. Thus, in subjects "stabilized" on 60 mg/70 kg of morphine four times daily, single doses of 60 or 120 mg/70 kg of morphine produced much smaller changes in the respiratory minute volume–carbon dioxide partial pressure curves than did 15 or 30 mg/70 kg of morphine in the nontolerant state. Inasmuch as there is no evidence of increased destruction or inactivation of morphine in the tolerant state, and as already noted, morphine continues to exerts its depressant actions on respiration during tolerance, the data can be explained by assuming that in the tolerant state, the primary pathway was blocked maximally by morphine but respiration was maintained by hypertrophied, morphine-insensitive, redundant pathways. The data obtained during morphine withdrawal are also consistent with this view. Thus, 20 hr after the last dose of morphine, the slope of the respiratory minute volume–carbon dioxide partial pressure curve, the mean of which was 1.5 in the nontolerant control state (and which did not change significantly in the tolerant state) rose to 3.1 (difference significant), whereas the pCO_2 for respiratory minute volumes of 10 liters/min fell to 52.7 (not significantly different from the nontolerant control value of 51.7).

Other evidence for existence of redundant pathways has been acquired by Martin and Eades (1967) and Martin (1970) in the chronic spinal dog. In this preparation, the flexor reflex is unaffected by phenoxybenzamine (alpha-adrenergic antagonist) or chlorpromazine (alpha-adrenergic and tryptaminergic antagonist); atropine does have a small but significant depressant effect. Nevertheless, facilitation of the flexor reflex and production of stepping ("running") movements by the adrenergic agonists methoxamine and amphetamine are antagonized by phenoxybenzamine and chlorpromazine. On the other hand, the same effects (facilitation of the flexor reflex and production of stepping movements) of tryptaminergic drugs (tryptamine, LSD, psilocin, mescaline, DOM) are not antagonized by phenoxybenzamine, but they are by chlorpromazine and cyproheptadine (a tryptaminergic antagonist). Again, facilitation of the flexor reflex and production of stepping movements by the cholinergic agonists physostigmine and oxotremorine are not antagonized by phenoxybenzamine but are by atropine. These phenomena can be explained by assuming that the segmental reflex arc for the flexor reflex is neither adrenergic, nor tryptaminergic, nor cholinergic (except possibly at the ventral horn ganglion synapse), but that there are redundant suprasegmental adrenergic, tryptaminergic, and cholinergic facilitatory pathways to the internuncial cells in the spinal cord subserving the flexor reflex, which can be activated by appropriate agonists. Atropine, but not phenoxybenzamine, has been found to depress the flexor reflex in the morphine-abstinent chronic spinal dog, suggesting that hypertrophy of redundant cholinergic neurons may occur during the development of chronic tolerance and physical dependence in this preparation.

Perhaps also explicable in terms of pharmacological redundancy are the observations of Collier *et al.* (1972), who found that in rats made physically dependent rapidly by subcutaneous injection of morphine (150 mg/10 ml/kg in a sustained-release preparation), certain antineurotransmitter drugs exerted selective actions of different combinations of signs of the abstinence syndrome precipitated by naloxone (up to 1.0 mg/kg subcutaneously) depending on whether these drugs were given after the morphine or before. For each drug test, the abstinence signs precipitated by naloxone were compared with those in rats treated similarly, except that they received normal saline instead of the antineurotransmitter drugs. Thus, when given 23.0 or 23.5 hr *after* morphine and 0.5–1.0 hr before naloxone, atropine (a cholingergic antagonist), 40 mg/kg subcutaneously, significantly decreased jumping, diarrhea, and chewing but increased irritability and head shakes; parachlorophenylanine (pCPA, which blocks the hydroxylation of tryptophan and hence depletes the brain of serotonin), 86–172 mg/kg intraperitoneally, decreased jumping, diarrhea and head shakes; indomethacin (which blocks the production of prostaglandins), 25 mg/kg orally, increased irritability and decreased chewing. However, some opposite effects were observed when these antineurotransmitter drugs were given in the same dose 1–24 hr (depending on the drug) *before* the induction of physical dependence on morphine and the precipitation of morphine abstinence with naloxone. Thus, atropine significantly increased jumping and head shakes and decreased irritability to touch and diarrhea. Collier *et al.* concluded "that morphine dependence is multipartite and that acetylcholine, 5-hydroxytryptamine and prostaglandins play intimate parts in various elements of dependence." The "multipartite" nature of dependence on morphine may be explained in terms of the pharmacological redundancy theory if it is assumed that a given sign of morphine abstinence can be mediated by more than one redundant circuit; if hypertrophy of the cholinergic redundant circuit is prevented by atropine, another noncholinergic redundant circuit may hypertrophy, in large part taking over the function of jumping.

For acute tolerance to and physical dependence on morphine, Martin (1968, 1970) postulated that while hypertrophy of redundant pathways may play some role, the more important mechanism appears to be partial restoration of autonomic functioning through responses of homeostatic regulatory systems to the abnormal internal environmental conditions (hypothermia, hypercapnia) created by the actions of morphine on "homeostats" (raising or lowering their "set points"). If, after the new state of homeostatic equilibrium has been established, a narcotic antagonist is administered, the set points of the homeostats are immediately restored to normal levels, and the homeostatic regulatory systems now respond vigorously to the still-persisting abnormal internal environmental conditions (acute precipitated abstinence syndrome) until these are dissipated.

New Receptors

In 1930, Sakel proposed a theory of tolerance to and physical dependence on morphine based on Ehrlich's "side-chain" concept of cellular receptors. According to Sakel's theory, sympathetic neurons in the "vegetative nervous system" are normally activated by combinations of their "side chains" with a circulating hormone, tentatively identified with adrenaline (epinephrine). Morphine also combines with these side chains, but the drug–receptor combination does not activate the sympathetic neuron. Inasmuch as there are now fewer side chains that can combine with circulating hormone, the sympathetic neuron is partially inactivated ("euphoria"). Inactivation of some side chain by morphine constitutes a biological stimulus for formation of new side chains in greater abundance than before. These excessive newly formed side chains combine with circulating hormone, producing overactivity of the sympathetic neuron and requiring larger amounts of morphine to displace the circulating hormone from the newly formed side chains and to inactivate the sympathetic neuron to the level required for euphoria (tolerance). This cycle is repeated again and again until the sympathetic neuron is covered with side chains, all but those required for maintenance of a normal or subnormal level of activation (by combination with circulating hormone) being combined with morphine. When morphine is suddenly withdrawn, all the old and newly formed side chains become free to combine with circulating hormone, thereby intensely overexciting the sympathetic neuron (abstinence syndrome) over a time course that corresponds to that of the "falling away" of the excess side chains, which are not regenerated since the biological stimulus of inactivation by morphine is lacking.

A more elaborate theory of "new receptors" in the development of tolerance and physical dependence was proposed independently by Collier (1965, 1966). As in Sakel's (1930) theory, Collier postulated that prolonged exposure to a drug or to increase or decrease of a neurotransmitter may change the number of its receptors. Collier distinguished between *silent* and *pharmacological* receptors. A "silent" receptor is

> ... one that interacts with a chemical substance without directly producing a pharmacological response. Such interaction might take the form of storage, excretion or enzymatic conversion of the substance to inactive products. (Collier, 1966, p. 176)

It should be noted that in a sense, an increase in the number of silent receptors does produce a pharmacological response, namely, diminution or absence of the pharmacological effects of the substance with which the silent receptors combine. Conversely, a decrease in the number of silent receptors also produces a pharmacological response, namely, augmentation of the pharmacological effects of that portion of the substance that remains free from combination with silent receptors because of the diminution in their number. A pharmacological receptor is one that interacts with a drug molecule to produce (directly) a pharmacological response, or with an endogenous substance (e.g., a neurotransmitter) to give a physiological response.

The development of tolerance *without* physical dependence ("metabolic" or "dispositional" tolerance) is explained in Collier's theory in two ways: (1) an increase in the number of silent receptors, for example, the activation of liver microsomal nonspecific oxidative enzymes, by phenobarbital, that catabolize phenobarbital itself (Conney, 1967) or, by ethanol, that catabolize ethanol itself (Lieber & DeCarli, 1968) as well as other substances; or (2) a decrease in the number of pharmacological receptors, for example, progressive decrease in N-demethylation of morphine and other opioids by rat liver *in vitro* as the animals acquire tolerance to morphine *in vivo*, and diminution of both of these changes when nalorphine is administered with morphine chronically *in vivo*; these data were interpreted by Axelrod (1956a,b) as indicating that N-demethylating enzyme receptor sites are inactivated by continuous interaction with opioids and become "unavailable" for such drugs. It may be remarked that N-demethylating enzyme receptors may be regarded as pharmacological ones, if it is assumed that the N-demethylated product (e.g., normorphine) is responsible for the agonistic effects of morphine, and similarly for other opioids.

To explain the development of tolerance *with* physical dependence, Collier (1966, p. 180) postulated an increase or decrease in the number of receptors for an endogenous neurotransmitter that is affected by the drug in various ways:

1. "Drug reduces the supply of an endogenous excitatory transmitter, causing the pharmacological receptors to increase in number. After withdrawal of the drug, the supply of transmitter rises to a normal level faster than the surplus receptors are removed" (Collier, 1966, p. 180). An example of reduction in supply of an endogenous excitatory neurotransmitter is the blocking of release of acetylcholine by morphine in the coaxially stimulated guinea pig ileum, to which tolerance develops rapidly (Paton, 1957; Schaumann, 1957). The development of "acute tolerance" (tachyphylaxis) to this effect is associated with greatly increased sensitivity of the guinea pig ileum to exogenous acetylcholine (Shoham & Weinstock, 1974); such "disuse supersensitivity" could be explained in terms of Collier's theory that in consequence of the decrease in release of endogenous acetylcholine, the number of pharmacological receptors for acetylcholine increases. However, Shoham and Weinstock (1974) did not observe a consistent increase in the height of electrically induced contractions (above that of premorphine controls) after replacing the morphine solution in the bath with normal Krebs–Hensleit solution; they offered two possible explanations for the absence of the expected "withdrawal syndrome": the fact that in their experiments the guinea pig ileum was always stimulated supramaximally, and that the morphine in the guinea pig ileum may not have been washed out completely by the Krebs–Hensleit solution. On the other hand,

Paton (1957) found a curious type of morphine dependence in the morphine-tolerant guinea pig ileum. After washing morphine out, the twitch response to coaxial electrical stimulation *decreased*, but it could be *restored* by adding morphine to the bath. This type of "morphine dependence" is reminiscent of the phenomena observed by Kuyer and Wijsenbeek (1913); they found that when a number of nonopioid drugs (including physostigmine, pilocarpine, and muscarine) were added to isolated smooth muscle preparations in a bath, the characteristic effects of each of these drugs subsided after a time but reappeared when the drug was washed out. At any rate, it appears that if suppression of release of acetylcholine and its consequences for "new receptors" plays a role in the central nervous system, such effects must be localized, as Jóhanneson and Long (1964) found no differences in the concentration of acetylcholine in the total brains of morphine-tolerant rats and nontolerant rats that had received no doses or just one dose of morphine.

    2. "Drug increases the supply of an endogenous inhibitory transmitter, causing the pharmacological receptors for the transmitter to decrease in number. After withdrawal of the drug, the supply of transmitter falls to its normal level faster than the receptors are restored" (Collier, 1966; p. 180). If the catecholamines (norepinephrine and dopamine) are regarded as inhibitory neurotransmitters (Collier, 1966, p. 182), then some evidence exists that they may be involved in the development of tolerance to and physical dependence on morphine in a manner consistent with Collier's postulate (quoted at Number 2, above). In the dog, brain norepinephrine concentrations remain unchanged in the morphine-tolerant state but fall markedly (along with brain dopamine concentrations) in the early morphine-abstinence period (following morphine withdrawal or nalorphine precipitation), when the dog is exhibiting marked excitement and hyperthermia (Gunne and Lewander, 1967). In the rat, brain norepinephrine concentrations (and adrenal epinephrine concentrations) increase as tolerance to the depressant effects of morphine develop and excitant effects of the drug predominate, but no change occurs in the concentrations of these catecholamines during the early morphine-abstinence period, when the rat is exhibiting certain excitant phenomena such as increased frequency of "wet-dog" shakes and hyperalgesia (Gunne & Lewander, 1967; Sloan *et al.*, 1963, Maynert & Klingman, 1962; Maynert, 1968). In both the dog and the rat, the output of norepinephrine and epinephrine is greately increased during the early morphine-abstinence period, returning to normal in two weeks (Gunne & Lewander, 1967; Sloan & Eisenman, 1968), but in the rat, the output of norepinephrine falls to subnormal levels for several months thereafter (Sloan and Eisenman, 1968). Results more consistent

with Collier's postulate (Number 2 above) were obtained by Smith and his associates (1970, 1972) on ^{14}C-catecholamine synthesis in mouse brain after single and repeated (every 6 hr) doses of morphine and following abrupt withdrawal of morphine. They found that single doses of morphine (100 mg/kg intraperitoneally) in nontolerant mice greatly increased the incorporation of intravenously injected ^{14}C-tyrosine into ^{14}C-norepinephrine and ^{14}C-dopamine in excised brain (cerebral cortex, diencephlon, brain stem, and cerebellum; striatum for dopamine only) and adrenals but not in heart or spleen; this effect was antagonized by naloxone (3 mg/kg). Morphine did not affect the free tyrosine or ^{14}C-tyrosine content of mouse brain, indicating that morphine increases both the synthesis and the turnover of ^{14}C-norepinephrine and ^{14}C-dopamine in mouse brain. d-Amphetamine (10 mg/kg) had no affect on the incorporation of ^{14}C-tyrosine into ^{14}C-catecholamines in brain, adrenals, or spleen, but it decreased that in the heart. After seven successive injections of morphine, tolerance developed to the increased incorporation of ^{14}C-tyrosine into ^{14}C-epinephrine and ^{14}C-dopamine. Similar changes were observed with levorphanol (30 mg/kg); when levorphanol-tolerant mice were switched to morphine, cross-tolerance was observed. Rosenman and Smith (1972) found that after the withdrawal of morphine from morphine-tolerant mice, incorporation of ^{14}C-tyrosine into ^{14}C-epinephrine and ^{14}C-dopamine in the brain decreased progressively to well below control values, the maximum fall occurring at the 36th hour of morphine abstinence; by the 66th hour, the incorporation of ^{14}C-tyrosine into ^{14}C-catecholamines barely returned to control values. From the 18th to the 54th hours after abrupt withdrawal of morphine, administration of single doses of morphine restored the incorporation of ^{14}C-tyrosine into ^{14}C-catecholamines in the brain to values equal to or higher than control values and, after the 66th hour, to values equal to those of brains of nontolerant mice after the same dose of morphine, indicating that continued morphine administration is necessary for fully tolerant mice to incorporate normal amounts of labeled tyrosine into labeled noradrenaline and dopamine in the brain. These investigators also reported that during the morphine-abstinence period, the specific activity of ^{14}C-tyrosine did not change, whereas that of ^{14}C-norepinephrine and ^{14}C-dopamine decreased significantly, reaching a minimum at the 36th hour of morphine abstinence. This finding indicates that during morphine abstinence, the rate of synthesis of ^{14}C-catecholamines decreases. Complementing these studies, in part, is that of Clouet and Ratner (1970), who reported that morphine increases the incorporation of ^{14}C-tyrosine into ^{14}C-dopamine in the hypothalamus and the striatum; however, no tolerance to this effect was observed.

Also, Pérez-Cruet (1976) reported that single doses, not only of morphine (10 mg/kg) but also of methadone (10 mg/kg) or bulbocapnine (50 mg/kg) given intraperitoneally, increased the conversion of intravenously administered ^{3}H-tyrosine into ^{3}H-dopamine in the rat striatum; these drugs did not alter striatal levels of dopamine but increased the levels of striatal homovanillic acid, indicating an increase in metabolism of dopamine. These pharmacologcal effects could be classically conditioned to a buzzer noise (30 sec) followed by injection of the drug as an unconditioned stimulus. In the rat, morphine and methadone, like haloperidol, reduce "social aggression" in the early (Puri & Lal, 1973) or protracted (Gianutros et al., 1974) morphine-abstinence syndrome. Also, like haloperidol, morphine (Puri et al., 1973) and methadone (Sasame et al., 1972) reduce stereotopy induced in rats by amphetamine or apomorphine and increase dopamine turnover in the striatum. From these data, it appears that morphine (and methadone) block receptors for dopamine, the increase in dopamine synthesis and turnover being due to positive feedback loops from the postsynaptic neuron, deprived of its inhibitory neurotransmitter, as has been postulated for haloperidol and some other psychotropic drugs (Carlsson and Lindqvist, 1963; Nybäck et al., 1968). If it is assumed that such feedback activation of dopamine synthesis continues with chronic drug administration, then from Collier's postulate (Number 2 above), the number of dopamine receptors at the postsynaptic neuron would decrease; after abrupt withdrawal of morphine, the supply of dopamine would fall to its normal level faster than the (inhibitory) receptors are restored, with resultant excitation (morphine-abstinence syndrome). As already noted (Rosenman and Smith, 1972), tolerance does develop to the morphine-induced increase in the synthesis of dopamine (and norepinephrine) from tyrosine, but after abrupt withdrawal of morphine, the synthesis of catecholamines from tyrosine falls *below* control levels; the deficiency in inhibitory neurotransmitter could account for the morphine-abstinence syndrome without invoking a deficiency in the number of inhibitory postsynaptic receptors.

If, as in peripheral tissues (Gaddum & Picarelli, 1957), morphine blocks receptors for serotonin (5-hydroxytryptamine, 5-HT) in the central nervous system, and if, in the central nervous system, serotonin is assumed to be an inhibitory neurotransmitter, then this monoamine may fill the role in the development of tolerance to and physical dependence on morphine in accordance with Collier's postulate (Number 2 above). Although steady-state levels of brain serotonin remain unchanged in morphine-tolerant and morphine-abstinent dogs, rats, rabbits, and mice (Gunne, 1962, 1963; Maynert et al., 1962; Sloan & Eisenman, 1968; Sloan et al., 1963; Way et al., 1968), it has been reported that the turnover (synthesis and catabolism) of brain serotonin is increased by morphine in the mouse. Thus, Way et al. (1968), Loh and Way (1968), and Loh et al. (1969) found that the concentration of brain serotonin increased greatly after administration of pargyline (a monoamine oxidase inhibitor) in mice made tolerant to morphine by repeated morphine injections or by morphine-pellet implantation, but not in nontolerant control mice; such increased turnover of serotonin reverted to normal two weeks after the withdrawal of morphine in the morphine-tolerant mice. Also, one or a few doses of p-chorophenylalanine (which inhibits hydroxylation of tryptophan and reduces the formation of serotonin) antagonized the analgesic effects of single doses of morphine, the development of tolerance to this effect, and the jumping response to naloxone (a morphine-abstinence sign). If the increased turnover of serotonin (presumed to be an inhibitory neurotransmitter) declines rapidly after withdrawal of morphine, the morphine-abstinence syndrome could be explained on the assumption of a persisting deficiency in receptors for the inhibitory neurotransmitter, the deficiency having been created during the period of increased turnover of serotonin in the development of tolerance. However, the role of serotonin in the development of tolerance to and physical dependence on opioids is still unclear in view of the conflicting data obtained by other investigators (see Wikler, 1972, especially the footnote to pp. 367–368).

3. "Drug occupies the receptors for an endogenous excitatory transmitter, causing the pharmacological receptors for the transmitter to increase in number. After withdrawal of the drug, its molecules leave the receptors for the transmitter faster than the surplus receptors are removed" (Collier, 1965, p. 180). In this postulate, no change in concentration of the (excitatory) neurotransmitter is predicated; tolerance to the blocking effects of the drug is ascribed to increase in the number of postsynaptic pharmacological receptors; the surplus receptors are presumed to persist for some time after the drug is withdrawn, and now that there is no blockade, the receptors respond to the normal concentration of neurotransmitter by excitation (abstinence syndrome). Noting that morphine blocks serotonin in peripheral tissues and regarding serotonin as an excitatory neurotransmitter because its precursor, 5-hydroxytrytophan, "causes central excitation somewhat like that of morphine withdrawal," Collier (1966, pp. 183–184) suggested that this monoamine may fulfill the requirements for the postulate (Number 3 above). If it is assumed that the turnover of serotonin is increased but blockade of (excitatory) serotonin postsynaptic receptors persists to some extent during morphine tolerance, the predicated increase in receptors would still be tenable and their persistence for some time after

morphine withdrawal could account for the morphine-abstinence syndrome.

Enzyme Expansion

Shuster (1961) and Goldstein and Goldstein (1961, 1968) have proposed theories of tolerance to and physical dependence on morphine that are very similar to each other. According to Shuster's theory, an enzyme E, which catalyzes the conversion of a precursor into a neurotransmitter, is itself being continually degraded and resynthesized; the rate of resynthesis is held in check by a "natural repressor." Morphine inhibits the activity of enzyme E, thereby reducing the concentration of the neurotransmitter, or it blocks the effects of the neurotransmitter on receptors, producing morphine-agonistic actions. At the same time, repeated doses of morphine result in "derepression" of resynthesis of enzyme E through interference with the actions of the "natural repressor"; or alternatively, repeated doses of morphine may repress the synthesis of an enzyme that destroys the neurotransmitter. In either case, the concentration of the neurotransmitter rises, requiring more morphine to produce agonistic effects (tolerance). When morphine is suddenly withdrawn, the unopposed high concentrations of neurotransmitter produce the morphine-abstinence syndrome. According to the Goldsteins' theory, the rate of resynthesis of enzyme E is governed by the concentration of the neurotransmitter in a negative manner; that is, the higher the concentration of the neurotransmitter, the greater is the repression of resynthesis of enzyme E. Inhibition of enzyme E by morphine reduces the concentration of the neurotransmitter, thereby producing morphine-agonistic actions. The reduction in concentration of the neurotransmitter results in derepression of resynthesis of enzyme E (or morphine inhibits the degradation of enzyme E), resulting in increased formation of the neurotransmitter from its precursor (tolerance) and the appearance of abstinence phenomena when morphine is suddenly withdrawn. Some of the data already discussed in connection with the new-receptor theory are also consistent with the enzyme-expansion theory. Indeed, the two theories differ from each other mainly in that the former postulates postsynaptic changes (new receptors) and the latter presynaptic changes (neurotransmitter-synthesizing enzyme expansion) during morphine dependence. The basic problem in differentiating the two would seem to be determining whether it is the turnover of cellular receptor-synthesizing enzyme protein or transmitter-synthesizing enzyme protein that is increased in the morphine-tolerant state.

That increase in protein synthesis is involved in the development of tolerance to and physical dependence on morphine is indicated by the inhibition of the development of these phenomena by actinomycin D (Cohen *et al.*, 1965; Cox *et al.*, 1968), an inhibitor of DNA-dependent RNA synthesis, by 8-azaguanine (Yamamoto *et al.*, 1967), a purine antagonist that produces a nonfunctional RNA, and by cycloheximide (Way *et al.*, 1968), which, according to Siegel and Sisler (1964), affects protein synthesis (in *Saccharomyces pastorianus*) by inhibiting the transfer of amino acid from soluble-RNA to the ribosomes and their subsequent polymerization into protein. Furthermore Loh *et al.* (1969) reported that cycloheximide blocked not only the development of tolerance to and physical dependence on morphine in mice but also the increased turnover of brain serotonin (as determined by the "pargyline method") that normally accompanies morphine tolerance. In the dose of cycloheximide used, no acute overt pharmacological effects and, when repeated, no toxic manifestations were apparent for one week. Thereafter, the cumulative mortality of chronically morphinized animals was enhanced considerably by cycloheximide treatment.

Immune Mechanisms

In 1964, Cochin and Kornetsky (1964) found that in the rat, tolerance to the analgesic action of morphine could last up to one year after a single injection or after several irregularly spaced doses. They noted that earlier, Eddy (1953) reported that tolerance to a second dose of morphine developed in mice if a 72- or 96-hr interval elapsed between injections, but not if the interval was 24 hr. They noted also that Fraser and Isbell (1952) found evidence of tolerance to the nauseant and emetic and temperature-lowering effects of a single dose of morphine in man, 6 months after chronic morphine administration. On the basis of such data and other evidence, Cochin and Kornetsky (1964) suggested that some sort of immune mechanism may be induced by the administration of morphine. Consistent with this suggestion were the observations of Kornetsky and Bain (1967, 1968), who, employing the electric shock-attenuation procedure for measuring analgesia, found that tolerance was not present when only three days intervened between two doses of morphine but was present when seven or more days intervened. Likewise, Cochin and Mushlin (1970) found, with the hot-plate method, that tolerance to a single dose of morphine was greatest if the interval between the first injection and the test dose was three weeks, less but still significant if the interval was two weeks, and not significant if the interval was one week. Evidently, tolerance to a single dose of morphine takes a considerable time to develop, as would be expected if it were due to an "immune mechanism." Further pursuit of this hypothesis by investigations of possible transferable factors in tolerant animals (serum factors, tissue extracts) and the effects of immunosuppressors on tolerance has led to contradictory or inconclusive results; these investigations have been reviewed by Cochin and Kornetsky (1968) and by Cochin (1971).

Learning Factors

In the theories of tolerance to (and physical dependence on) morphine considered so far, biochemical–neurophysiological mechanisms are postulated to explain how enzymes (Shuster, 1961; Goldstein & Goldstein, 1961, 1968), cells (Collier, 1965, 1966) or central neuronal circuits (Martin, 1968) may be involved in compensating for a disturbance in function produced by the agonistic effects of a drug. In such theories, it is tacitly assumed that the initial disturbance in function is actually present (i.e., it is not merely potential), and that the disturbed function is vital to the organism. Thus, morphine depresses respiratory rate and the organism must breathe; on repeated administration of morphine, compensatory mechanisms come into play, and respiratory rate is partially restored to its premorphine control value (tolerance). Though described in biochemical–neurophysiological terms, the elaboration of such compensatory mechanisms over time (pharmacological tolerance) can be regarded as a type of nonassociative "learning."

In "psychological" experiments, however, the function initially disturbed by morphine may not actually be present unless the organism attempts to perform that function under the influence of morphine. Thus, a common method for testing the analgesic action of morphine is measurement of the latency to paw lick or jumping after placing a rat on the hot plate. Rats tested on the hot plate *after* each dose of morphine develop greater tolerance to morphine than rats tested on the hot plate *before but not after* each dose of morphine, for an identical number of morphine injections (Adams *et al.*, 1969). Evidently, some sort of learning is involved in this phenomenon, but whether it is nonassociative (as in pharmacological tolerance) or is an example of "behavioral tolerance" (Hayes and Mayer, 1978) or of Pavlovian conditioning (Siegel, 1976, 1978) is currently disputed.

That the testing procedure is involved in the development of tolerance to morphine has been demonstrated by many investigators. Kayan *et al.* (1969) reported that rats that had been given a series of subcutaneous injections of morphine (5 mg/kg), each followed by testing for analgesia on the hot plate, developed significantly greater tolerance than rats given an identical series of morphine injections without testing until the day of the final dose of morphine, after which they were tested on the hot plate. Interestingly, on the day of the final dose of morphine, premorphine control reaction times to paw lick or jumping (algesimetric response) were significantly shorter in the group that had been tested on the hot plate after each morphine injection than in the group that had not been tested, and this was also true of comparable tested and non-tested groups that had received an identical series of saline injections until the final day, when they were given morphine (5 mg/kg subcutaneously) and tested on the hot plate. Inasmuch as such "control hyperalgesia" developed in both the morphine-tested and saline-tested groups, but tolerance developed only in the morphine-tested group, it would appear that control hyperalgesia cannot, itself, account for the development of tolerance. Apparently, tolerance to morphine in these experiments was dependent on some other consequence of interaction between the effects of morphine and the analgesic-testing procedure.

That the hot plate need not be "hot" for the development of tolerance was demonstrated by Adams *et al* (1969). Their investigations showed that tolerance to morphine developed in rats that had been exposed to a hot plate (55°C) or to a *cold plate* (25°C) *before and after* morphine (5 mg/kg subcutaneously) on repeated occasions, all rats being tested on the hot plate before and after morphine on the final day of the experiments. No tolerance was observed on the final day of the experiments in groups that had received an identical series of morphine injections but were *never tested* or that were tested on the hot plate or the cold plate *before but not after* each morphine injection. Likewise, no tolerance developed in comparable groups that had received saline injections instead of morphine. As the rat makes no algesimetric response (paw lick or jumping) when exposed to the cold plate, the development of tolerance to morphine in the drug–test interaction cannot be explained on the basis of learning to make the response.

Siegel (1975) has proposed that the development of tolerance to morphine is based on an associative (Pavlovian) learning process. According to his scheme, the unconditioned stimulus (US) is morphine (5 mg/kg subcutaneously); the unconditioned response (UR) is analgesia; the conditioned stimulus (CS) is the complex of "environmental cues" in the *particular* algesimetric procedure employed; and the conditioned response (CR) is "hyperalgesia," which accounts for the shortening of the latency to the algesimetric response (i.e., tolerance to morphine). As already noted, identifying hyperalgesia as the CR that accounts for tolerance is questionable, but Siegel has adduced data indicating that the hyperalgesic CR undergoes extinction when elicited repeatedly without injection of morphine, and that the degree of tolerance developed to morphine is related to the specific CSs in the drug–test interactions. Thus, Siegel (1975) reported that as Adams *et al* (1969) showed previously, rats given morphine (5 mg/kg subcutaneously) every other day for a total of four injections, each followed by testing on the hot plate or the cold plate, developed tolerance compared with rats given morphine in their homes cages but not tested until the day of the last morphine injection (these rats did develop tolerance after three additional morphine injections, each of which was followed by testing on the hot plate). On the fifth day, the latency (reaction time) of the paw-lick response to the hot plate after an injection of *saline* was measured in the morphine-tested group, in a comparable saline-tested group, and in a group that had received morphine (5 mg/kg subcutaneously) every other day for a total of four injections in their home cages without testing. The latencies of the latter two groups were not significantly different (9.1–10.3 sec), but the latency of the previously morphine-tested group was significantly shorter (4.4 sec, $p < 0.002$). In another experiment, Siegel (1975) demonstrated that in rats that had become tolerant after four subcutaneous injections of morphine (5 mg/kg) every other day, each followed by testing on the hot plate, the hyperalgesic response to the hot plate after a *saline* injection was retained after two weeks' rest in the home cage without injections or testing. On further saline injections every other day, each followed by testing on the hot plate, the hyperalgesic response extinguished rapidly (disappeared by the third saline injection). Unfortunately, no data have been published to date on the latencies of the paw-lick responses to the hot plate in rats that had received morphine injections followed by exposure to the *cold plate*. Inasmuch as such rats also develop tolerance to morphine, it would be crucial for Siegel's "conditioned hyperalgesic anticipatory response" hypothesis of morphine tolerance to test whether or not such a conditioned response also develops in previously morphine-(cold-plate)-tested rats. In further studies, Siegel (1976) tested the development of tolerance to the analgesic effect of morphine in rats given repeated injections of morphine, each of which was followed by testing on a hot plate that was functional for one group and nonfunctional (on the cold plate) for another group. For each of the four morphine-injected groups, there were saline-injected control groups tested similarly. Finally, tests on each of the eight groups were made with both the functional and the nonfunctional paw-pressure apparatus and the functional hot plate and nonfunctional cold plate, after injection of the same agent (morphine or saline) used previously. The threshold paw-withdrawal response (grams of pressure) in the functional paw-pressure apparatus and the response latencies to the hot plate did not change significantly in the saline-injected rats (no tolerance). In the morphine-injected rats, tolerance was *greater* when tested with the *same* technique than with the different analgesimetric technique, regardless of whether in acquisition of tolerance, the paw-pressure apparatus or the hot plate was *functional or nonfunctional.* Siegel concluded that an association with (specific) environmental cues and the systemic effects of morphine is crucial to tolerance development.

REFERENCES

Adams, W. J., Yeh, S. Y., Woods, A., and Mitchell, C. L., 1969, Drug-test interaction as a factor in the development of tolerance to the analgesic effect of morphine, *J. Pharmacol. Exp. Ther. 168*:251–257.

Axelrod, J., 1956a, The enzymatic N-demethylation of narcotic drugs, *J. Pharmacol. Exp. Ther. 117*:322–330.

Axelrod, J., 1956b, Possible mechanism of tolerance to narcotic drugs, *Science 124*:263–264.

Bergel, F., 1951, Parasympathomimetics and anticholinesterases, *J. Pharmacol. 3*:385–399.

Carlsson, A., and Lindqvist, M., 1963, Effect of chlorpromazine or haloperidol on formation of 3-methoxytryramine and normetanephrine in mouse brain, *Acta Pharmacol. Toxicol. 20*:140–144.

Clouet, D. H., and Ratner, M., 1970, Catecholamine biosynthesis in brains of rats treated with morphine, *Science 168*:854–856.

Cochin, J., 1971, Role of possible immune mechanisms in the development of tolerance, in *Narcotic Drugs: Biochemical Pharmacology* (D. H. Clouet, Ed.), pp. 432–448. Plenum Press, New York.

Cochin, J., and Kornetsky, C., 1964, Development and loss of tolerance to morphine in the rat after single and multiple injections, *J. Pharmacol. Exp. Ther. 145*:1–10.

Cochin, J., and Kornetsky, C., 1968, Factors in blood of morphine-tolerant animals that attenuate or enhance effects of morphine in nontolerant animals, in *The Addictive States: Research Publications of the Association for Research in Nervous and Mental Disease,* Vol. 46 (A. Wikler, Ed.), pp. 263–269. Williams & Wilkins, Baltimore, Maryland.

Cochin, J., and Mushlin, B. E., 1970, The role of dose-interval in the development of tolerance to morphine, *Fed. Proc. 29*:685.

Cohen, M., Keats, A. S., Kirvoy, W., and Ungar, G., 1965, Effect of actinomycin D on morphine tolerance, *Proc. Soc. Exp. Biol. Med. (N.Y.) 119*:381–384.

Collier, H. O. J., 1965, A general theory of the genesis of drug dependence by induction of receptors, *Nature 205*:181–182.

Collier, H. O. J., 1966, Tolerance, physical dependence and receptors: A theory of the genesis of tolerance and physical dependence through drug-induced changes in the number of receptors, in *Advances in Drug Research* (N. J. Harper and A. B. Simmonds, Eds.), pp. 171–188. Academic Press, London.

Collier, H. O. J., 1973, Pharmacological mechanisms of drug dependence, in *Pharmacology and the Future of Man. Proc. 5th Int. Congr. Pharmacol., San Francisco, 1972,* Vol. 1 (J. Cochin, Ed.), pp. 65–76. Karger, Basel, Switzerland.

Collier, H. O. J., Francis, D. L., and Schneider, C., 1972, Modification of morphine withdrawal by drugs interacting with humoral mechanisms: Some contradictions and their interpretation, *Nature 237*:220–223.

Conney, A. H., 1967, Pharmacological implications of microsomal enzyme induction, *Pharmacol. Rev. 19:*317–353.

Cox, B. M., Ginsburg, M., and Osman, O. H., 1968, Acute tolerance to narcotic analgesic drugs in rats, *Brit. J. Pharmacol. Chemotherap. 33:*245–256.

Eddy, N. B., 1953, The hot-plate method for measuring analgesic effect in mice, in *Minutes of the 12th Meeting of the Committee on Drug Addiction and Narcotics,* NAS-NRC, pp. 603–618. Boston, Massachusetts.

Emmelin, N., and Murén, A., 1952, The sensitivity of submaxillary glands to chemical agents studied in cats under various conditions over long periods, *Acta Physiol. Scand. 26:*221–231.

Fleming, W. W., and Trendelenburg, U., 1961, The development of supersensitivity to norepinephrine after pretreatment with reserpine, *J. Pharmacol. Exp. Ther. 133:*41–51.

Fraser, H. F., and Isbell, H., 1952, Comparative effects of 20 mgm. of morphine sulfate on non-addicts and former morphine addicts, *J. Pharmacol. Exp. Ther. 105:*498–502.

Friedman, M. J., and Jaffe, H. J., 1969, A central hypothermic response to pilocarpine in the mouse, *J. Pharmacol. Exp. Ther. 167:*34–44.

Friedman, M. J., Jaffe, H. J., and Sharpless, S. K., 1969, Central nervous system supersensitivity to pilocarpine after withdrawal of chronically administered scopolamine, *J. Pharmacol. Exp. Ther. 167:*45–55.

Gaddum, J. H., and Picarelli, A. P., 1957, Two kinds of tryptamine receptors, *Brit. J. Pharmacol. Chemotherap. 12:*323–328.

Gebhart, G. F., Sherman, A., and Mitchell, C. L., 1971, The influence of learning on morphine analgesia and tolerance development in rats tested on the hot plate, *Psychopharmacol. 22:*295–304.

Gianutros, G., Hynes, M. D., Puri, S. K., Drawbaugh, R. B., and Lal, H., 1974, Effect of apomorphine and nigrostriatal lesions on aggression and striatal dopamine turnover during morphine withdrawal: Evidence for dopaminergic supersensitivity in protracted abstinence, *Psychopharmacol 34:*37–44.

Goldstein, A., and Goldstein, D. B., 1968, Enzyme expansion theory of drug tolerance and physical dependence, in *The Addictive States: Research Publications of the Association for Research in Nervous and Mental Disease,* Vol. 46 (A. Wikler, Ed.), pp. 265–267. Williams & Wilkins, Baltimore, Maryland.

Goldstein, D. B., and Goldstein, A., 1961, Possible role of enzyme inhibition and repression in drug tolerance and addiction, *Biochem. Pharmacol. 8:*48.

Gunne, L. M., 1962, Catecholamine metabolism in morphine withdrawal in the dog, *Nature 195:*815–816.

Gunne, L. M., 1963, Catecholamines and 5-hydroxytryptamine in morphine tolerance and withdrawal, *Acta Physiol. Scand. 58* (Suppl. 204):1–91.

Gunne, L. M., and Lewander, T., 1967, Long-term effects of some dependence-producing drugs on the brain monoamines, in *Molecular Basis of Some Aspects of Mental Activity,* Vol. 2 (O. Wallaas, Ed.), pp. 75–81. Academic Press, New York.

Hampel, C. W., 1935, The effect of denervation on the sensitivity to adrenine of the smooth muscle in the nictitating membrane of the cat, *Amer. J. Physiol. 111:*611–621.

Hayes, R. L., and Mayer, D. J., 1978, Morphine tolerance: Is there evidence for a conditioning model? *Science 200:*343–344.

Himmelsbach, C. K., 1941, Studies on the relation of drug addiction to the autonomic nervous system: Results of cold pressor tests, *J. Pharmacol. Exp. Ther. 73:*91–97.

Himmelsbach, C. K., 1942, Clinical studies on drug addiction: Physical dependence, withdrawal and recovery, *Arch. Intern. Med. 69:*766–772.

Himmelsbach, C. K., 1943, With reference to physical dependence, *Fed. Proc. 2:*201–203.

Jaffe, J. H., and Sharpless, S. K., 1965, The rapid development of physical dependence on barbiturates, *J. Pharmacol. Exp. Ther.* 150:140–145.

Jaffe, J. H., and Sharpless, S. K., 1968, Pharmacological denervation supersensitivity in the central nervous system: a theory of physical dependence, in *The Addictive States: Research Publications of the Association for Research in Nervous and Mental Disease*, Vol. 46 (A Wikler, Ed.), pp. 226–243. Williams & Wilkins, Baltimore, Maryland.

Jasinski, D. R., Martin, W. R., and Haertzen, C. A., 1967, The human pharmacology and abuse potential of N-allylnoroxymorphone (naloxone), *J. Pharmacol. Exp. Ther.* 157:420–426.

Jóhanneson, T., and Long, J. P., 1964, Acetylcholine in the brain of morphine tolerant and nontolerant rats, *Acta Pharmacol. Toxicol.* 21:192–196.

Kayan, S., Woods, L. A., and Mitchell, C. L., 1969, Experience as a factor in the development of tolerance to the analgesic effect of morphine, *Eur. J. Pharmacol.* 6:333–339.

Kornetsky, C., and Bain, G., 1967, Single dose tolerance to morphine, *The Pharmacologist* 9:219.

Kornetsky, C., and Bain, G., 1968, Morphine: Single-dose tolerance, *Science* 162:1011–1012.

Kuyer, A., and Wijsenbeek, I. A., 1913, Über Entgiftungserregung und Entgiftungshemmung, *Arch. Ges. Physiol.* 154:16–38.

Lieber, C. S., and DeCarli, L. M., 1968, Ethanol oxidation by hepatic microsomes: Adaptive increase after ethanol feeding, *Science* 162:917–918.

Loh, H. H., and Way, W. L., 1968, Brain serotonin turnover and tolerance development to morphine, *The Pharmacologist* 10:211.

Loh, H. H., Shen, F. H., and Way, E. L., 1969, Inhibition of morphine tolerance and physical dependence development and brain serotonin synthesis by cycloheximide, *Biochem. Pharmacol.* 18:2711–2721.

Martin, W. R., 1967, Opioid antagonists, *Pharmacol. Rev.* 19:463–521.

Martin, W. R., 1968, A homeostatic and redundancy theory of tolerance to and dependence on narcotic analgesics, in *The Addictive States: Research Publications of the Association for Research in Nervous and Mental Disease*, Vol. 46 (A. Wikler, Ed.), pp. 206–223. Williams & Wilkins, Baltimore, Maryland.

Martin, W. R., 1970, Pharmacological redundancy as an adaptive mechanism in the central nervous system, *Fed. Proc.* 29:13–18.

Martin, W. R., and Eades, C. G., 1967, Pharmacological studies of spinal cord adrenergic and cholinergic mechanisms and their relation to physical dependence on morphine, *Psychopharmacologia* 11:195–223.

Martin, W. R., and Jasinski, D. R., 1969, Physiological parameters of morphine dependence in man—Tolerance, early abstinence, protracted abstinence, *J. Psychiat. Res.* 7:9–17.

Martin, W. R., Wikler, A., Eades, C. G., and Pescor, F. T., 1963, Tolerance to and physical dependence on morphine in rats, *Psychopharmacologia* 4:247–260.

Martin, W. R., Jasinski, D. R., Sapira, J. D., Flanary, H. G., Kelly, O. A., Thompson, A. K., and Logan, C. R., 1968, The respiratory effects of morphine during a cycle of dependence, *J. Pharmacol. Exp. Ther.* 162:182–189.

Maynert, E. W., 1968, Catecholamine metabolism in the brain and adrenal medulla during addiction to morphine and in the early abstinence period, in *The Addictive States: Research Publications of the Association for Research in Nervous and Mental Disease*, Vol. 46 (A. Wikler, Ed.), pp. 89–95. Williams & Wilkins, Baltimore, Maryland.

Maynert, E. W., and Klingman, G. I., 1962, Tolerance to morphine. I. Effects on catecholamines in the brain and adrenal glands, *J. Pharmacol. Exp. Ther.* 135:285–295.

Maynert, E. W., Klingman, G. I., and Kaji, H. K., 1962, Tolerance to morphine. II. Lack of effects on brain 5-hydroxytryptamine and gamma-amino-butyric acid, *J. Pharmacol. Exp. Ther.* 135:296–299.

Nybäck, H., Borzecki, Z., and Sedvall, G., 1968, Accumulation and disappearance of catecholamines formed from tyrosine ^{14}C in mouse brain: Effect of some psychotropic drugs, *Europ. J. Pharmacol.* 4:395–403.

Paton, W. D. M., 1957, The action of morphine and related substances on contraction and on acetylcholine output of the coaxially stimulated guinea pig ileum, *Brit. J. Pharmacol. Chemotherap.* 12:119–127.

Paton, W. D. M., 1963, Cholinergic transmission and acetylcholine output, *Canad. J. Biochem. Physiol.* 41:2637–2653.

Pérez-Cruet, J., 1976, Conditioning or striatal dopamine metabolism with methadone, morphine or bulbocapnine as an unconditioned stimulus, *Pavlovian J. Biol. Sci.* 11:237–250.

Puri, S. K., and Lal, H., 1973, Effect of dopaminergic stimulation or blockade on morphine-withdrawal aggression, *Psychopharmacologia* 32:113–120.

Puri, S. K., Reddy, C., and Lal, H., 1973, Blockade of central dopaminergic receptors by morphine: Effect of haloperidol, apomorphine or benztropine, *Res. Comm. Chem. Path. Pharmacol.* 5:389–401.

Rosenman, S. J., and Smith, C. B., 1972, ^{14}C-catecholamine synthesis in mouse brain during morphine withdrawal, *Nature* 240:153–155.

Sakel, M., 1930, Theorie der Sucht, *Z. Ges. Neurol. Psychiat.* 129:639–646.

Sasme, H., Pérez-Cruet, J., DiChiara, G., Tagliamonte, A., Tagliamonte, P., and Gessa, G. L., 1972, Evidence that methadone blocks dopamine receptors in the brain, *J. Neurochem.* 19:1953–1957.

Schaumann, W., 1957, Inhibition by morphine of the release of acetylcholine from the intestine of the guinea pig, *Brit. J. Pharmacol. Chemotherap.* 12:115–118.

Seevers, M. H., and Deneau, G. A., 1961, A critique of the "dual action" hypothesis of morphine physical dependence, *Arch. Int. Pharmacodyn. Thérap.* 140:514–520.

Shoham, S., and Weinstock, M., 1974, The role of supersensitivity to acetylcholine in the production of tolerance to morphine in stimulated guinea-pig ileum, *Brit. J. Pharmacol.* 52:597–603.

Shuster, L., 1961, Repression and derepression of enzyme synthesis as a possible explanation of some aspects of drug action, *Nature* 189:314–315.

Siegel, S., 1975, Evidence from rats that morphine tolerance is a learned response, *J. Comp. Physiol. Psychol.* 89:498–506.

Siegel, S., 1976, Morphine analgesic tolerance: its situation specificity supports a Pavlovian conditioning model, *Science* 193:323–325.

Siegel, S., 1978, Morphine tolerance: Is there evidence for a conditioning model? *Science* 200:344–345.

Siegel, M. R., and Sisler, H. D., 1964, Site of action of cycloheximide in cells of *saccharomyces pastorianus*. II. The nature of inhibition of protein synthesis in a cell free system, *Biochem. Biophys. Acta* 87:83–89.

Sloan, J. W., and Eisenman, A. J., 1968, Long persisting changes in catecholamine metabolism following addiction and withdrawal from morphine, in *The Addictive States: Research Publications of the Association for Research in Nervous and Mental Disease,* Vol. 46 (A Wikler, Ed.), pp. 96–105. Williams & Wilkins, Baltimore, Maryland.

Sloan, J. W., Brooks, J. W., Eisenman, A. J., and Martin, W. R., 1963, The effect of addiction to and abstinence from morphine on rat tissue catecholamine and serotonin levels, *Psychopharmacologia* 4:261–270.

Smith, C. B., Villareal, J. E., Bednarczyk, J. H., and Sheldon, M. I., 1970, Tolerance to morphine-induced increases in (^{14}C) catecholamine synthesis in mouse brain, *Science* 170:1106–1108.

Smith, C. B., Sheldon, M. I., Bednarczyk, J. H., and Villareal, J. E., 1972, Morphine-induced increases in the incorporation of ^{14}C-tyrosine into ^{14}C-dopamine and ^{14}C-norepinephrine in the mouse brain: Antagonism by naloxone and tolerance, *J. Pharmacol. Exp. Ther.* 180:547–557.

Tatum, A. L., Seevers, M. H., and Collins, K. H., 1929, Morphine addiction and its physiological interpretation based on experimental evidences, *J. Pharmacol. Exp. Ther.* 36:447–475.

Way, E. L., Loh, H. H., and Shen, F. H., 1968, Morphine tolerance, physical dependence, and synthesis of brain 5-hydroxytryptamine, *Science* 162:1290–1292.

Weeks, J. R., 1962, Experimental morphine addiction: Method for automatic intravenous injections in unrestrained rats, *Science* 138:143.

Wikler, A., 1953, *Opiate Addiction: Psychological and Neurophysiological Aspects in Relation to Clinical Problems.* Charles C Thomas, Springfield, Illinois.

Wikler, A., 1972, Theories related to physical dependence, in *The Chemical and Biological Aspects of Drug Dependence* (S. J. Mulé and H. Brill, Eds.), pp. 359–377. Chemical Rubber Co. Press, Cleveland, Ohio.

Wikler, A., and Carter, R. L., 1953, Effects of single doses of N-allynormorphine on hindlimb reflexes of chronic spinal dogs during cycles of morphine addiction, *J. Pharmacol. Exp. Ther.* 109:92–101.

Wikler, A., and Frank, K., 1948, Hindlimb reflexes of chronic spinal dogs during cycles of addiction to morphine and methadone, *J. Pharmacol. Exp. Ther.* 94:382–400.

Wikler, A., and Rayport, M., 1954, Lower limb reflexes of a chronic "spinal" man in cycles of morphine and methadone addiction, *Arch. Neurol. Psychiat.* (Chicago) 71:160–170.

Yamamoto, I., Inoki, R., Tamari, Y., and Iwatsubo, K., 1967, Inhibitory effect of 8-azaguanine on the development of tolerance in the analgesic action of morphine, *Jap. J. Pharmacol.* 17:140–142.

CHAPTER 7

Conditioning Processes in Opioid Dependence and in Relapse

Although conditioning may play a role in the development of tolerance to opioids (see Chapter 6), this phenomenon and physical dependence are basically unconditioned; that is, they can be demonstrated in animal preparations virtually incapable of acquiring classically conditioned responses. Thus, Wikler and Frank (1948) reported the development of tolerance to the depressant effects of morphine and methadone on the flexor reflex in the chronic spinal dog, as well as well-defined abstinence syndromes after abrupt withdrawal of these drugs (hyperexcitability of the flexor reflex and spontaneous "running" movements of the paralyzed hind limbs). Earlier, Shurrager and Culler (1938, 1940) and Shurrager and Shurrager (1946) reported that a semitendinosus twitch could be conditioned in acute spinal preparations; Dykman and Shurrager (1956) also described spinal conditioning in chronic preparations. However, Kellogg et al. (1947) and Deese and Kellogg (1949) were unable to obtain spinal conditioning in recent chronic preparations. Reinvestigating this question, Lloyd et al. (1969) were unable to demonstrate classical conditioning of the flexor reflex in three drug-free chronic spinal dogs even after a maximum of 2500 conditioning and 500 test trials; they concluded that at least in the adult dog, classical conditioning of a skeletal motor response requires the functional integrity of supraspinal as well as intraspinal pathways. Hence, classical conditioning could have played no role in the development of tolerance to and physical dependence on morphine or methadone in chronic spinal dogs.

Wikler (1950) described in detail the behavior of two chronic decorticated dogs that survived 12 and 18 months after complete surgical removal of all neocortex (and portions of the archicortex, amygdalae, and thalami). Over many months, the decorticated dogs did display some rudimentary learning, such as backing out of corners, eating pig's liver from the center (only!) of a bowl into which their snouts were thrust, ceasing "obstinate progression," and ceasing to abrade their skin while perambulating along the periphery of a large, circular, linoleum-lined tub. In a Pavlovian conditioning chamber, no classical conditioned response (CR) was observed after about 1000 pairings of a conditioned stimulus (US) consisting of a light or tone (which evoked orienting responses) with an unconditioned stimulus (US) consisting of brief electric shocks to one hind limb, which always evoked an unconditioned response (UR), namely, flexion of the hind limb. However, after about 600 pairings of a tactile CS, consisting of 10 strokes of a comb over the lower back with the US, clear-cut CRs began to appear; these were extinguished by presenting the tactile CS repeatedly without the US and were promptly reinstated by renewed pairing of the CS with the US. It appears, therefore, that in these chronically decorticated dogs, the capacity to acquire classically conditioned responses was drastically reduced, though not completely eliminated. Yet in subsequent studies on cycles of addiction to morphine and methadone (Wikler, 1952b), both chronic decorticated dogs readily developed marked tolerance to the depressant effects of these opioids on "sham rage" and locomotor activity and exhibited striking abstinence syndromes after abrupt withdrawal of morphine or methadone (e.g., ceaseless locomotor activity followed by prostration, fever, and, in one, death).

Despite such evidence of the basic unconditioned nature of tolerance and physical dependence, the possibility remained that in the intact animal or man, opioid-abstinence phenomena and opioid-seeking behavior could become conditioned and thereby strongly dispose to relapse, given appropriate stimulus and reinforcement conditions. Hints that such a process occurs in human addicts were obtained in a long-term psychodynamic study of a postaddict during self-regulated readdiction to morphine, conducted in 1947 (Wikler, 1952a). Under the terms of the study, the subject was permitted to ask for and self-administer or have an aide administer any drug by any route, in any amount (up to a safe level), at any time of day or night, for an unspecified period of time, which, however, would not be less than one month; also the subject would be informed, one month in advance, of the termination of this agreement. In addition, the subject agreed to psychoanalytic-type interviews two or three times a week and occasional electroencephalograms during the entire study. It was stressed that the experimenter had no interest in the subject's getting himself "hooked," but if he should, the experimenter would be glad to advise the subject on how to withdraw himself from whatever drug he was taking with a minimum of discomfort. The subject assured the experimenter that he would not get hooked and elected to take 30 mg of morphine intravenously as his first dose. Two hours later, he took another 30-mg dose of morphine intravenously, and over the next three and one-half months, he took morphine by the intravenous route exclusively every day, gradually increasing the daily frequency and dose in stepwise fashion, attaining an average level of about 1100 mg/day in 12 divided doses just before the "one month's notice" date. After about 2 weeks at this daily morphine-dosage level, he asked for and was given advice on the methadone substitution and withdrawal method, which he adopted initially; however, 3 days before the termination of the study, he reverted to morphine intravenously, taking about 1000 mg of morphine (plus 30 mg of methadone) in divided doses during the last day, following which a rather severe but typical morphine-abstinence syndrome ensued. The self-regulated morphine (and methadone) daily dose schedule is shown graphically in Figure 2.

From the patient's "free associations," manifest dream content, and observation of his behavior during this study, a number of conclusions were drawn:

1. The "euphoric" effects of morphine (verbally in keeping with the Morphine-Benzedrine Group (MBG) scale items, though the "energized" patient spent most of his time "nodding" and "coasting" in bed) disappeared within a few days (except for the momentary "thrill" produced by the intravenous injection of morphine) and was replaced by a prevailing mood of dysphoria, which continued throughout the remainder of the study.

2. The major motivational variable for continuation of the self-administration of morphine was not fear of the withdrawal syndrome (the patient denied such fear and, in fact, elected to withdraw himself abruptly at the termination date of the study) but the gratification achieved through the suppression, by each dose of morphine, of the mild abstinence changes (perceived by the patient as a "need" or "craving") that ensued a few hours after the last previous dose; as the patient put it, "A steak tastes good any time, but if you are a little hungry, it tastes even better."

3. With the development of physical dependence, all other

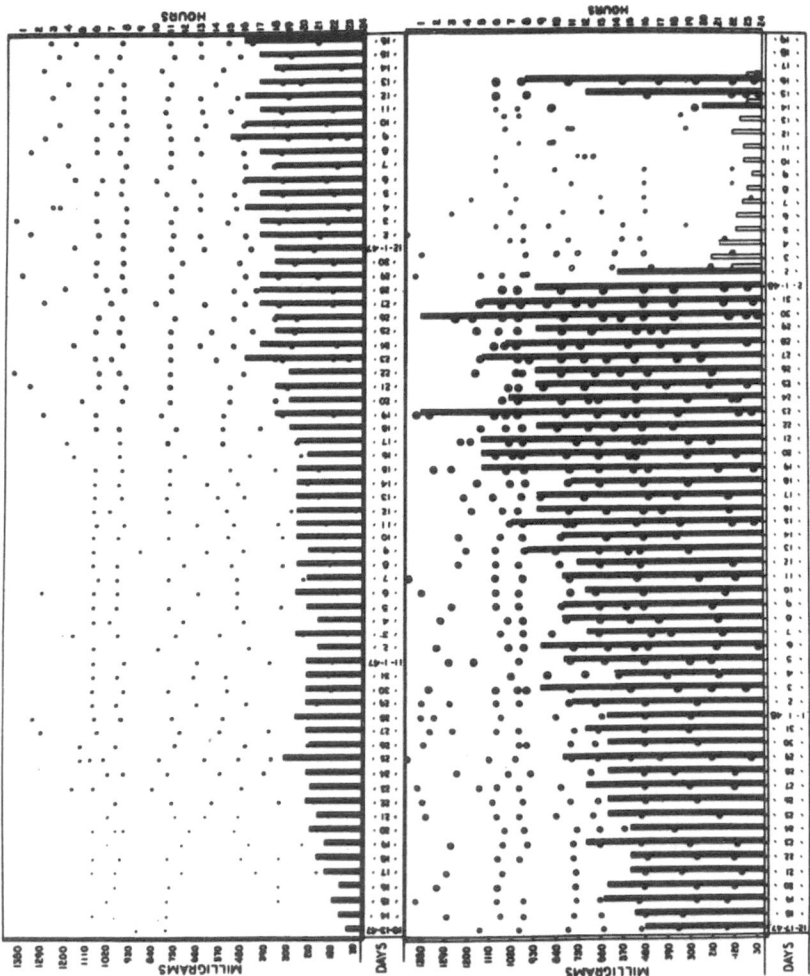

FIGURE 2. Self-regulated readdiction to morphine, 13 October 1947–16 February 1948. Subject No. 765. Left ordinate: mg of drug (morphine or methadone). Right ordinate: hour of day (24 hr, beginning at midnight). Abscissa: date. Bars: total daily amount of morphine (black) or methadone (outline). Dots: amount of each dose, size in proportion to dose, ranging from 30 mg to 115 mg. Reprinted with permission from Wikler (1952a).

motivational variables (family ties, interpersonal relations, work assignments) became subsidiary to and often conflictful with the overriding preoccupation with morphine self-administration, engendering feelings of guilt and resentment. Also, strongly suggested by the patient's recollections in free associations were that "hustling" (operant behavior directed toward obtaining drugs) was reinforcing in its own right (i.e., it brought about reinforcements in addition to the acqusition of drugs), and that episodes of relapse after "cure" in the past, attributed by the patient to unexplained "sickness" or feelings of "disgust" at times of chance encounters with other addicts may, in fact, have been due to evocation by the latter of conditioned abstinence phenomena. These conclusions furnished a basis for construction and testing of a conditioning theory of drug dependence and relapse in animals (see below).

OPERANT CONDITIONING
OF OPIOID-ACQUISITIVE BEHAVIOR

Whatever the reasons for self-administration of a drug may be, the term *operant conditioning* refers to the increase in probability of renewed drug self-administration if the effects of this response-contingent event are "rewarding." In man, the rewarding effects of a given drug may be inferred from the subject's verbal report ("good feeling," "high"). In animals, if it is observed that the probability of renewed drug self-administration has been increased, it is inferred that the effects of the drug are rewarding or, less anthropomorphically, reinforcing. In cases where the probability of renewed drug self-administration or other behavior has been decreased, the effects of the response-contingent event are said to be "punishing." Reinforcing effects of a drug are often qualified by the adjective, *positive*, to indicate positive pleasure, or by the adjective, *negative*, to indicate negative pleasure (relief from or avoidance of discomfort). In this usage, response-contingent opioid-euphoria is considered positive reinforcement (analogous to food-reinforcement after food-deprivation), while opioid-relief of opioid-abstinence phenomena is considered "negative reinforcement" (analogous to escape from, or avoidance of, electric shock). However, food-reinforcement after food-deprivation may be viewed as *escape* from hunger (negative reinforcement), and by manipulation of the history of schedules of reinforcement, electric shock can be used for positive reinforcement (see Chapter 2). Moreover, the terms "positive" and "negative" have also been used to refer to presentation or withholding of reinforcement (Pavlov, 1927). To avoid such ambiguities, Wikler *et al.* (1971) defined *appetitive reinforcement* as a response-contingent event that results in the subject's getting more of the reinforcer, and *aversive reinforcement* was defined as a response-contingent event that results in the subject's getting less of the reinforcer; "positive" or "negative" may be used to qualify either type of reinforcement to indicate whether the reinforcement was a consequence of presenting or withholding the reinforcer.

In a review of the literature, Schuster and Thompson (1969) cited numerous examples of rats and monkeys, equipped with intravenous cannulae for self-injection, which readily took and maintained themselves on morphine, amphetamines, cocaine, or pentobarbital. In such species (rats and monkeys), one cannot speak of "relapse," in view of the alacrity with which self-injection of these drugs is initiated by the previously drug-naive animal. Most drug-naive beagle dogs will not initiate self-injection of morphine (though they will initiate self-injection of amphetamines); however, Jones and Prada (1973) found that after inducing physical dependence by passive injection of morphine, all six beagle dogs in their study learned to maintain their addiction by intravenous self-injection of morphine, and one to six months following removal from the operant chamber and withdrawal of morphine, they all relapsed promptly to intravenous self-injection of morphine when they were replaced in the operant chamber.

In the rat (Weeks & Collins, 1968) and the monkey (Woods & Schuster, 1968; Deneau *et al.*, 1969), the reinforcing properties of morphine are manifested even in self-administered doses that are too small to produce physiological or behavioral signs of physical dependence. However, that the development of physical dependence can augment the process of operant conditioning and facilitate relapse has been demonstrated in numerous studies (Schuster & Villareal, 1968). Perhaps the earliest formulation of what would now be called *operant conditioning* in the genesis of relapse in man was expressed by Kolb (1939):

> The addict, even if he has sufficient narcotics, becomes uncomfortable several times a day when the last dose wears down. If another dose is not available, he suffers acute distress in about 18 hours. Over a period of years, he relieves such discomfort or distress thousands of times by injection of morphine. During the same period he enjoys the drug in pleasurable association with friends and by taking it to get the effect that many of them describe by the statement, "It makes my troubles roll off my mind." By thus building up a strong association between pleasure and pain and the taking of a narcotic he becomes conditioned to taking one in response to most any situation that may arise. (pp. 398–399)

Experimentally, the earliest demonstration of operant conditioning based on reduction of morphine-abstinence distress (physical dependence) was reported by Spragg (1940) in chimpanzees. Prior to passively induced morphine addiction, the chimpanzees solved rather complicated stick-and-box problems, the solution of which yielded access to food, and they scored poorly in the solution of similar problems that yielded access to a syringe containing morphine solution, which was subsequently administered to the animals by the investigator. However, when the drug was withheld after the chimpanzees had become tolerant to morphine, performance scores in the food-reinforced and morphine-reinforced problem-solving tasks were reversed. When morphine was withheld for a time sufficiently long to permit the appearance of well-marked abstinence signs (which resembled strikingly those seen in man), the chimpanzees assumed postures similar to those they assumed in receiving morphine injections. However, no evidence of relapse was noted: after permanent withdrawal of morphine and subsidence of the morphine-abstinence syndrome, behavior patters reverted to those of the preaddiction period.

In 1955, Headlee et al. reported that head turning in a particular direction could be reinforced in morphine-dependent and -abstinent rats by making intraperitoneal injections of morphine contingent on this operant. The interrelation of physical dependence and operant conditioning in facilitating relapse was demonstrated by Nichols et al. (1956), who found that physically dependent rats that had been forced (by prior fluid deprivation) to drink morphine solution (0.5 mg/ml) during acute morphine abstinence ingested more of the morphine solution in choice tests (morphine solution versus water) up to seven weeks following morphine withdrawal than rats that had not been forced to drink morphine solution while physically dependent and acutely abstinent, or had been forced to drink quinine or alum solutions, "equiaversive" to the morphine solution.

Beach (1957) trained physically dependent rats to run to the "preferred" goal box in a T-maze, where they remained one hour after receiving a saline injection, and to run to the "nonpreferred" goal box, where they remained one hour after receiving a morphine injection, both injections being given in another room after the rats had reached the preferred or the nonpreferred goal box. Choice trials (both alleys open) were run at intervals after the physically dependent rats had received an injection of morphine or of saline *prior* to the choice trial. In the choice trials, both the morphine- and the saline-preinjected groups developed a preference for the previously nonpreferred goal box ($p <$ 0.001). Beach concluded that not only "drive reduction" (suppression of morphine-abstinence phenomena) but also "euphoria" (continuing effect of morphine after suppression of abstinence had been achieved) reinforced morphine-seeking behavior. To test this hypothesis, Beach trained nondependent rats to run to the preferred goal box after saline injections, and to the nonpreferred goal box after single injections of morphine (insufficient to produce physical dependence). Comparisons of choice trials before and after training revealed that a significant preference had developed for the previously nonpreferred goal box, indicating that morphine euphoria alone was sufficient to reinforce morphine-seeking behavior. However, in a third series of experiments, choice trials were made *three weeks after termination of morphine injections* on three groups of rats, two of which had been addiction-trained (as in the first series of experiments described above), while the third had been only euphoria-trained (as in the second series of experiments). It was found that significant preference for the originally nonpreferred goal box was exhibited by the addiction-trained but not by the euphoria-trained rats. Therefore, Beach concluded that "in rats, the euphoric effects of morphine do not constitute reinforcement which makes for a durable habit, while drive-reduction effects do" (p. 110).

Kumar and Stolerman (1972) reported that even 110 days after enforced abstinence from morphine, previously morphine-dependent rats resumed oral self-administration of morphine solution. Originally, the morphine solution was aversive to these rats, but they had been operantly trained to drink it by a form of modified water deprivation, and they eventually became physically dependent.

The interrelations of physical dependence, operant conditioning, and environment were demonstrated by Thompson and Ostlund (1965). They found that rats made physically dependent on morphine by forced oral self-administration and retained in the "addiction" environment for 30 days after morphine was withdrawn ingested more morphine solution in choice tests (morphine versus water) conducted in the "addiction" environment than in a completely different environment. Likewise, physically dependent rats that were removed to a completely different environment for 30 days after morphine withdrawal ingested more morphine solution in choice tests conducted in the original addiction environment than in the different environment. It should be noted that operant conditioning (morphine reinforcement contingent on drinking the morphine solution) *while physically dependent* took place only in the addiction environment, which thereby acquired the properties of a conditioned (discriminative) stimulus for the drinking of the morphine solution.

With the intravenous self-injection technique that they originally developed, Weeks and Collins (1968) prepared five groups of rats: post-addict (morphine by self-injection, then abstinence from morphine for four weeks); morphine pretreated (morphine by passive injection, then abstinence from morphine for four weeks); water-conditioned (trained on lever pressing for water, then no lever presentations for four weeks); combined morphine pretreated plus training on lever pressing for water; and normal (naive, untreated, untrained). Upon replacement in the operant chambers where lever pressing produced intravenous morphine injections, the postaddict group and the group that had had combined morphine pretreatment plus training on lever pressing for water promptly resumed lever pressing at high and equal rates, while the water-conditioned, normal, and morphine pretreated groups responded at lower rates, in that descending order. In all groups except the morphine pretreated group, the average number of daily self-injections of morphine increased over the seven days of relapse testing. These investigators concluded that

> Prior exposure to morphine is only a minor factor in the etiology of relapse; a more important factor seems to be conditioning, established during active addiction by repeated incipient abstinence and its relief by lever-pressing for morphine. Then, when returned to the experimental cage with access to morphine, a powerful drive to press the lever is activated and this is reduced by morphine. (p. 297)

This conclusion is quite appropriate for the postaddict group, which had been operantly trained while presumably physically dependent, but it is difficult to understand how it applies to the group that had had combined morphine pretreatment plus training on lever pressing for water, which had not been operantly trained to suppress incipient morphine-abstinence phenomena.

Schuster and Woods (1968) investigated the efficacy of a secondary (conditioned) reinforcer in maintaining morphine-lever responding both during temporary acute morphine abstinence (first extinction) and 15 days after permanent withdrawal of morphine (second extinction), when, presumably, the acute morphine-abstinence syndrome had subsided. During this 15-day period, the animals were removed from the experimental situation to rest cages. In the experimental situation, the conditioned reinforcer was a red light plus saline for intravenous self-injection, which had acquired conditioned reinforcing properties through association of the red light with morphine for intravenous self-injection in physically dependent monkeys. During the first extinction period (acute morphine abstinence), morphine-lever responding for the red light plus saline was much higher than morphine-lever responding which had no programmed consequences for the first 5–7 days of such extinction. During the second extinction period (15 days after permanent withdrawal of morphine) morphine-lever responding for the red light plus saline exceeded morphine-lever responding that had no programmed consequences over the first 5 days of extinction. These investigators argued that the conditioned reinforcing properties of red light plus saline had been acquired during the initial period of self-injection of morphine, which was accompanied by the red light, not through association with suppression of morphine abstinence but through association with an independent reinforcing action of morphine. This hypothesis may account for the short duration of "relapse" to the conditioned reinforcer.

That conditioned reinforcers may be established through repeated temporal contiguity with primary morphine reinforcement in rats that presumably are not physically dependent was demonstrated by Davis and Smith (1974, 1976). Rats with intravenous catheters were shaped to self-inject morphine sulfate for 4 days in doses per infusion of 60 μg/kg by pressing a lever; each morphine self-injection was accompanied by a buzzer contingent on the lever press. Changing the morphine solution to saline and removing the buzzer resulted in extinction of responding. Reinstating the buzzer resulted in a large increase in responding for the saline solution, indicating that the buzzer had acquired secondary (conditioned) reinforcing properties. Varying the infusion doses of morphine from 3.2 to 320 μg/kg during the acquisition of morphine self-injection (accompanied by the buzzer) and subsequently testing responding to the buzzer plus self-injection of saline showed that the strength of the secondary (conditioned) reinforcer (total lever-press responses) varied directly with the dosage of the primary reinforcer. Substituting normal saline solution for the morphine solution while retaining presentation of the buzzer with each lever press resulted in extinction of lever pressing over a period of 3 days. Substituting normal saline for morphine without the buzzer also resulted in extinction of lever pressing over a period of 2–3 days; however, reinstating the buzzer now restored lever pressing (for saline) to quite high levels on the first day, with eventual extinction by the third day. Exactly the same results were obtained when, instead of substituting normal saline for morphine, the rats continued to self-inject morphine, but in extinction trials (with and without the buzzer present), they were pretreated with the narcotic antagonist naloxone (25 mg/kg subcutaneously): if such extinction was carried out with the buzzer removed, then lever-press responding reappeared when the buzzer was reinstated; such restored responding rapidly extinguished. These experiments have direct relevance to therapeutic problems in extinguishing opioid-acquisitive behavior in addicts: if extinction (e.g., under narcotic antagonist blockade) is carried out in the absence of conditioned reinforcers (other addicts; drug-related paraphernalia), then opioid-acquisitive behavior is likely to recur in the presence of such conditioned reinforcers; extinction of opioid-acquisitive behavior should be carried out in the presence of the conditioned reinforcers. Davis and Smith (1976) further showed that passive, subcutaneous injections of morphine sulfate (5 mg/kg) could restore lever-press responding for saline in the presence of the buzzer after such responding had been extinguished by substituting saline for morphine. Similar results were obtained when d-amphetamine (2 mg/kg), a different primary reinforcer, was given subcutaneously instead of morphine (5 mg/kg), and analagous data were obtained when the primary reinforcing agent was d-amphetamine (50 μg/kg/infusion) and, after saline-extinction in the presence of the buzzer, morphine (5 mg/kg) was given subcutaneously. Interestingly, such restored lever-press responding (for saline, in the presence of the buzzer) was higher than that seen previously for the primary reinforcer (morphine or d-amphetamine) and did not extinguish by the last extinction trial (third day). These data indicate that in addition to the therapeutic extinction of drug-seeking behavior in the presence of exteroceptive conditioned reinforcers, extinction should be carried out in the presence of the interoceptive stimuli produced by the primary reinforcer. Conceivably, such interoceptive stimuli could have acquired secondary (conditioned) reinforcing properties of their own; in the experiments of Davis and Smith, subcutaneous injection of the primary reinforcer restored lever pressing for saline to some extent in the absence of the buzzer, though such restored lever pressing extinguished over a 3-day period.

It should be noted that in the extinction procedures of Davis and Smith (1974, 1976), initial increase in responding did not occur (i.e., rats that had acquired high rates of lever pressing for intravenous self-administration of morphine decreased their lever-pressing rates immediately and progressively when normal saline was substituted for morphine in the infusion system); the same was true when, instead of substituting saline for morphine, the rats were pretreated with the narcotic antagonist naloxone. Carnathan et al. (1977) observed identical phenomena but concluded that their rats did not extinguish but decreased responding because morphine was not "available." This conclusion is ambiguous because operationally, experimental extinction is defined as the change in strength of a conditioned response consequent on omission of a previously effective reinforcer (e.g., by substitution of saline for morphine); the "nonavailability" of morphine is a subjective (anthropomorphic) interpretation of the fact of extinction. Apparently, initial increase in responding is not a *sine qua non* of experimental extinction.

CLASSICAL CONDITIONING OF THE OPIOID AGONIST-ABSTINENCE CYCLE AND INTEROCEPTIVE CONDITIONING OF OPIOID-SEEKING BEHAVIOR

In studies on operant conditioning, attention is focused on environmentally directed behavior, the reliable consequence of which is some "reward" or "punishment." Concomitantly, however, autonomic (and probably motor) responses are classically conditioned to the same environmental stimuli or components thereof (Shapiro, 1960). If the critical reinforcing event in both operant and classical conditioning is regarded as the delayed activation of rewarding or punishing centers in the limbic system, then both types of conditioning may be regarded as varieties of classical (Pavlovian) conditioning, as Stein (1964) has suggested:

> Pairing an operant response with reward may be viewed as an instance of Pavlovian conditioning. Response-related stimuli (environmental as well as internal) are the conditioned stimulus and reward is the unconditioned stimulus. By virtue of the pairing, the medial forebrain "go" mechanism is conditioned to response related stimuli. Thus, on future occasions, any tendency to engage in the previously rewarded behavior initiates facilitatory feedback by activation of the "go" mechanism and thereby increases the probability that the response will go off to completion. In the case of punishment, periventricular activity is conditioned to stimuli associated with the punished operant. This decreases the probability that the operant will be emitted in the future because feedback from the "stop" mechanism will tend to inhibit the behavior. (p. 94)

From another point of view, classically conditioned reflex autonomic and motor responses together with delayed activation of rewarding and punishing centers in the limbic system may be regarded as "emotions" creating a problem that the organism attempts to solve by conditioned operant responding. Therefore, investigation of classically conditioned reflex autonomic and motor responses produced by single doses of opioids and during the development of tolerance and physical dependence is of central importance in the study of the genesis of addiction and relapse.

Classical conditioning of morphine salivation (also, in some experiments, vomiting and sleep) in dogs appears to have been first reported by Collins and Tatum (1925) and by Kleitman and Crisler (1927), though it is mentioned by Pavlov (1927) that "quite recently" this phenomenon had been observed by Krylov. Levitt (1964) reported that morphine sleep could be classically conditioned in dogs, but not in rats. Discussing these and many other studies on classical conditioning of single-dose effects of drugs other than opioids, Wikler (1948, 1973) concluded that what becomes classically conditioned are unconditioned central reflex ("adaptive") responses to the initial drug–receptor combinations in cells of the *afferent* arms of neural circuits that include not only the afferent arm but also central processing and peripheral effector arms. Thus, in the case of morphine, salivation and vomiting are reflex responses to the initial morphine– receptor combination in cells of the medullary chemoreceptor trigger zone; morphine sleep is a reflex mediated through central processing and centrifugal pathways in response to the initial morphine–receptor combination in cells of the ascending (centripetal) reticular activating system. At first, atropine produces drying of the mouth by blockade of cholinergic receptors peripherally in the salivary glands, but on chronic administration, classically conditioned salivation and mydriasis occur, which appear to be a conditional physiological adaptation mediated through a central sympathetic reflex with efferent alpha and beta adrenergic pathways (Korol *et al.*, 1966).

Kun and Horvath (1947) reported that oral administration of saccharin to human subjects produced a significant *fall* in blood sugar concentration; they suggested that this phenomenon is due to the sweet taste, which may act as a reflex mechanism to induce insulin secretion. More formally, hypoglycemic response to saccharin may be regarded as a second-order classically conditioned adaptive (reflex) response to its taste, similar to that of sugars, which, through a lifetime of conditioning, have come to evoke insulin secretion, an adaptive (reflex) response to postprandial hyperglycemia.

In line with this concept of the "adaptive" nature of classically conditioned reflexes, one would expect that the classically conditioned response to repeated injections of insulin would be (conditioned) *hyperglycemia*. However, the data are conflicting. Woods *et al.* (1968) reported that insulin-induced *hypoglycemia* could be conditioned to a complex conditional stimulus in rats. On the other hand, Siegel (1972, 1975) found that repeated intraperitoneal injections of insulin in rats reliably produced hypoglycemia as an unconditioned response, but subsequently, when saline was substituted for insulin, the classically conditioned response was *hyperglycemia*, which extinguished on successive daily intraperitoneal injections of saline over the next three days.

The unconditioned opioid-abstinence syndrome (indicative of physical dependence) may be regarded as a further unconditional coun-teradaptation to the adaptive responses evoked by the initial effects of opioids, that is, the opioid–receptor combinations in the afferent arms of central reflex circuits. Therefore, classically conditioned responses in the opioid-tolerant and physically dependent addict are likely to differ from those in the nontolerant, nonphysically dependent individual. In the tolerant and physically dependent addict, the agonistic effects of an opioid (e.g., morphine or heroin) are greatly attenuated (because of tolerance) and are followed, within a number of hours, by morphine- or heroin-abstinence phenomena, which increase in intensity with time and are suppressed by the next dose of the opioid, if it is obtained. This cycle of events (attenuated opioid-agonistic effects followed by pro-gressively increasing opioid-abstinence phenomena, or the reverse se-quence) occurs repeatedly in the environment in which the physically dependent addict "hustles" for and self-administers his opioids. In con-sequence, this cycle of events comes to be elicited as a classically con-ditioned response to the drug environment, which now has become a conditioned stimulus.

In 1948, Wikler proposed a theory that holds that, in part, relapse after "cure" (detoxification) is due to evocation by drug-related con-ditioned stimuli (home environment of the "street addict," encounters with other addicts and "pushers") of fragments of the opioid-abstinence syndrome as a classically conditioned response that has *not* been extin-guished by mere removal of the addict from his drug environment to a jail or a hospital and withdrawal of the opioid drug. Operant condition-ing (hustling for opioids) also becomes conditioned to the drug envi-ronment (Wikler, 1961) and is likewise not extinguished by removal of the addict to a jail or a hospital and detoxification. This concept of the role of conditioning factors in opioid addiction and relapse has been schematized most recently as shown in Figure 3.

In support of this concept are statements made by addicts who had long been detoxified that on returning to their home environment, they felt sick, craved a fix, and immediately hustled for heroin. Some former addicts described the "sickness" in more detail: running nose, watery eyes, sweating, chills, nausea, and vomiting—"like the flu, Doc." One former addict, a physician, remarked that the sickness resembled heroin-abstinence phenomena, but he dismissed that interpretation as preposterous. On two separate occasions, psychiatrists at the Lexington hospital related that in group therapy with long detoxified addicts, the patients would suddenly blow their noses, wipe their eyes, and yawn incessantly when the subject under discussion turned to dope. The psy-chiatrists, unaware of the conditioning theory of relapse, were puzzled

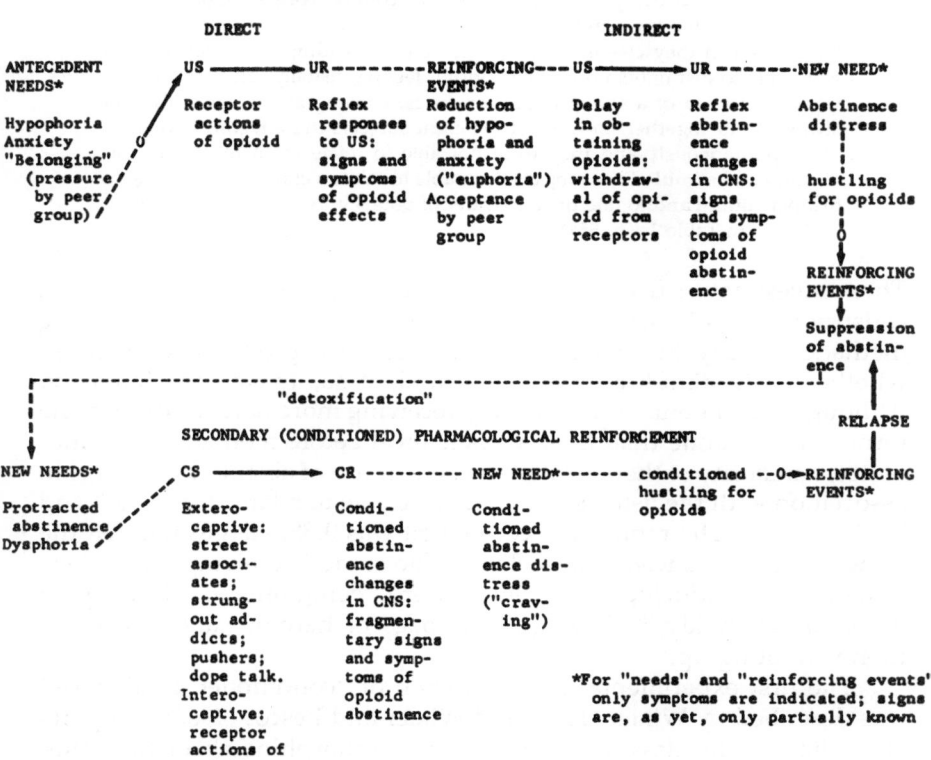

FIGURE 3. Conditioning theory of opioid addiction and relapse. O = self-administration of an opioid (e.g., heroin). US = unconditioned stimulus. UR = unconditioned response. CS = conditioned stimulus. CR = conditioned response. The events under "Secondary (conditioned) pharmacological reinforcement" are generated in street addicts during "Primary pharmacological reinforcement" (unconditioned) but are depicted separately as they continue to operate after the opioid has been withdrawn when the former street addict returns to his drug-infested environment, thereby leading to relapse. Reprinted with permission from Wikler (1975).

by the reappearance of opioid-abstinence phenomena three to six months after detoxification. Likewise, Teasdale (1973) reported that scores on the Addiction Research Center Opiate Withdrawal Scale were significantly higher in former narcotic addicts after visual presentation of opioid-related slides than after neutral slides. O'Brien (1976) interviewed eight former heroin addicts who had been drug-free for 2–15 months:

All subjects described periodic episodes of discomfort consisting of tightness in the throat, tearing, yawning, rhinorrhea, abdominal pain, back pain, or nausea which they classified under the general heading of "sickness." All were able to distinguish this from another feeling, usually called "craving," which consisted of a strong desire for drugs. Craving and sickness did not always occur together. In three of the eight subjects these feelings occurred only spontaneously and they were not able to relate them to specific environmental stimuli. Five subjects were able to relate sickness and craving to distinct stimuli and to rate them in order of potency. A representative rating is shown in Table 1. (p. 534)

These investigators used the stimuli reported by the drug-free addicts to construct a questionnaire that they submitted to 100 patients receiving methadone daily in a methadone maintenance program to ascertain whether such stimuli affected them and, if so, to rate the intensity. Although the patients were probably receiving more narcotic drug in the form of methadone than their average level before methadone maintenance, a majority of them related the occurrence of abstinence feelings in association with the listed stimuli; 62 were able to relate "sickness," and 58, "craving". The rank-order correlation was 0.88, suggesting that the same stimuli produced both feelings. The stimuli receiving the highest rankings for producing both feelings were "Being offered a taste by an old copping buddy," "Seeing a few bags of heroin," and "Seeing a friend shooting up."

The first experimental demonstration of "conditioned abstinence" was described by Wikler (1965) and Wikler and Pescor (1967) in reports of studies on the classical conditioning of a morphine-abstinence phe-

TABLE 1. Hierarchy of Stimuli Provoking "Sickness" and/or "Craving"[a]

Patient No. 5

1. Being offered a "taste" by an old copping buddy.
2. Seeing a friend in the act of "shooting up."
3. Talking about drugs on copping corner.
4. Standing on copping corner.
5. Seeing a successful pusher—making lots of money, envy.
6. Socially awkward situations: job interview, family criticism, feeling like an outsider at a party.
7. Talking about drugs in group therapy.
8. Seeing a few bags of heroin.
9. Seeing someone's "works."
10. Seeing pictures of drugs and "works."
11. Seeing antidrug poster with "good veins" and somebody "shooting up."

[a] Ranked from most potent down to least potent. From O'Brien (1976).

nomenon, reinforcement of opioid-drinking behavior, and "relapse" in morphine-addicted rats. Basic to these studies are earlier ones on the characteristics of tolerance to and physical dependence on morphine in rats (Martin et al., 1963) and on factors regulating oral consumption of an opioid (etonitazene) by morphine-addicted rats (Wikler et al., 1960, 1963).

In the studies of Martin et al. (1963), white, male albino Wistar rats were experimentally addicted to morphine given intraperitoneally over a period of 42 days, beginning with 5 mg/kg twice daily and increasing the dose twice a week until the rats were receiving 320 mg/kg/day (in two divided doses) by the 35th day; the rats were stabilized at this dose level for another week, and then morphine was withdrawn abruptly. Another group of rats, which served as controls, received normal saline (0.9% aqueous solution of sodium chloride) intraperitoneally at the same times and the same volumes as the rats receiving morphine. Throughout the entire study, food (Purina Chow bars) and tap water were available ad libitum in the home cages. The most striking difference between nontolerant and morphine-tolerant rats was their responses to a large dose of morphine. In the nontolerant rat, 100 mg/kg of morphine (intraperitoneally) produced cyanosis (not necessarily associated with decrease in respiratory rate) and almost total absence of spontaneous activity, together with slight depression of body (colonic) temperature and metabolic rate. In rats receiving morphine chronically to levels of 80 or 320 mg/kg/day, single doses of morphine (100 or 140 mg/kg) produced a marked increase in body temperature and metabolic rate and, after a short initial period of inactivity, a marked increase in activity, with much standing, walking, circling, exploring, and gnawing of the paw pads. On abrupt withdrawal of morphine, abstinence phenomena proceeded in two phases: an early (or acute, or primary) abstinence syndrome lasting about 72 hr, followed by a protracted (or chronic, or secondary) abstinence syndrome qualitatively different in several respects and of lower intensity, which continued for at least 6 months. The first detectable sign of early abstinence was an increase in frequency of "wet-dog" shakes (so-called because of their resemblance to a dog shaking water off its back (Wikler et al., 1960). These were accompanied by obviously increased frequency of head shakes, which, however, were too fast to count. In normal rats, the average frequency of wet-dog shakes measured under standard conditions (i.e., removal from the home cage; weighing; placement in individual tall, wide cylindrical glass observation jars; and counting the number of wet-dog shakes during the first 15 min) is less than one. In rats under the influence of single or chronic doses of morphine, wet-dog shakes are almost never seen. The striking increase in wet-dog shakes in morphine-addicted rats following abrupt withdrawal of morphine became apparent at about the twelfth hour of abstinence. From the sixteenth to the twenty-fourth hours, the early morphine-abstinence syndrome became almost fully developed. In addition to further increase in wet-dog shakes, tap-water intake dropped to subnormal levels; body (colonic) temperature and metabolic rate fell to normal or subnormal levels; spontaneous activity changed to much scratching, preening, and licking or gnawing of the nails and the tail; and most strikingly, the rats in early morphine abstinence showed a decreased tendency to sleep: they remained in a sitting posture with their heads up during the entire hour of observation in the cylindrical glass jar, instead of eventually going to sleep after an initial period of exploration, as normal rats do. In addition, the rats in early morphine abstinence showed more soft stools and urine and more hostility than normal rats, and they lost a significant amount of weight (maximal at 48 and 72 hr of abstinence). As the early morphine-abstinence syndrome subsided, the protracted abstinence syndrome emerged. The abstinent rats began to gain weight rapidly, body temperature and metabolic rate became considerably elevated, and water consumption was approximately 30% above that of the control rats. Activity and wet-dog shakes, after subsiding to the levels in the control rats during the first week of abstinence, rose again slightly but not significantly above control levels and remained elevated for 4–6 months.

Roffman *et al.* (1973) reported that like morphine itself, a conditional stimulus (bell) paired with each intraperitoneal injection of morphine (four times daily, increasing gradually from 10 mg/kg to 200 mg/kg) could *prevent* the hypothermia that followed abrupt withdrawal of morphine for 72 hr. This conditioned effect of the bell could be *blocked* by injection of naloxone (2 mg/kg) given 10 min after the bell (Drawbaugh & Lal, 1974), a phenomenon suggesting that morphine produces its central effects through release of endogenous opioid peptides; if this is so, then the bell would exert its effects through conditioned release of endogenous opioid peptides (reversing withdrawal hypothermia), and naloxone would block such reversal by displacing endogenous opioid peptides from opioid receptors (Lal *et al.*, 1976).

In the studies of Wikler *et al.* (1960, 1963), very dilute solutions of etoniazene were investigated as possible oral reinforcers for morphine-abstinent rats *without prior water deprivation*, which would avoid the complications in interpretation of results introduced by the initial water deprivation required to force rats to drink dilute solutions of morphine. Etonitazene is a benzimidazole derivative with morphinelike properties, which subcutaneously is about 1000 times as potent as morphine for analgesia in the rat (Gross & Turrian, 1957; Hunger *et al.*, 1957; CIBA Pharmaceutical Co., Ltd., 1958). In man, Fraser *et al.* (1960) found that etonitazene was effective orally, 1 mg by this route being equivalent to about 60 mg of morphine subcutaneously in suppressing morphine abstinence in physically dependent addicts. It then occurred to Wikler and his collaborators (Wikler *et al.*, 1960) that without prior water deprivation, rats might drink a very dilute aqueous solution of etonitazene that was yet sufficiently potent to produce morphinelike effects rapidly. As a first guess, an aqueous solution of 5 μg/ml (the taste threshold of one of the investigators) was tried in water-deprived normal rats; they drank the 5-μg/ml solution avidly, and within 3 min, exophthalmos, tail rigidity, and quick, jerky, darting movements of the rats were noted. Then non-water-deprived normal rats were tested for consumption of water from 4:00 P.M. to 8:00 A.M. one day, and consumption of etonitazene (5 μg/ml) from 4:00 P.M. to 8:00 A.M. the subsequent day in single-tube drinking tests (note: rats being nocturnally active animals, eat and drink far more during the night than in an equivalent period during the daytime). No significant difference was found between water and etonitazene consumption under these conditions (when the order of water and etonitazene availability was reversed— that is, etonitazene, 5 μg/ml, the first day and the water the next day— the consumption of water was far less than that of etonitazene, indicating a prolonged pharmacological effect of etonitazene on water drinking). From these data it was concluded that for *normal* rats, etonitazene (5 μg/ml) is neither *appetitively nor aversively reinforcing.* In contrast, rats 7–24 hr abstinent from morphine (stabilization dose, 200 mg/kg, given intraperitoneally once daily at 7:30 A.M.) consumed significantly *less* water than normal rats when only water was available for drinking, but significantly *more* etonitazene (5 μg/ml) than normal rats (drinking water) when only etonitazene was available for drinking. From these data, it was concluded that etonitazene (5 μg/ml) was *appetitively reinforcing for rats in early morphine abstinence;* that is, in such rats, orally ingested etonitazene increased the probability of continuing to drink the etonitazene solution. The physiological basis of such reinforcement was revealed in measurements of wet-dog shakes, body (colonic) temperature, and metabolic rate: such consumption of etonitazene (5 μg/ml) ameliorated signs of morphine abstinence other than decreased water intake, namely, increased frequency of wet-dog shakes, hypothermia, and fall in metabolic rate; however, the morphine-abstinent rats still showed soft stools and wallowed in their urine. When the concentration of etonitazene was increased to 10 μg/ml, rats in early morphine abstinence also drank the etonitazene solution in volumes significantly greater than normal rats (drinking water), and such drinking completely abolished all morphine-abstinence phenomena without producing observable signs of opioid intoxication. When the concentration of etonitazene was increased to 20 or 40 μg/ml, rats in early morphine abstinence drank volumes of etonitazene that were not significantly different from those of normal rats drinking water, but such drinking of etonitazene produced signs of opioid intoxication: elevated body temperature and metabolic rate (compared to normal rats) and exophthalmos, tail rigidity, and quick, darting movements. The patterns of fluid consumption and physiological changes (body temperature and metabolic rate) as functions of drinking water and 5, 10, 30, and 40 μg/ml of etonitazene in early morphine-abstinent rats compared to normal rats drinking water only are shown, respectively, in Figures 4 and 5.

The data obtained by Martin *et al* (1963) and by Wikler *et al.* (1960, 1963) were utilized in designing a series of studies on conditioning factors in opioid addiction and relapse. In all these studies, male, albino Wistar rats were given intraperitoneal injections of morphine beginning with 5 mg/kg twice daily, the dosage being increased at intervals until,

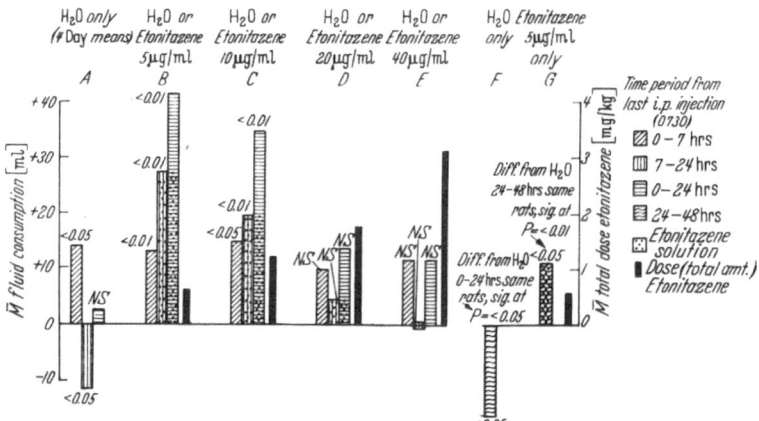

FIGURE 4. Mean *differences* in consumption of fluids between morphine-tolerant and physically dependent rats receiving 200 mg/kg of morphine intraperitoneally at 7:30 A.M. and control rats receiving normal saline intraperitoneally at 7:30 *A.M.* at various times from the last injection (0–7 hr, 7–24 hr, 0–24 hr, and 24–48 hr) when the drinking fluids offered were water for both morphine-addicted and control rats (A,F) or etonitazene (5, 10, 20, or 40 μg/ml) for morphine-addicted and water for control rats (B, C, D, E, and G). Left ordinate: mean volumes of fluid consumption (ml). Right ordinate: mean total dose of etonitazene (mg/kg) for morphine-addicted rats. *P* values indicated above or below bars were derived from *t* tests for independent groups (A–E) or for replicate comparisons (F, G). Reprinted with permission from Wikler *et al.* (1963).

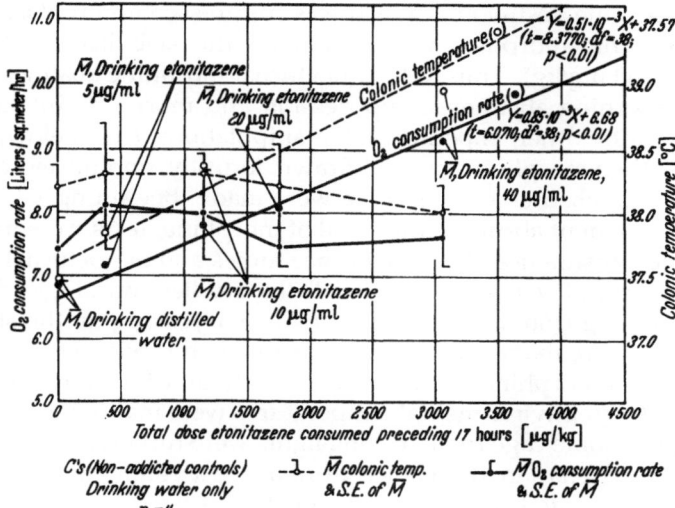

FIGURE 5. Regression lines for oxygen consumption (heavy, continuous) and colonic temperature (heavy, dashed) as functions of total amounts of etonitazene consumed during preceding 17 hr by addicted rats 24 hr abstinent from morphine, 200 mg/kg given intraperitoneally at 7:30 A.M.; the points plotted (with standard errors of the means) are for such morphine-addicted rats drinking 5, 10, 20, and 40 μg/ml of etonitazene (large dots for oxygen consumption and large circles for colonic temperature). Also plotted are corresponding means of concurrently observed control rats drinking water only, 24 hr after last previous intraperitoneal injection of normal saline, indicated by smaller dots for oxygen consumption and smaller circles for colonic temperature (both with standard errors of the means), connected, respectively, by lighter continuous and lighter dashed lines. Left ordinate: oxygen consumption (liters/square meter/hour). Right ordinate: colonic temperature (°C). Abscissa: total dose of etonitazene (μg/kg) consumed during preceding 17 hr (morphine-addicted rats only). Reprinted with permission from Wikler *et al.* (1963).

after about 4 weeks, it reached 100 mg/kg twice daily; then, over the next 2 weeks, the morning dose was increased and the afternoon dose was decreased until the rats were receiving 200 mg/kg/day given in a *single* dose each morning at about 8:00 A.M., after which they were maintained on this dose schedule ("stabilization level") for variable periods, depending on other features of the experimental design. While on the stabilization level of morphine, the rats exhibited signs of chronic morphine intoxication for about 7 hr following the injection of morphine at 8:00 A.M.; then, after about 12 hr following the morning injection, they began to exhibit signs of the early morphine-abstinence syndrome (increased frequency of wet-dog shakes, decreased water intake, hypothermia), which increased progressively in intensity until the 24th hour of morphine abstinence, which was suppressed and replaced with signs of chronic morphine intoxication by the stabilization dose of morphine (200 mg/kg). This cycle of nocturnal morphine abstinence followed by morning abstinence suppression and morphine intoxication continued until other experimental manipulations (see below) were completed; then morphine was withdrawn abruptly, and measurements of the terminal abstinence syndrome were made. Beginning 1–2 weeks after the permanent abrupt withdrawal of morphine, tests were made of "conditioned abstinence" in some of the studies and of nocturnal choice in the drinking of various fluids in all the studies, on single days at intervals ranging from about 6 weeks to over 1 year. In all the studies, comparisons were made with control rats that had received saline injections instead of morphine on the same time schedule but were otherwise treated similarly. Environmental temperatures were maintained at about 23.3°C. In the home cage room, ceiling lights were turned on at 8:00 A.M. and off at 4:00 P.M. In the choice drinking-test room, dim overhead lighting was provided throughout the nocturnal testing period.

In the first studies on conditioning and relapse, rats "stabilized" on 200 mg/kg of morphine given intraperitoneally at 8:00 A.M. each morning (M group) and rats receiving saline injections on the same schedule (S group) were transferred from their individual home cages to individual "linear mazes" (73.7 × 17.8 × 17.8 cm) constructed of solid metal (except for hardware cloth floors and removable tops), which were permanently divided into three equal compartments by two transverse portals (7.6 × 7.6 cm), either or both of which could be closed completely by insertion of solid metal panels. Over a 2-week period, measures were made of total daily distilled-water consumption from two 100-ml graduated glass drinking tubes placed respectively in the end compartments with both transverse portals open, and food (Purina Chow bars) was always available in both end compartments. These measurements served to establish the preferred end compartment for each rat. For 6 weeks thereafter, the procedure was as follows. On Mondays, Wednesdays, and Fridays, the drinking tubes in both end compartments contained distilled water from 8:00 A.M. to 2:00 P.M., and each rat had free access to both end compartments during that time; from 2:00 P.M. to 7:30 A.M., the drinking tube in the preferred end compartment still contained distilled water, and access to the nonpreferred end compartment was barred by shutting the portal to it at 2:00 P.M. On Saturdays, all rats had access only to the preferred end compartment (distilled water) from 8:00 P.M. to 7:30 A.M., and on Sundays, from 8:00 A.M. to 8:00 P.M. On Tuesdays and Thursdays, all rats had free access to both end compartments (distilled water) from 8:00 A.M. to 8:00 P.M.; on these days and also on Sundays, access to the preferred end compartment was barred from 8:00 P.M. to 7:30 A.M. by shutting the portal to it at 8:00 P.M., leaving free access to the nonpreferred end compartment or (on Sundays) providing such free access by opening the portal to it. In the nonpreferred end compartment, from 8:00 P.M. to 7:30 A.M., the distilled water in the drinking tube was flavored by passing it through a filter on which a few drops of anise oil had been placed; for half the rats in the M group, the anise-flavored distilled water also contained etonitazine, 10 μg/ml (MFET, or morphine-addicted, flavored etonitazene-trained subgroup), while for half the rats in the S group, the concentration of etonitazene was 5 μg/ml (SFET, or saline control, flavored etonitazene-trained subgroup) for the other half of the M group (MFPT, or morphine-addicted flavor pseudotrained subgroup) and the half of the S group (SFPT, or saline control flavor pseudotrained subgroup), the drinking tube in the nonpreferred end compartment contained only anise-flavored distilled water from 8:00 P.M. to 7:30 A.M. For other details, see Wikler and Pescor (1967). This 6-week training procedure provided repeated opportunities for classical conditioning of morphine abstinence phenomena to the preferred end compartment, where all rats had resided during unrelieved nocturnal morphine abstinence from 2:00 P.M. to 7:30 A.M. (only distilled water available for drinking), and for operant conditioning of opioid-seeking behavior to the nonpreferred end compartment, where the MFET and SFET subgroups had anise-flavored etonitazene for drinking (presumably, such operant conditioning would be much stronger in the MFET than in the SFET subgroup because etonitazene drinking suppresses morphine-abstinence phenomena only in the former); for the MFPT and SFPT subgroups, no such operant conditioning would be expected, as in other experiments anise-flavored distilled water had no reinforcing effects.

After completion of the 6-week training period, morphine (and saline) injections were abruptly discontinued, and all rats were transferred to their home cages. Frequency of wet-dog shakes was selected as an easily quantifiable morphine-abstinence phenomenon, the classical conditioning of which could be tested by comparing the frequency of wet-dog shakes in the home cage, where the rats resided permanently after morphine withdrawal, and in the preferred end compartment of the linear maze, to which they had been confined during unrelieved morphine abstinence from 2:00 P.M. to 7:30 A.M. on repeated occasions. The first "relapse" test was conducted in this study 9 days after abrupt withdrawal of morphine (or saline) and subsequently at intervals of 2 or more weeks. On each relapse test, the procedures were as follows. At 8:00 A.M., wet-dog-shake frequency counts were made in two ways for each rat: after removing from the home cage, weighing, and replacing in the home cage, and after removing from the home cage, weighing and placing in the preferred end compartment of the linear maze (portal to the nonpreferred end compartment closed). Within each subgroup, the order of home-cage and linear-maze wet-dog counts was reversed for successive rats. After completion of wet-dog counting, those rats remaining in their home cages were also transferred to the preferred end compartments of the linear mazes (portals to the nonpreferred end compartments closed), and all rats stayed there (with food and distilled water *ad libitum*) until 8:00 P.M. At 8:00 P.M., a drinking tube containing anise-flavored etonitazene (5 μg/ml) was placed in the nonpreferred end compartment of the linear maze for each rat (all subgroups), and the portal to that compartment was also opened, permitting the rat the choice of drinking distilled water or anise-flavored etonitazene (5 μg/ml) until 8:00 A.M. the next morning, after which all the rats were returned to their home cages. After the seventh relapse test (94th day after withdrawal of morphine) procedures for "etonitazene extinction" followed by "etonitazene and anise-flavor extinction" were carried out by substituting anise-flavored water for anise-flavored etonitazene for several days, and then distilled water for anise-flavored water in the nonpreferred end compartments for 21 days (distilled water always in the preferred end compartment) and allowing the rat the free choice of drinking from the tube in either end compartment continuously, 24 hr each day. Tests for etonitazene extinction and for etonitazene plus anise-flavor extinction were interpolated before, during, and after these extinction procedures in exactly the same manner as in the relapse tests. The last relapse test was conducted 142 days after the withdrawal of morphine, with the choice of drinking distilled water in the originally preferred end compartment and the anise-flavored etonitazene (5 μg/ml) in the originally nonpreferred end compartment. In addition, wet-dog-shake frequencies were measured in the home cages and in the originally preferred end compartment of the linear mazes on the 145th, 148th, and 155th days after the withdrawal of morphine, as in the relapse tests.

The results for both formerly morphine-addicted groups (combined) and both saline control groups (combined) are shown graphically in Figures 6 and 7. At 24 and 48 hr after abrupt withdrawal of morphine (early morphine-abstinence syndrome), wet-dog-shake frequencies were higher in the preferred end compartment of the linear maze (24 hr abstinent) and in the home cage (48 hr abstinent) in the previously morphine-addicted subgroups (MFET and MFPT) than in the previously saline-injected subgroups (SFET and SFPT). Over the period 9–72 days after morphine withdrawal (Figure 6, relapse tests I–V), the higher

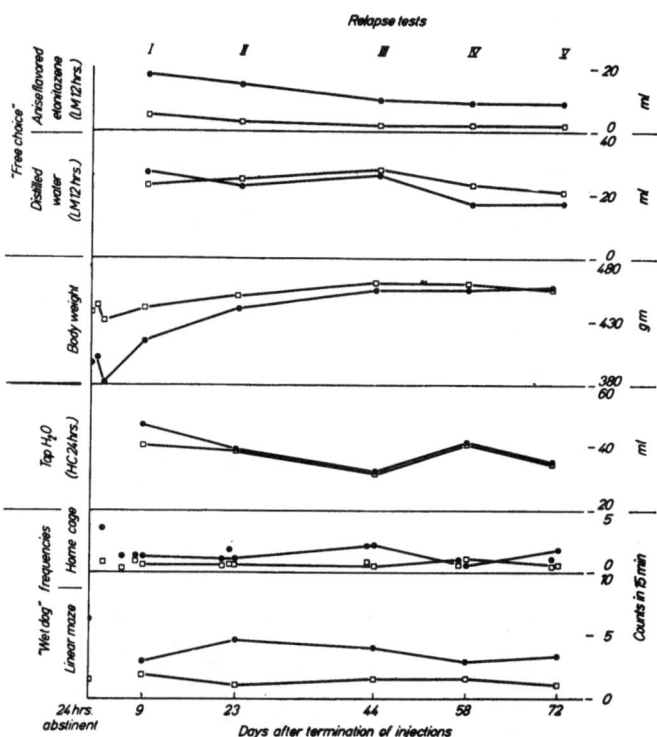

FIGURE 6. Behavior of formerly morphine-addicted and saline control rats on five "relapse" tests conducted 9, 23, 44, 58, and 72 days after termination of morphine or saline injections with regard to choice of drinking distilled water (preferred end compartment) or anise-flavored etonitazene, 5 μg/ml (nonpreferred end compartment), body weight, 24-hr consumption of tap water in home cage, and wet-dog-shake frequencies in linear maze (classical conditioning environment) or in home cage. (●) formerly morphine-addicted rats (groups MFET and MFPT combined, see text); (□) saline control rats (groups SFET and SFPT combined, see text). Reprinted with permission from Wikler and Pescor (1967).

wet-dog-shake frequencies in the previously morphine-addicted subgroups compared with the previously saline-injected subgroups were much more prominent and consistent in the linear maze than in the home cage. Thereafter, 85–155 days after morphine withdrawal (Figure 7, relapse tests VI–VIII), these differences persisted, though less consistently. Analysis of variance (Table 2) showed that wet-dog-shake frequencies (home cage and linear maze) were significantly greater for the previously morphine-addicted than for the previously saline-injected subgroups on relapse tests II, III, and V and on the mean of 12 tests 84–155 days after withdrawal of morphine; wet-dog-shake frequencies

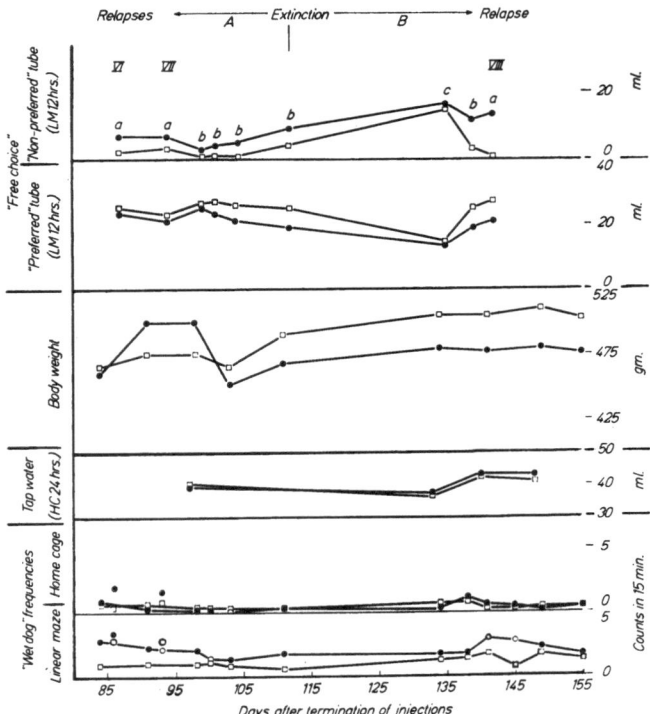

FIGURE 7. Behavior of formerly morphine-addicted and saline control rats after termination of morphine or saline injections, continued. "Relapse" tests VI, VII, and VIII, consisting of choice of drinking distilled water (preferred end compartment) or anise-flavored etonitazene, 5 μg/ml (nonpreferred end compartment), denoted by the symbol "a" were conducted 87, 94, and 142 days, respectively, after termination of morphine or saline injections. "A" and "B" denote the periods of etonitazene extinction and etonitazene-plus-anise-flavor extinction, respectively; the symbol "b" denotes choice drinking tests of water versus anise-flavored water, and "c" of water versus water. Circled points on wet-dog frequency graphs refer to counts made 24 hr after forced drinking of anise-flavored etonitazene (5 μg/ml) for 12 hr on two occasions between the 85th and 95th days after termination of injections. See legend for Figure 6 and text for explanation of animal groups. Reprinted with permission from Wikler and Pescor (1967).

were higher in the linear maze than in the home cage (all subgroups combined) on all tests, 9–155 days after morphine withdrawal; and the interaction, previously morphine-addicted versus previously saline-injected × linear maze versus home cage was significant on relapse II, IV, and the mean of 12 tests 84–155 days after withdrawal of morphine. These results indicate that given repeated temporal contiguities between a specific environment and the occurrence of early morphine-abstinence

TABLE 2. Analysis of Variance (Mixed Type) for "Wet Dog" Shake Frequencies after Termination of Injections[a]

Relapse test no.	I		II		III		I'		V		Mean of 12 tests	
Days after end of injections	9		23		44		58		72		84–155	
Source	df	MS	df	MS	df	MS	df	MS	df	MS	df	MS
M vs. S	1	11.69	1	48.17[b]	1	51.40[c]	1	2.47	1	37.50[c]	1	3.58[b]
Error, between subjects	23	4.93	23	6.22	23	6.47	23	5.36	22	4.21	22	0.65
Between subjects	24	5.21	24	7.97	24	8.34	24	5.24	23	5.66	23	0.78
Within subjects	25	2.70	25	5.30	25	2.32	25	2.70	24	2.00	24	0.99
LM vs. HC	1	19.22[c]	1	40.50[c]	1	18.02[c]	1	16.82[c]	1	10.29[b]	1	14.46[c]
Interaction (M vs. S × LM vs. HC)	1	0.15	1	26.88[c]	1	1.15	1	8.51[b]	1	3.82	1	2.86[c]
Error (LM vs. HC × subjects)	23	2.09	23	2.83	23	1.69	23	1.83	22	1.54	22	0.30
Total	49	3.93	49	6.61	49	5.27	49	3.94	47	3.79	47	0.89

[a] From Wikler & Pescor (1967).
M = rats previously injected with morphine ("trained," MFET, + "pseudotrained," MFPT).
S = rats previously injected with saline ("trained," SFET, + "pseudotrained," SFPT).
LM = linear maze. HC = home cage.
[b] $p < 0.05$.
[c] $p < 0.01$.

phenomena, the latter can become classically conditioned to the former, and that "conditioned abstinence" can be evoked by that specific environment for 155 days after morphine withdrawal, at least in the rat.

Free-choice consumption of distilled water (preferred end compartment) and of anise-flavored etonitazene, 5 µg/ml (nonpreferred end compartment) by the previously morphine-addicted subgroups (MFET and MFPT) and the previously saline-injected subgroups (SFET and SFPT) on all relapse tests are shown in Figures 6, 7, 8, and 9. The mean volumes of distilled water consumed by the previously morphine-addicted and the previously saline-injected subgroups were not different, or the previously morphine-addicted subgroups drank somewhat less. In contrast, the previously morphine-addicted subgroups consumed greater volumes of etonitazene (5 µg/ml) than the previously saline-injected subgroups in all relapse tests (I–VIII, 9–142 days after morphine withdrawal). By the Mann–Whitney U test (Table 3) the mean percentage of total fluids (distilled water plus etonitazene, 5 µg/ml) consumed in the form of etonitazene (5 µg/ml) was significantly greater in the previously morphine-addicted subgroups than in the previously

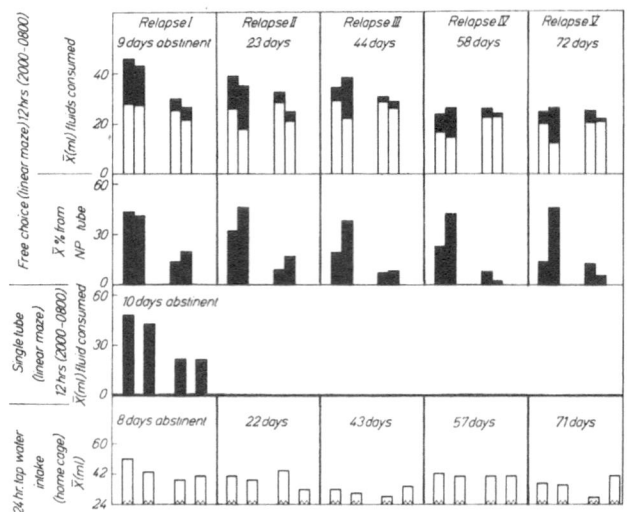

FIGURE 8. Drinking behavior of individual subgroups of rats 9–72 days after termination of morphine or saline injections. In all quartets of bar graphs, data are shown for subgroups in the following order (left to right): MFET, MFPT, SFET, SFPT (see text for explanations of animal subgroups). Fluids available in free-choice tests were as specified in legend for Figures 6 and 7 on corresponding days after termination of injections. (■) anise-flavored etonitazene (5 µg/ml); (□) water. Reprinted with permission from Wikler and Pescor (1967).

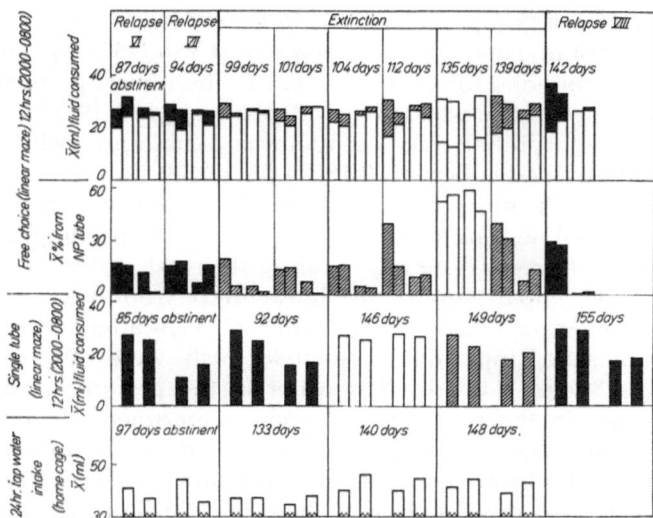

FIGURE 9. Drinking behavior of individual subgroups of rats 87–142 days after termination of morphine or saline injections. See legend for Figure 8 for explanation of sequence of animal subgroups in bar graphs, of fluids available in free-choice tests, and of the symbols thereof; also, (▨) anise-flavored water. Reprinted with permission from Wikler and Pescor (1967).

TABLE 3. Drinking Behavior of Rats in "Free Choice" Relapse Tests[a]

	Mean percentage total fluids (water + anise-flavored etonitazene, $5 \mu g/ml$) ingested in form of anise-flavored etonitazene, $5 \mu g/ml$							
"Relapse" test no.	I	II	III	IV	V	VI	VII	VIII[b]
Days after termination of injections	9	23	44	58	72	87	94	142
Groups: MFET + MFPT[c]	40.5	38.4	24.1	31.5	28.2	17.1	16.9	29.2
SFET + SFPT[d]	16.2	12.9	7.3	5.2	8.7	6.7	10.9	1.0
Mann–Whitney U test	34.5[e]	28.5[f]	38.5[e]	33.5[f]	48.0	35.0	45.0	18.0[f]

[a] From Wikler and Pescor (1967).
[b] After successive etonitazene and anise-flavor extinction periods.
[c] $N = 11$ on all relapse tests.
[d] $N = 14$ on relapse tests I–IV, 13 on V, 12 on VI and VII, and 11 on VIII. See Table 2 and text for explanation of groups.
[e] $p < 0.05$.
[f] $p < 0.02$.

saline-injected subgroups on relapse tests I–IV (9–58 days after withdrawal of morphine) and again on relapse test VIII (142 days after withdrawal of morphine). However, contrary to theoretical prediction, this difference was better sustained in relapse tests I–V (9–72 days after withdrawal of morphine) in the pseudotrained subgroup (MFPT) than in the operantly trained subgroup (MFET) (Figure 8). In a separate anise-flavor control study, morphine-addicted (200 mg/kg in a single dose each morning) and saline-injected (saline injection each morning) rats were pseudotrained (forced drinking of anise-flavored water in the non-preferred end compartment of the linear maze from 8:00 P.M. to 8:00 A.M. on repeated occasions); then 9 and 23 days after termination of morphine or saline injections, free-choice tests were conducted from 8:00 P.M. to 8 A.M. with distilled water in the preferred, and anise-flavored water in the nonpreferred end compartment. In these free-choice tests, the previously saline-injected rats drank about half of their total fluids in the form of anise-flavored water, while the previously morphine-addicted rats drank only about one-third of their total fluids in the form of anise-flavored water in both tests. These results indicate that anise flavor *per se* has no appetitive or aversive reinforcing properties for normal rats, but it may be mildly aversive for postaddict rats (though insufficient to counteract the relative reinforcing effects of etonitazene, if added to the anise-flavored water). This finding does not explain the less-sustained increased consumption of anise-flavored etonitazene (5 μg/ml) in the MFET than in the MFPT subgroup compared with those of the SFET and SFPT subgroups in relapse tests I–V (see above); nevertheless, the anise-flavor discriminative cue could have introduced an aversive factor in the training of morphine-addicted rats that revealed itself in relapse testing after morphine was withdrawn.

Therefore, the study was repeated (Wikler and Pescor, 1967, Study 2), eliminating the anise-flavor discriminative cue entirely and substituting untrained for the pseudotrained rats. Provision of cues for discriminating the drinking tube containing etonitazene (5 μg/ml) from that containing distilled water in the linear mazes was accomplished by painting the inner walls of one end compartment black and fitting it with a graduated glass drinking tube outside, the spout of which protruded inside; the inner walls of the other end compartment were painted white, as was a strip of corrugated aluminum fixed to the floor extending from the portal to a smooth metal ramp leading to a metal spout inside, which was connected with a graduated glass drinking tube outside. The middle compartment was fitted with a large custard bowl containing tap water. Food (Purina Chow bars) were freely available in all three compartments at all times. For each trained rat, assignment of etonitazene (5

μg/ml) to one end compartment and of distilled water to the other end compartment was made permanently according to a table of random numbers. Trained rats consisted of two groups: MT, addicted to morphine, 200 mg/kg per day given in a single dose each morning at 8:00 A.M., and ST, saline-injected, on the same time schedule. MT and ST rats were confined to the middle compartment (portals to both end compartments closed) throughout the training period except on training nights (8:00 P.M. to 8:00 A.M.), when they were confined to one or the other end compartment (thus providing repeated opportunities for classical conditioning of nocturnal morphine abstinence in the end compartment with only distilled water available and of operant conditioning of opioid drinking behavior in the end compartment with etonitazene 5 μg/ml, available). After abrupt withdrawal of morphine (and saline), the MT and ST groups were removed to their home cages, and relapse testing was conducted exactly as in the first study, except that the free choice in drinking was between distilled water and etonitazene, 5 μg/ml (anise flavor replaced by visual–tactile discriminative cues). Untrained rats were likewise of two groups: MU, addicted to morphine, 200 mg/kg per day given in a single dose each morning at 8:00 A.M., and SU, saline-injected, on the same time schedule. MU and SU groups resided in their home cages without any training while receiving morphine or saline injections. After abrupt withdrawal of morphine or saline, relapse testing was conducted exactly as in the MT and ST groups, assignment ˙of etonitazene (5 μg/ml) to one end compartment and of distilled water to the other end compartment being made permanently for each rat according to a table of random numbers.

Analysis of variance of wet-dog-shake frequencies on relapse tests I–VIII (9–142 days after withdrawal of morphine or saline) revealed that the critical interaction, "previous addiction × abstinence place (linear maze for MT and home cage for MU)," was significant on relapse tests I–III (9–44 days after withdrawal of morphine), thus confirming the results of the first study, indicating that conditioned abstinence can be evoked by environmental stimuli that are temporally contiguous with the occurrence of morphine abstinence on repeated occasions, long after withdrawal of morphine. Likewise consistent with the results of the first study were the free-choice drinking patterns of the various groups in the relapse tests. Although in these tests, MT and MU consumed about the same volumes of distilled water as ST and SU, each of the postaddict groups drank much more of the etonitazene solution than their respective normal controls, and for MT versus ST, their difference was significant on every relapse test through the 142nd day after withdrawal of morphine or saline (for MU versus SU, this was true on relapse tests II and III, 23 and 44 days after withdrawal of morphine, and by a one-tailed test only on relapse tests IV–VIII combined, 58–142 days after withdrawal of morphine.) However, in regard to mean percentage of total fluids consumed in the form of etonitazene (5 μg/ml) there was no significant difference between MT and MU on any of the relapse tests. It appears, therefore, that postaddict rats relapse, regardless of whether or not they have been operantly trained, although in the second study, there was some evidence that operant training increased the degree of relapse (MT versus ST, compared with MU versus SU).

The duration of the relapse tendency of untrained postaddict rats was investigated further by Wikler and Pescor (1970). As in the previous studies, one group (M) was addicted to morphine (stabilization level, 200 mg/kg per day, given intraperitoneally in a single dose at 8:00 A.M. each morning), while another group (S) received normal saline injection on the same time schedule. All rats were housed in individual home cages with food and water plentifully available. After 4 months, morphine and saline injections were terminated abruptly. On each of the first 5 postinjection days, measurements on all rats included body weight, 24-hr tap-water consumption, and wet-dog-shake frequency counts. At intervals of 1 or more weeks following the first 5-day post-injection period, all of these measurements were repeated, and in addition, relapse tests were conducted in the following manner. From 8:00 P.M. on the day after measurement of 24-hr tap-water consumption and wet-dog-shake frequency in the home cage until 8:00 A.M. the next morning, each rat was placed in a narrow corridor between apposing cages, the inside of one of which was painted black, and the other, white. Access to both cages was then furnished simultaneously by removal of the apposing, sliding walls. Each half of the double cage thus formed contained Purina Chow bars in plentiful amounts and a graduated glass drinking tube, the spout of which protruded inside the wall opposite to the entrance. One of these tubes contained etonitazene (5 μg/ml) and the other, distilled water. Prior to the first relapse test, the half-cage (black or white) provided with the etonitazene tube was assigned to a given rat according to a sequence of random numbers applied to each group (M or S), and this assignment was retained for each rat throughout all the relapse tests, which continued for more than one year. The relapse-testing cages were located in a laboratory room separate from that housing the home cages. In both rooms, environmental temperature was maintained at about 23.3°C, and ceiling lights were turned on at 8:00 A.M. and off at 4:00 P.M.; in the relapse-testing room, dim overhead lighting was provided throughout the testing period (8:00 P.M. to 8:00 A.M.). After completion of each free-choice drinking period, the volumes of fluid consumed (etonitazene, 5 μg/ml, and distilled water) were measured, and all rats were returned to their home cages.

The results of the relapse tests are summarized in Table 4. The mean volumes of distilled water consumed by postaddict (M) and normal (S) rats did not differ significantly on any of the relapse tests, but the mean volume of etonitazene (5 μg/ml) consumed by the M group was significantly greater than that consumed by the S group on every relapse test for about a year (p value of the difference, M $-$ S, < 0.05 on relapse test VIII, 336 days after termination of morphine and saline injection, NS on relapse test IX, 372 days, and again < 0.05 on relapse test X, 406 days). Although the differences in consumption of distilled water were nonsignificant, it is interesting to note that on the first six relapse tests (7–140 days after termination of injections), the M group consumed slightly less water than the S group, and slightly more water thereafter. Computation of the data in terms of percentage of total fluids (etonitazene, 5 μg/ml, plus distilled water) consumed in the form of etonitazene in each relapse test also revealed that the relapse tendency of the M group lasted approximately one year.

One conceivable explanation of the apparent, long-persisting tendency of untrained postaddict rats to relapse is the possible persistence of the protracted morphine-abstinence syndrome, implying a derange-

TABLE 4. Drinking Behavior of Untrained Postaddict (M) and Normal (S) Rats in 12-Hr (8:00 P.M. to 8:00 A.M.) Free Choice (Etonitazene, 5 μg/ml versus Distilled Water) Relapse Tests[a]

		N		Etonitazene			Water		
Test no.	Days after termination of injections (morphine or saline)	M	S	Diff. M $-$ S (ml)	t	p $<$	Diff. M $-$ S (ml)	t	p
I	7	11	11	34.4	3.376	.01	−4.2	0.386	NS
II	14	11	11	35.7	4.223	.01	−5.5	0.590	NS
III	23	11	11	38.5	3.907	.01	−10.5	0.871	NS
IV	71	11	11	18.7	2.803	.02	−3.0	0.382	NS
V	92	11	11	9.8	2.215	.05	−2.0	0.291	NS
VI	140	11	11	11.6	2.657	.05	−5.1	0.540	NS
VII	161	11	11	10.9	2.911	.02	6.7	0.883	NS
VIII	336	11	11	10.2	2.312	.05	1.7	0.281	NS
IX	372	10	10	2.4	1.175	NS	9.7	1.563	NS
X	406	10	10	4.5	2.374	.05	4.3	0.595	NS
XI	434	10	9	1.7	0.982	NS	5.4	0.814	NS

[a] From Wikler and Pescor (1970).

ment of physiological homeostasis. However, measurements of body weight, 24-hr consumption of tap water, and wet-dog-shake frequencies lent support to such an explanation only for the first 23 days after the termination of morphine and saline injections. Thus, on relapse tests I–III (7–23 days abstinent), the mean 24-hr tap-water intake of the M group was 59.2 ml and that of the S group 35.9 ml, the difference being significant at the $p < 0.01$ level, while the mean (unconditioned) wet-dog frequency count of the M group was 0.6 and that of the S group 0.0, the difference being significant at the $p < 0.05$ level by a one-tailed test; the difference in mean body weight (M, 512 g; S, 503 g) was nonsignificant. On relapse tests IV–VII (71–336 days abstinent), neither the differences in mean 24-hr tap-water consumption nor the differences in wet-dog-shake frequency was significant; however, the mean body weight of the M group (637 g) was significantly greater than that of the S group (565 g) at the $p < 0.05$ level.

Another conceivable explanation that has not been formally investigated is the persistence of residual cross-tolerance of postaddict rats to etonitazene, in view of the long persistence of tolerance to morphine in rats that had received single or multiple injections of this drug (Cochin & Kornetsky, 1964).

However, a third possible explanation, which has been investigated, is that of *interoceptive conditioning*. Thus, in all the studies on relapse to etonitazene, the experimental rats, trained or untrained, had been previously stabilized on morphine, 200 mg/kg per day given intraperitoneally in a single dose each morning; hence, they were morphine-abstinent each night, and this morphine abstinence was suppressed by the scheduled dose of morphine the next morning; and the cycle of morphine abstinence and its suppression was continued daily for several weeks before injections of morphine were abruptly terminated. It may be presumed that while the rats were stabilized on morphine (200 mg/kg per day), the first effects of each morning injection of morphine were the interoceptive sensorial effects of this drug on such receptors as the medullary chemoreceptor trigger zone, the aortic body, and the thermoregulatory centers, as well as the interoceptive sensorial effects of feedback impulses from smooth muscles directly affected by morphine. Occurring coincidentally with or shortly after such interoceptive sensorial effects were those central actions of morphine that are responsible for the dramatic suppression of morphine-abstinence syndrome (certainly a "rewarding" effect), thus providing an ideal condition for acquisition of secondary (conditioned) reinforcing properties by the interoceptive sensorial effects of morphine, regardless of whether or not the morphine-addicted rats are operantly conditioned by the experimenter. After abrupt the termination of morphine injection, the secondary (conditioned) reinforcer is withheld for a week or so, but in subsequent relapse tests, it is provided again in the form of etonitazene solution, which, after absorption from the gut, has the same interoceptive sensorial effects as morphine given intraperitoneally. Ingesting a few milliliters of the etonitazene solution by chance in the first relapse test, the postaddict rat, trained or untrained, is likely to continue to drink the etonitazene solution because of its secondary (conditioned) reinforcing properties, whereas the normal rat is not. Provision of gustatory–olfactory (anise flavor) or visual–tactile cues for the etonitazene solution and for water facilitates choice learning in subsequent relapse tests. One might expect that extinction would supervene eventually (as indeed it does) in the absence of conditions such as physical dependence that would allow etonitazene to act as a primary (unconditioned) reinforcer. If the morphine-abstinence syndrome had been classically conditioned to the environment in which relapse testing is conducted, then conditioned abstinence may provide the basis for etonitazene to act as a primary (unconditioned) reinforcer and thus explain the long persistence of relapse tendencies in such rats. However, such an explanation cannot hold for untrained rats that had not been subjected to classical conditioning of the morphine-abstinence syndrome to the relapse-testing environment; in these rats, etonitazene must act as a secondary (conditioned) reinforcer, and the long persistence of its reinforcing properties is, to say the least, remarkable.

The long-persisting potency of a pharmacologically inert interoceptively conditioned secondary reinforcer following withdrawal of morphine from physically dependent rats was demonstrated by Wikler et al. (1971). In that study, two groups of rats, one maintained on 200 mg/kg of morphine given intraperitoneally in a single dose at 8:00 A.M. each morning, and another receiving saline injections intraperitoneally on the same time schedule, were transferred from their home cages to individual training–testing cages on nine nights (8:00 P.M. to 8:00 A.M.) during the last 25 days of morphine or saline injection. In the training–testing cages, one subgroup of the morphine-addicted and one subgroup of the saline-injected rats had only anise-flavored etonitazene (5 μg/ml) to drink, while the other subgroup of morphine-addicted and the other subgroup of saline-injected rats had only anise-flavored water to drink. Thus, theoretically, anise flavor (a pharmacologically inert, *exteroceptive*, gustatory–olfactory discriminative stimulus) could acquire *interoceptively* conditioned secondary reinforcing properties only in the morphine-addicted (and, from 8:00 P.M. to 8:00 A.M., morphine-abstinent) subgroups to which anise-flavored etonitazene (5 μg/ml) was

provided for drinking. One day after completion of the nine conditioning trials, morphine and saline injections were terminated abruptly (all
rats in their home cages). The next morning, the 24-hr morphine-
abstinence syndrome was measured (compared with the normal rats,
the postaddict rats had significantly elevated mean wet-dog-shake frequencies, $p < 0.001$, and significant falls in colonic temperature, $p <$
0.001). Beginning on the third day after termination of morphine and
saline injections, nocturnal (8:00 P.M. to 8:00 A.M.) choice drinking tests
were made on all rats in their individual training–testing cycles on 18
occasions at variable intervals through the 287th postinjection day. In
these choice drinking tests, two graduated glass drinking tubes, identical with those used in the conditioning trials, were placed in each cage,
one containing *anise-flavored water* and the other, *plain water* (position
reversed from one testing trial to the next). Analysis of variance revealed
that the postaddict subgroup that had had anise-flavored etonitazene to
drink during the conditioning trials consumed significantly greater volumes of *anise-flavored water* in the testing trials than any of the other
three subgroups for the first 137 days after termination of morphine and
saline injections, whereas there were no significant differences among
the four subgroups with respect to consumption of *plain water*, confirming the theoretical prediction. Thus, it was shown that an *exteroceptive,*
pharmacologically inert substance (anise flavor) could acquire long-
persisting secondary reinforcing properties through *interoceptive* conditioning.

However, a definitive investigation remained to be done to test the
hypothesis that *interoceptive* actions of morphine could similarly acquire
long-persisting, interoceptively conditioned secondary reinforcing properties at the same time that it acts as a primary (unconditioned) reinforcer in cyclically morphine-intoxicated and morphine-abstinent rats.
This study (Dougherty *et al.*, 1979; Miller *et al.*, 1979) involved three
groups of rats, all provided with permanent intravenous catheters for
administration of morphine or saline:

1. *Infusion* rats, which received morphine by continuous intravenous infusion, 24 hr each day, 7 days each week, in gradually increasing
daily doses to a maintenance level of 200 mg/kg/day, at which they were
maintained for 2–3 weeks before morphine was withdrawn abruptly;
until the terminal withdrawal of morphine, these rats were *never abstinent* from morphine, and hence the hypothesized interoceptive conditioning should not take place.

2. *Injection* rats, receiving continuous intravenous infusion of saline
24 hr a day, 7 days a week, and in addition, morphine by injection
through the intravenous catheter in gradually increasing daily doses to

200 mg/kg given in a single injection at 10 A.M., on which they were maintained for 2–3 weeks before morphine was withdrawn abruptly; before the terminal withdrawal of morphine, such rats were *morphine-abstinent each night, and this morphine abstinence was suppressed by the scheduled intravenous injection of morphine at 10 A.M. the next morning;* hence, the hypothesized interoceptive conditioning should occur.

3. *Saline* rats, which received normal saline solution by continuous intravenous infusion, 24 hr each day, 7 days each week, for the same number of weeks as the infusion and injection rats before intravenous saline was withdrawn abruptly. It was predicted that in relapse tests (operant responding for etonitazene, 5 µg/ml, and for water, see below), conducted from 4:00 P.M. to 8:00 A.M. at intervals of two weeks over a period of several months following terminal cessation of intravenous morphine and saline administration, relapse would be more persistent in the *injection* than in the *infusion* group, compared with each other or with the *saline* group.

Prior to intravenous catheterization, rats (male, Wistar, 4 months old) were trained in an operant chamber to obtain access to one of two drinking tubes containing water alternately, as follows. A rat was placed in the operant chamber at 4:00 P.M. During the first 15 min, no levers were present in the chamber. Then a lever was presented on the right side (RL) for one-half hour. The first lever press resulted in presentation of a drinking tube containing water for 10 sec. Thereafter, for the remainder of that one-half-hour period, the drinking tube was presented for 10 sec, after level presses on the average of every 60 sec (i.e., a variable-interval 60-sec reinforcement schedule). After the initial half-hour period, the RL was retracted and no levers were in the operant chamber for 15 min (time-out, or TO). Then the left lever (LL) was presented for one-half hour, the first press on this lever resulted in presentation of the other drinking tube, also containing water, for 10 sec, and thereafter, for the remainder of the half-hour period, the drinking tube was presented for 10 sec on the average of every 60 sec (variable-interval 60-sec reinforcement schedule). Following a 15-min TO period, the sequence was repeated on the right and left sides with TO periods in between alternately until 8:00 A.M. Hence, between 4:00 P.M. and 8:00 A.M., there were 10 RL and 10 LL presentations. This method provided the following measures: over each half-hour period from 4:00 P.M. to 8:00 A.M., response (lever-pressing) rates on the RL and LL continuously, latencies (time from presentation of a lever to the first press), and number of response-contingent right and left drinking-tube presentations; also, the total volumes of water consumed from the right and left drinking tubes from 4:00 P.M. to 8:00 A.M.

The aim of the training procedure was to select rats that showed, as closely as possible, an equal distribution of water consumed from the right and left drinking tubes in the operant chamber. In actual practice, rats that showed unequal distributions up to 60%–40% were retained for further experiments, the remainder being discarded. After reaching this criterion, each rat was anesthetized, and a permanent indwelling silicon catheter was inserted through the facial vein in the neck into the superior vena cava (the tip close to the heart) and fixed in place. The external end of the catheter was passed subcutaneously around to the back, where it emerged through a slit in the skin and was attached to a short piece of metal tubing anchored in place in a metal "backpiece" that had been sutured to the subcutaneous tissues and muscles some time before. The other end of the short piece of metal tubing was connected to a long polyvinyl tube (surrounded by a tightly wound spring coil), which was connected to a fixed overhead "swivel" that connected to a multibarreled continuous infusion pump and a reservoir (at first, containing heparinized normal saline solution for all rats). Continuous saline infusions were started and continued for a week or more until healing of the cutaneous surgical wounds and patency of the infusion system were evident. Because of serious problems due to infection at the site of the backpiece during subsequent addiction to morphine, this procedure was modified eventually in that the external end of the intravenous catheter was passed subcutaneously around to the base of the back of the neck (instead of to the backpiece, which was eliminated) and was converted to a short piece of metal tubing in a headpiece, fixed to the skull by screws and dental acrylic.

Following completion of these preparatory procedures, continuous infusions of morphine (*infusion* group), continuous infusions of saline plus daily morning injections of morphine through the intravenous catheter (*injection* group), and continuous infusions of saline (*saline* group) were started, as already described (see above). For various reasons, the daily dose of morphine did not reach 200 mg/kg in a few rats, while in a few others, the number of days on 200 mg/kg of morphine was less than two weeks. After the approximately 6-week period of morphine and/or saline intravenous administration, the latter was abruptly discontinued, the metal spring coil was removed, and the polyvinyl tube encased therein was snipped. Two weeks after abrupt withdrawal of morphine and/or saline, each rat was placed in the operant chamber from 4:00 P.M. to 8:00 A.M., and the sequences of RL, LL, TO, and drinking-tube presentations (*water* on both sides) were carried out exactly as described above to determine whether each rat had retained the equal or at least 60%–40% distribution it had previously acquired. If it had, the data obtained (see above) constituted the "water baseline." If it had not, the rat was replaced in the operant chamber the next day (4:00 P.M. to 8:00 A.M.), and the same sequences were carried out. Regardless of the distribution attained on this second day, the data obtained constituted the water baseline for that rat. Most rats displayed an equal or at least a 60%–40% distribution, but some showed more pronounced preferences on the water-baseline test. Thereafter, every 2 weeks for 20 weeks, relapse tests were conducted in exactly the same manner as the water-baseline tests, except that the drinking tube on the *nonpreferred* side contained *etonitazene, 5 μg/ml,* while that on the preferred side contained water. At appropriate times throughout the study, measurements were made of colonic temperature, body weight (including, when present, the backpiece or headpiece and the metal spring coil with the encased polyvinyl tubing), and water consumption from a drinking bottle always available in the home cage, from 8:00 A.M. to 4:00 P.M. and from 4:00 P.M. to 8:00 A.M. In addition, each morphine-treated rat was observed and compared with saline-treated rats at the appropriate times for nonmeasurable signs of morphine abstinence (diarrhea, irritability, and hyperalgesia). Wet-dog shakes were not counted, as such counts would be unreliable because of the presence of backpieces, headpieces, and metal spring coils encasing the polyvinyl tubing. Room temperature was maintained at about 24.4°C. A masking noise was continuously present. Room lights were turned on at 7:00 A.M. and off at 7:00 P.M.

During the approximately 6-week period of morphine and/or saline infusions, the *injection* rats showed, as expected, "inversion" of their water-drinking patterns in their home cages; that is, whereas *saline* (normal) rats drank water in their home cage at a faster rate (ml/hr) from 4:00 P.M. to 8:00 A.M. than from 8:00 A.M. to 4:00 P.M., *injection* rats drank water at a faster rate from 8:00 A.M. to 4:00 P.M. (subtending the effects of the morning intravenous injection of morphine) than from 4:00 P.M. to 8:00 A.M. (development of the morphine-abstinence syndrome). For the *infusion* rats, water-drinking rates in the two periods tended to equalize. Compared with the *saline* rats, the colonic temperatures of the *infusion* rats were the same or higher. Surprisingly, the morning (premorphine-injection) temperatures of the *injection* rats were consistently higher than those of the *saline* rats; that is, the expected hypothermia at 23 hr of morphine abstinence did not occur. After permanent abrupt termination of intravenous morphine and/or saline administration, the *infusion* and *injection* rats lost weight on the first 3 days, and their water consumption in the home cages dropped below that of the *saline* rats at 20 to 46 hr of abstinence; again, no initial morphine-abstinence hypothermia was observed. After the second day of permanent morphine abstinence, the *infusion* and *injection* rats drank more water in the home cages than the *saline* rats (a sign of protracted abstinence). In general, it appeared that the *infusion* and *injection* rats were physically dependent on morphine to an approximately equal degree. The absence of hypothermia before the daily morning injection of morphine in the *injection* rats suggested the possibility that in previous studies in which such preinjection hypothermia was consistently observed, this hypothermia was an anticipatory or conditioned counteradaptive (or opponent-process) response to the unconditioned hyperthermic effects of morphine in morphine-tolerant rats. The expected transient, initial morphine-withdrawal hypothermia in the *infusion* and *injection* rats may have been missed because of the time schedule of measurements of colonic temperature after the last dose of morphine (not earlier than the twentieth hour of abstinence from morphine).

Nine relapse tests were made on all animals, but data were incomplete on the 10th test; hence, only the results of the first nine tests were analyzed statistically. In consonance with the interoceptive conditioning hypothesis, it was found that, by a groups × blocks (three blocks of three relapse tests each) analysis of variance with blocks as a repeated measure, etonitazene consumption by the *injection* group was significantly greater than by the *infusion* group ($F = 4.03$, $p = 0.06$), whereas the two groups did not differ in water consumption ($F = 0.75$, NS). This finding gains added significance from the results of an analysis of variance performed on the "baseline" tests (water versus water) prior to the first relapse test, which revealed no significant difference between the *injection* and *infusion* groups in consumption of water from the drinking tube on either side ($F = 0.84$, NS). However, in the relapse tests, there were no significant differences in etonitazene consumption between the *injection* and the *saline* or between the *infusion* and the *saline* groups. Groups × blocks analyses of variance on response rates, latencies to the first response, and number of drinking tube presentations in *each* half-hour period of lever availability for etonitazene revealed no significant intergroup differences, though means of the *injection* group for response rates were greater than those of the *infusion* or the *saline* group, and means of the *injection* group were shorter for latencies than those of the *infusion* group. The most crucial findings in support of the interoceptive conditioning hypothesis were yielded by groups × blocks analyses of variance of etonitazene and water drinking-tube presentations (taken as an indirect measure of the volumes of fluids consumed) during the *first* half-hour period of lever availability, when the *conditioned* reinforcing properties of etonitazene would be least likely to be confounded with its pharmacological actions, including any primary reinforcing properties that the drug may have. This analysis of variance revealed that across all blocks of relapse tests, the *injection* group produced significantly more etonitazene drinking-tube presentations than the *infusion* group ($F = 5.82$, $p = 0.03$), and there was no significant difference in numbers of water drinking-tube presentations. Similar analyses of variance comparing etonitazene and water drinking-tube presentations for the *injection* versus *saline* and for the *infusion* versus *saline* groups showed no significant differences. However, in the *first block,* both etonitazene and water drinking-tube presentations were greater for the *injection* than for the *saline* group; therefore, an analysis of variance was made on the baseline test and the first three relapse tests with tests as a repeated measure. This procedure revealed that the *injection* group produced significantly more etonitazene drinking-tube presentations than either the *infusion* group ($F = 6.24$, $p = 0.02$) or the *saline* group ($F = 6.28$, $p = 0.02$), and there were no significant intergroup differences in water drinking-tube presentations. A similar "main-effects" analysis of variance of the interaction for the *injection* versus *saline* group revealed no significant difference on the baseline test or the second and third relapse tests, but on the *first relapse test,* the *injection* group produced many more etonitazene drinking-tube presentations than the *saline* group ($F = 19.38$, $p = 0.001$).

Such evidence of experimentally produced conditioned interoceptive reinforcing effects of an opioid (etonitazene) in the rat (Dougherty *et al.*, Miller *et al.*, 1979) applies especially to the street addict, who typically has experienced, many times, the cycle of opioid (heroin) abstinence and its suppression. In such a person, the reinforcing properties of a single dose of an opioid, given for whatever reason after "cure" (detoxification), are likely to be far greater than in a nonaddict, and thereby they facilitate renewed opioid-acquisitive behavior (relapse). Therapeutically, extinction of such interoceptively conditioned responses to opioid stimuli is needed (Davis & Smith, 1976; Wikler, 1977).

CLASSICAL CONDITIONING OF THE OPIOID-ANTAGONIST-PRECIPITATED OPIOID-ABSTINENCE SYNDROME

In the course of the original investigations on precipitation of opioid-abstinence syndromes by single doses of nalorphine in man (Wikler *et al.*, 1953), some evidence was obtained that such precipitated abstinence syndromes could be classically conditioned (unpublished observations; see Wikler, 1974). Five postaddicts who volunteered for the experiments were made tolerant to morphine, methadone, or heroin (40–400 mg/day in divided doses subcutaneously). On an irregular schedule, single doses of nalorphine always evoked typical opioid-abstinence phenomena within 2 or 3 min after subcutaneous injection. Later, subcutaneous saline injections were occasionally substituted for nalorphine. During the first 2–3 weeks of such trials, saline evoked complaints of "hot and cold all over," "cramps," "nausea," or "gagging," and frequently, objective responses including yawning, lacrimation, rhinorrhea, and mydriasis within 30 min after subcutaneous injection of saline. Then such responses to saline (but not to nalorphine) declined rapidly. Up to that time, the author kept away from the ward, the test injections (nalorphine on one day and saline on another day) being administered to all five subjects by an aide, who also recorded the subjects' subjective and objective responses. When the conditioned responses to saline suddenly declined, the author unobtrusively watched the behavior of the subjects while the aide was administering the test injection that day (saline). It turned out that while one of the subjects, in bed, received the test injection, the others stood about watching the proceedings. After about 5 min following the subcutaneous injection (of saline), when the subject who received it made no complaints, the others clamored for the aide to give them the "blank" injection immediately, without going through the "ritual" of lying down in bed for observations of pupil size, respiratory rate, lacrimation, rhinorrea, etc. Asked how they knew the test injection that day was a blank, the subjects informed the author that they had noticed that on some days, they would get "sick" within 2 or 3 min after the test injection (nalorphine), while on other days, the onset of "sickness" following the test injection (saline) would be delayed up to half an hour. Evidently, such decoding of the stimulus conditions was sufficient in man to extinguish the experimentally conditioned opioid-abstinence syndrome. Although, in retrospect, the design of this study of experimental conditioning of the opioid-abstinence syndrome was faulty (test injections of nalorphine or saline should have been randomized across subjects and days to make it impossible for the subjects to decode the stimulus conditions), the discovery that "cognitive labeling" of the proper sort can hasten extinction of classically conditioned opioid abstinence may have therapeutic applications (see below).

In monkeys physically dependent on morphine, Goldberg and Schuster (1967) paired a tone with the intravenous injection of nalorphine. The unconditioned response to nalorphine was a precipitated morphine-abstinence syndrome, including transitory suppression of food-reinforced lever pressing, excessive salivation, emesis, and tachycardia. After a number of tone–nalorphine pairings, presentation of the tone and an intravenous injection of normal saline solution or the tone alone evoked a similar conditioned morphine-abstinence syndrome except for bradycardia (instead of tachycardia). Extinction of the conditioned abstinence changes in these physically dependent monkeys was accomplished by presenting the tone plus an intravenous injection of saline over 40–45 sessions, but they could be reinstated by a few pairings of the tone with intravenous nalorphine injections. In a subsequent study, Goldberg and Schuster (1970) classically conditioned an identical nalorphine-precipitated morphine-abstinence syndrome to a red light (instead of a tone) in physically dependent monkeys. After 10 red-light–nalorphine pairings, morphine administration was permanently discontinued, and the monkeys were tested once monthly for persistence of the conditioned responses. The conditioned stimulus (red light plus intravenous saline injection) continued to suppress food-reinforced lever pressing and to produce bradycardia for 60–120 days after permanent morphine withdrawal. Subsequently, daily presentations of the red-light–saline conditional stimulus resulted in rapid extinction of the conditioned responses, but they could be rapidly reinstated by nalorphine injections, even though, presumably, the monkeys were no longer physically dependent on morphine. Discussing this surprising finding, Goldberg and Schuster noted that Irwin and Seevers (1956) described similar reinstatement of conditioned responses by nalorphine in postaddict monkeys in which nalorphine had previously precipitated morphine abstinence during maintained physical dependence on morphine, and they suggested that the responses to nalorphine long after withdrawal of morphine was a conditioned effect resulting from past experience with unconditioned nalorphine-precipitated morphine abstinence. However, an alternative explanation —namely, that increased nalorphine-sensitivity may result from persistence of physiological changes after periods of physical dependence on morphine—was supported by the findings of Goldberg and Schuster (1969) that postaddict monkeys with no history of nalorphine-precipitated morphine abstinence showed an increased sensitivity to nalorphine, when compared with nondependent monkeys. The nature of such persistent physiological changes in postaddict monkeys is unclear. Perhaps it reflects a protracted morphine-abstinence syndrome, but this has not been studied in monkeys, and in any case, the protracted abstinence syndrome alone would not explain the increased sensitivity to nalorphine. Conceivably, recovery from the early morphine-abstinence syndrome is hastened by renewed synthesis and release of endophins or enkephalins masking the still-persisting central counteradaptive changes that are responsible for the morphine-abstinence syndrome; nalorphine could then percipitate abstinence phenomena by antagonizing the endorphins.

Complementing these studies, Goldberg *et al.* (1969, 1971) found that morphine-dependent monkeys increased the rate of intravenous self-injection of saline in the presence of a red light that had previously been paired repeatedly with passive intravenous injection of nalorphine; such conditioned increases in self-administration of saline extinguished eventually.

In eight former heroin addicts maintained on a constant daily dose of methadone (median, 40 mg) in a methadone-maintenance clinic, O'Brien *et al.* (1977) paired a tone and an odor (oil of peppermint), which served as a conditioned stimulus, with the time course (20–30 min) of the opioid-abstinence syndrome precipitated by the unconditioned stimulus, naloxone (0.1 mg intramuscularly), on 12 occasions, interspersed with test trials of the conditioned stimulus alone. Naloxone (the unconditioned stimulus) produced mydriasis, lacrimation, rhinorrhea, yawning, increased respiratory and cardiac rates, and decreased skin temperature. Of the measurable signs of opioid abstinence, classically conditioned responses (to the tone and odor alone) were observed for increased respiratory rate and for decrease in skin temperature by the second test trial and for increased cardiac rate (decreased cardiac rate in one subject) by the third test trial. When data on preconditioning and all conditioned test trials (except the last, when conditioned responses began to be extinguished) were pooled for all eight subjects, respiratory rate showed a significant ($p < 0.025$) increase and skin temperature a significant ($p < 0.05$) decrease in response to the conditioned stimulus. Cardiac rate (regardless of direction) also changed significantly ($p < 0.025$) in response to the conditioned stimulus. The frequency of "motor behaviors," indicative of nonmeasurable opioid-abstinence phenomena, such as touching the eyes (lacrimation) or nose (rhinorrhea) and yawning, also changed (almost significantly, p between 0.05 and 0.10) across blocks of 5 min for each test trial, compared with preconditioning test trials. Pupil diameter did not change significantly in response to the conditioned stimulus when data for all eight subjects were pooled, though four showed slight pupillary dilatation. Subjective reports of opioid-abstinence symptoms (awareness of lacrimation, rhinorrhea, sweating, tremors, feeling cold, anxiety, depression, and anger) were significantly ($p < 0.05$) greater for conditioning test trials than for preconditioning test trials. In two control subjects, who were exposed to exactly the same stimulus conditions except that they received intramuscular injections of normal saline solution instead of naloxone, no conditioned responses to the conditioned stimulus were observed.

OCCURRENCE OF CLASSICALLY CONDITIONED RESPONSES IN STREET ADDICTS

From the foregoing, it is clear that the opioid-abstinence syndrome or fragments of it can be classically conditioned experimentally to environmental stimuli in both animals and man. Also, retrospective reports by addicts or postaddicts (see above) strongly suggest that such conditioning takes place under natural conditions on the street. A crucial question is whether objective evidence of such natural conditioning can be demonstrated in street addicts.

In detoxified heroin addicts maintained on opioid-blocking doses of naltrexone (350 mg/wk), O'Brien et al. (1979) measured autonomic and behavioral changes during approximately 1 hr sessions in which the subjects injected themselves with either 2 mg of hydromorphone or saline, carrying out their customary cooking-up and shooting-up rituals. Each session was videotaped to permit observers to score the frequency of certain behavioral responses. In each session, verbal responses to taped questions were recorded, fingertip skin temperatures were measured continuously, and pupil size was measured intermittently by a video pupillometer. Under the conditions of the study (naltrexone blockade), each session constituted an extinction trial. These subjects were divided into three groups: Massed Extinction Trials Hydromorphone, four trials, daily; Spaced Extinction Trials Hydromorphone, three times weekly; and Spaced Extinction Trials Saline, three times weekly (the assignment of hydromorphone or saline to the Spaced Extinction Trials groups was double-blind). A nonexperimental group of detoxified heroin addicts on naltrexone (350 mg/wk) who did not participate in these extinction trials served as a No Extinction comparison group. In the majority of subjects in all extinction groups, the preinjection rituals of cooking-up and tying-off produced decreased fingertip skin temperatures and other physiological and behavioral signs of conditioned opioid-abstinence (O'Brien et al., 1979; O'Brien, personal communication, 1978) which increased in intensity as extinction trials continued, regardless of whether the agent self-injected was hydromorphone or saline. In some subjects, the responses on the initial extinction trials were opioid-like, but in succeeding extinction trials they became increasingly characteristic of opioid-abstinence. As the extinction trials proceeded, they became increasingly aversive to the subjects who stated that they "hated" them and refused to continue (thus leaving conditioned abstinence unextinguished). Nevertheless, on six-month follow-up (presumably after maintenance on naltrexone had been discontinued), the Massed Extinction Trials Hydromorphone group showed an unexpectedly favorable outcome compared with the No Extinction group; the Spaced Extinction Trials Hydromorphone group also had a favorable outcome, but the outcome in the Spaced Extinction Trials Saline group was less favorable than in the No Extinction group. In another study, Ternes *et al.* (1979) observed significant increases in heart rates and decreases in fingertip skin temperatures during 10 min presentations of drug-related slides, videotapes, and objects but not on presentations of neutral stimuli of the same sort in detoxified heroin addicts (not maintained on narcotic antagonists) and methadone maintenance patients, contrasting with no changes in a control group that had never used heroin. Scores on the Weak Opioid Withdrawal Scale tended to be higher after presentation of the drug-related than the neutral stimuli in the detoxified heroin addicts and in the methadone maintenance patients, but in the control group, the trend was in the opposite direction. Sideroff and Jarvik (1979) recorded heart rates, fingertip skin temperatures, galvanic skin reflexes (GSRs) and subjects' estimates of "craving" in 10 controls and in 12 heroin addicts at various stages of detoxification (or on methadone maintenance) while they viewed drug-related and neutral videotapes. The heroin addict group showed marked increase in "craving," heart rate and number of GSRs while viewing drug-related videotapes compared with neutral videotapes, while the control group reported no "craving" to either videotape and showed only slightly higher heart rate on viewing drug-related compared with neutral videotapes. In four of the heroin addicts viewing drug-related videotapes, systematic decreases in fingertip skin temperatures (0.3–1.3°C) on at least three of five trials were observed.

Common to all three of these reports is the finding that physiological signs of classically conditioned opioid-abstinence do indeed occur in detoxified heroin addicts in response to drug-related stimuli. The sequence of conditioned responses observed in the successive extinction trials conducted by O'Brien *et al.* (1979) may be interpreted as follows: in the heroin-tolerant subject prior to detoxification, each dose of heroin produced initial heroin-agonistic effects followed by heroin-abstinence phenomena. Early in the course of tolerance, the heroin-agonistic effects predominated after each dose, but as tolerance developed further, they became progressively attenuated while the heroin-abstinence phenomena increased in intensity. In the street addict, both the heroin-agonistic effects and the heroin-abstinence phenomena became classically conditioned (though not necessarily in their cyclic pharmacological order) to the specific drug-related environment and ritual practices. On the *first* reexposure to these conditioned stimuli, long after detoxification, the previous pharmacological events after a dose of heroin, as they had been *early* in the subject's history of tolerance, are now evoked as conditioned responses. In some subjects, the conditioned heroin-agonistic effects predominate, while in others the conditioned responses are more characteristic of heroin-abstinence. In either case, *succeeding* reexposures to the conditioned stimuli evoked as conditioned responses the previous pharmacological events following a dose of heroin as they had been *later* in the subject's history of tolerance, namely, increasing degrees of heroin-abstinence phenomena which predominate over heroin-agonistic effects. With the proviso of separate conditioning of the opioid-agonistic and opioid-abstinence changes during previous opioid-tolerance, and taking into account the subject's history of the development of tolerance, this interpretation of the extinction data of O'Brien *et al.* (1979) is in keeping with the theoretical formulation of classical conditioning of the cycle of opioid-agonistic and opioid-abstinence changes as it has been postulated to occur in street addicts (Wikler, 1961).

IMPLICATIONS OF CONDITIONING FACTORS FOR RELAPSE AND TREATMENT

If the occurrence of classically conditioned opioid-agonist and opioid-abstinence phenomena as well as operantly conditioned opioid-seeking behavior in street addicts is confirmed by further research, then opioid addiction and relapse in such persons must be regarded as a disease *sui generis*, and as such, its features must be eliminated by specific *extinction* procedures before, or concomitantly with, other therapeutic measures directed at presumed antecedent variables (e.g., premorbid personality abnormalities). Mere detoxification (withdrawal from heroin or other opioids) and retention of the addict for a long time in a drug-free hospital or prison with or without conventional individual or group psychotherapy do not extinguish such conditioned responses (if only because neither the patient nor the therapist is aware of them) any more than satiating a rat with food (i.e., reducing its hunger drive) and keeping it away from the operant chamber for a period of time "cures" it of its lever-pressing habit (Neuringer, 1969; Carder & Berkowitz, 1970). What

is needed after detoxification is active extinction of both classically conditioned opioid-agonist and opioid-abstinence changes, as well as operantly conditioned opioid-seeking behavior in the presence of such
"natural" conditioned stimuli and secondary reinforcers as self-injection
with all the street-addict rituals and opioid-related objects such as bags
of heroin and scenes of addicts shooting up under conditions in which
primary reinforcement (pharmacological effects of opioids) is not possible. The extinction procedures currently used by O'Brien *et al.* under
naltrexone blockade (see above) offer a model for such therapy, although some means must be found to retain the patients who usually
refuse to go on with the extinction procedures because of the discomfort
associated with unrelieved conditioned abstinence; in these patients,
conditioned responses have not been completely extinguished. Nevertheless, some of them agree to naltrexone-blockade maintenance on an
outpatient basis, without completing the formal extinction procedures.
If, under naltrexone blockade, they should hustle for heroin spontaneously, self-injection of heroin (or other opioid) would constitute an extinction trial, inasmuch as no primary reinforcing effect is likely to occur,
nor is physical dependence likely to be reestablished after repeated
self-injection. Should such "misbehavior" actually transpire, then the
chances for extinction of conditioned responses would be increased,
with a greater probability that the patients would remain opioid-free
after naltrexone maintenance has been discontinued.

In addition to naltrexone maintenance with or without formal extinction procedures, efforts at rehabilitation should be made. This includes job counseling, vocational retraining where needed, alteration of
lifestyle and possibly home environment, and psychotherapy with em-
phasis on "cognitive relabeling," that is, recognition by the patient of
the subjective aspects of conditioned abstinence and the circumstances
under which they occur. The efficacy of self-achieved cognitive relabeling in abolishing conditioned nalorphine-precipitated abstinence phenomena in man (see above, and Wikler, 1974) suggests that this may be
of some benefit if applied therapeutically.

Extinction of interoceptively conditioned opioid-seeking behavior
poses a very difficult problem. From the experimental studies of Davis
and Smith (1976) in the rat, which have already been discussed, it may
be inferred that despite successful completion of extinction procedures
under naltrexone blockade and termination of daily blocking doses of
naltrexone for many months, a former opioid addict will relapse
promptly if, for whatever reason (e.g., a medical or surgical contingency), he receives an injection of morphine or other opioid
analgesic. Wikler (1977) has suggested that during the period of nal-

trexone maintenance, the patient should be readmitted to the hospital from time to time, taken off the opioid antagonist, given an injection of morphine or other opioid, and then replaced on naltrexone before discharge from the hospital. Presumably, the interoceptive effects of the opioid given after removal of naltrexone blockade in the hospital will reinstate opioid-seeking behavior as a conditioned response, but reinforcement of this response will be blocked by resumption of naltrexone blockade after discharge from the hospital. Following an as-yet-to-be-determined number of such treatments, the interoceptively conditioned responses should extinguish. One problem that can be foreseen is whether the patient would consent to immediate resumption of naltrexone blockade after discharge from the hospital, where an unblocked dose of an opioid reinstituted his previously extinguished craving.

REFERENCES

Beach, H. D., 1957, Morphine addiction in rats, *Canad. J. Psychol.* 11:104–112.

Carder, B., and Berkowitz, K., 1970, Rats' preference for earned in comparison with free food, *Science* 167:1273–1274.

Carnathan, G., Meyer, R. E., and Cochin, J., 1977, Narcotic blockade, length of addiction, and persistence of intravenous morphine self-administration in rats, *Psychopharmacology* 54:67–71.

CIBA Pharmaceutical Co., Ltd., 1958, *An Introductory Report on Ciba 20'684-Ba: A New Benzimidazole Derivative with a Highly Potent Analgesic Action.* Basle.

Cochin, J., and Kornetsky, C., 1964, Development and loss of tolerance to morphine in the rat after single and multiple injections, *J. Pharmacol. Exp. Ther.* 145:1–10.

Collins, K. G., and Tatum, A. L., 1925, A conditioned salivary reflex established by chronic morphine poisoning, *Amer. J. Physiol.* 74:14–15.

Davis, W. M., and Smith, S. G., 1974, Naloxone use to eliminate opiate-seeking behavior: Need for extinction of conditioned reinforcement, *Biol. Psychiat.* 9:181–189.

Davis, W. M., and Smith, S. G., 1976, Role of conditioned reinforcers in the initiation and extinction of drug-seeking behavior, *Pavlovian J. Biol. Sci.* 11:222–236.

Deese, J., and Kellogg, W. N., 1949, Some new data on the nature of spinal conditioning, *J. Comp. Physiol. Psychol.* 42:157–160.

Deneau, G., Yanigita, T., and Seevers, M. H., 1969, Self-administration of psychoactive substances by the monkey, *Psychopharmacologia* 16:30–48.

Dougherty, J. A., Miller, D. B., and Wikler, A., 1979, Interoceptive conditioning through repeated suppression of morphine-abstinence. I. Basis for conditioning: Once-daily vs. continuous intravenous morphine infusion, *Pavlovian J. Biol. Sci.* 14:160–169.

Drawbaugh, R., and Lal, H., 1974, Reversal by narcotic antagonist of a narcotic action elicited by a conditioned stimulus, *Nature* (London) 247:65–67.

Dykman, R. A. and Shurrager, P. S., 1956, Successive and maintained conditioning in spinal carnivores, *J. Comp. Physiol. Psychol.* 49:27–35.

Fraser, H. F., Isbell, H., and Wolbach, A. N., Jr., 1960, Addictiveness of new synthetic analgesics, in *Minutes, 21st Meeting, Committee on Drug Addiction and Narcotics, NAS–NRC, January 11–12,* pp. 35–51. U.S. Government Printing Office, Washington, D.C.

Goldberg, S. R., and Schuster, C. R., 1967, Conditioned suppression by a stimulus associated with nalorphine in morphine-dependent monkeys, *J. Exp. Anal. Behav.* 10:235-242.

Goldberg, S. R., and Schuster, C. R., 1969, Nalorphine: Increased sensitivity of monkeys formerly dependent on morphine, *Science* 166:1548-1549.

Goldberg, S. R., and Schuster, C. R., 1970, Conditioned nalorphine-induced abstinence changes: Persistence in post morphine-dependent monkeys, *J. Exp. Anal. Behav.* 14:33-46.

Goldberg, S. R., Woods, J. H., and Schuster, C. R., 1969, Morphine: Conditioned increases in self administration in rhesus monkeys, *Science* 166:1306-1307.

Goldberg, S. R., Woods, J. H., and Schuster, C. R., 1971, Nalorphine-induced changes in morphine self-administration in rhesus monkeys, *J. Pharmacol. Exp. Ther.* 176:464-471.

Gross, R., and Turrian, H., 1957, Über Benzimidazolderivate mit starker analgetischer Wirking, *Experientia* 13:401-403.

Headlee, C. P., Coppock, H. W., and Nichols, J. R., 1955, Apparatus and technique involved in a laboratory method of detecting addictiveness of drugs, *J. Amer. Pharmaceut. Ass. Sci. Ed.* 44:229-231.

Hunger, A. J., Kebrle, J., Rossi, A., and Hoffmann, K., 1957, Synthese basisch substituierter, analgetisch wirksamer Bezimidazolderivate, *Experientia* 13:400-401.

Irwin, S., and Seevers, M. H., 1956, Altered response to drugs in the post addict *Macaca mulatta*, *J. Pharmacol. Exp. Ther.* 116:31-32.

Jones, B. E., and Prada, J. A., 1973, Relapse to morphine use in dogs, *Psychopharmacologia* 30:1-12.

Kellogg, W. N., Deese, J., Pronko, N. H., and Feinberg, M., 1947, An attempt to condition the chronic spinal dog, *J. Exp. Psychol.* 37:99-117.

Kleitman, N., and Crisler, G., 1927, A quantitative study of a salivary conditioned reflex, *Amer. J. Physiol.* 79:571-614.

Kolb, L., 1939, Drug addiction as a public health problem, *Sci. Monthly* 48:391-400.

Korol, B., Sletten, I. W., and Brown, M. L., 1966, Conditioned physiological adaptation to anticholinergic drugs, *Amer. J. Physiol.* 211:911-914.

Kumar, R., and Stolerman, I. P., 1972, Resumption of morphine self-administration by ex-addict rats: An attempt to modify tendencies to relapse, *J. Comp. Physiol. Psychol.* 78:457-465.

Kun, E., and Horvath, I., 1947, The influence of oral saccharin on blood sugar, *Proc. Soc. Exp. Biol. Med.* (N.Y.) 66:175-177.

Lal, H., Miksic, S., Drawbaugh, R., Numan, R., and Smith, N., 1976, Alleviation of narcotic withdrawal syndrome by conditional stimuli, *Pavlovian J. Biol. Sci.* 11:251-262.

Levitt, R. A., 1964, Sleep as a conditioned response, *Psychonom. Sci.* 1:273-274.

Lloyd, A. J., Wikler, A., and Whitehouse, J. M., 1969, Nonconditionability of flexor reflex in the chronic spinal dog, *J. Comp. Physiol.* 68:576-579.

Martin, W. R., Wikler, A., Eades, C. G., and Pescor, F. T., 1963, Tolerance to and physical dependence on morphine in the rat, *Psychopharmacologia* 4:247-260.

Miller, D. B., Dougherty, J. A., and Wikler, A., 1979, Interceptive conditioning through repeated suppression of morphine-abstinence. II. Relapse-testing, *Pavlovian J. Biol. Sci.* 14:170-176.

Neuringer, A. J., 1969, Animals respond for food in the presence of free food, *Science*, 166:399-401.

Nichols, J. R., Headlee, C. P., and Coppock, H. W., 1956, Drug addiction. I. Addiction by escape training, *J. Amer. Pharm. Ass., Sci. Ed.* 45:788-791.

O'Brien, C. P., 1976, Experimental analysis of conditioning factors in human narcotic addiction, *Pharmacol. Rev.* 27:533-543.

O'Brien, C. P., Testa, T., O'Brien, T. J., Brady J. P., and Wells B., 1977, Conditioned narcotic withdrawal in humans, *Science, 195*:1000-1002.

O'Brien, C. P., Testa, T., O'Brien, T. J., Brady, J. P., and Wells, B. Personal communication (letter), September 5, 1978.

O'Brien, C. P., Greenstein, R., Ternes, J., McLellan, A. T. and Grabowski, J., 1979, Unreinforced self-injections: Effects on rituals and outcome in heroin addicts in *Problems of Drug Dependence, 1979* (L. S. Harris, ed.). Proceedings of the 41st Annual Scientific Meeting of the Committee on Problems of Drug Dependence, Inc., Philadelphia, June 4–6, 1979 NIDA Research Monogr. 27, pp. 275–281. Superintendent of Documents, U.S. Government Printing Office, Washington, D.C.

Pavlov, I. P., 1927, *Conditioned Reflexes: An Investigation of the Physiological Activity of the Cerebral Cortex* (G. V. Anrep, Trans. and Ed.), pp. 34–35. Oxford University Press, London; Dover Publications edition, Dover Publications, Inc., New York, 1960.

Roffman, M., Reddy, C., and Lal, H., 1973, Control of morphine-withdrawal hypothermia by conditional stimuli, *Psychopharmacologia 29*:197–201.

Schuster, C. R., and Thompson, T., 1969, Self-administration of and behavioral dependence on drugs, *Annual Rev. Pharmacol. 9*:483–502.

Schuster, C. R., and Villareal, J. E., 1968, The experimental analysis of opioid dependence, in *Psychopharmacology: A Review of Progress 1957-1967* (D. H. Efron, Ed.), pp. 811–828. Publ. Health Service Publ. No. 1836, U.S. Government Printing Office, Washington, D.C.

Schuster, C. R., and Woods, J. H., 1968, The conditioned reinforcing effects of stimuli associated with morphine reinforcement, *Int. J. Addictions 3*:233–230.

Shapiro, M. M., 1960, Respondent salivary conditioning during operant lever pressing in dogs, *Science 132*:619–620.

Shurrager, P. S., and Culler, E. A., 1938, Phenomena allied to conditioning in the spinal dog, *Amer. J. Physiol. 123*:186–187.

Shurrager, P. S., and Culler, E. A., 1940, Conditioning in the spinal dog, *Exp. Psychol. 26*:133–159.

Shurrager, P. S., and Shurrager, H. C., 1946, The rate of learning measured at a single synapse, *J. Exp. Psychol. 36*:347–354.

Sideroff, S. I. and Jarvik, M. D., 1979, Conditioned heroin responses as an indication of readdiction liability in *Problems of drug dependence, 1979* (L. S. Harris, ed.). Proceedings of the 41st Annual Scientific Meeting of the Committee on Problems of Drug Dependence, Inc., Philadelphia, June 4–6, 1979 NIDA Research Monogr. 27, pp. 268–274. Superintendent of Documents, U.S. Government Printing Office, Washington, D.C.

Siegel, S., 1972, Conditioning of insulin-induced glycemia, *J. Comp. Physiol. Psychol. 78*:233–241.

Siegel, S., 1975, Conditioning insulin effects, *J. Comp. Physiol. Psychol. 89*:189–199.

Spragg, S. D. S., 1940, *Morphine Addiction in Chimpanzees, Comparative Psychology Monographs*, Vol. 15. John Hopkins Press, Baltimore.

Stein, L., 1964, Amphetamine and neural reward mechanisms, in *Ciba Foundation Symposium on Animal Behaviour and Drug Addition* (H. Steinberg, A. V. S. de Reuck, and J. Knight, Eds.), pp. 91–113. J. & A. Churchill, London.

Teasdale, J. D., 1973, Conditioned abstinence in narcotic addicts, *Int. J. Addictions 8*:273–292.

Ternes, J. S., O'Brien, C. P., Grabowski, J., Wellerstein, H. and Jordan-Hayes, J., 1979, Conditioned drug responses to naturalistic stimuli in *Problems of drug dependence, 1979* (L. S. Harris, ed.). Proceedings of the 41st Annual Scientific Meeting of the Committee on Problems of Drug Dependence, Inc., Philadelphia, June 4–6, 1979, NIDA Research

Monogr. 27, pp. 282–288. Superintendent of Documents, U.S. Government Printing Office, Washington, D.C.

Thompson, T., and Ostlund, W., 1965, Susceptibility to readdiction as a function of the addiction and withdrawal environment, *J. Comp. Physiol. Psychol. 59*:388–392.

Weeks, J. R., and Collins, R. J., 1968, Patterns of intravenous self-injection by morphine-addicted rats, in *The Addictive States: Research Publications of the Association for Nervous and Mental Disease*, Vol. 46: (A. Wikler, Ed.), pp. 288–298. Williams & Wilkins, Baltimore.

Wikler, A., 1948, Recent progress in research on the neurophysiologic basis of morphine addiction, *Amer. J. Psychiat. 105*:329–338.

Wikler, A., 1950, Adaptive behavior in long-surviving dogs without neocortex, *Arch. Neurol. Psychiat.* (Chicago) 64:29–41.

Wikler, A., 1952a, A psychodynamic study of a patient during experimental self-regulated re-addiction to morphine, *Psychiat. Quart. 26*:270–293.

Wikler, A., 1952b, Reactions of dogs without neocortex during cycles of addiction to morphine and methadone, *Arch. Neurol. Psychiat.* (Chicago) 67:672–684.

Wikler, A., 1961, On the nature of addiction and habituation, *Brit. J. Addiction 57*:73–79.

Wikler, A., 1965, Conditioning factors in opiate addiction and relapse, in *Narcotics* (D. M. Wilner and G. G. Kassebaum, Eds.), pp. 85–100. McGraw-Hill, New York.

Wikler, A., 1973, Conditioning of successive adaptive responses to the initial effects of drugs, *Conditional Reflex 8*:193–210.

Wikler, A., 1974, Requirements for extinction of relapse-facilitating variables and for rehabilitation in a narcotic-antagonist treatment program, in *Narcotic Antagonists Advances in Biochemical Psychopharmacology*, Vol. 8 (M. C. Braude, L. S. Harris, E. L. May, J. P. Smith, and J. E. Villareal, Eds.), pp. 399–414. Raven Press, New York.

Wikler, A., 1977, Methadone maintenance and narcotic blocking drugs, *Int. J. Addictions 12*:851–856.

Wikler, A., and Frank K., 1948, Hindlimb reflexes in chronic spinal dogs during cycles of addiction to morphine and methadone, *J. Pharmacol. Exp. Ther. 94*:382–400.

Wikler, A., and Pescor, F. T., 1967, Classical conditioning of a morphine abstinence phenomenon, reinforcement of opioid-drinking behavior and "relapse" in morphine-addicted rats, *Psychopharmacologia 10*:255–284.

Wikler, A., and Pescor, F. T., 1970, Persistence of "relapse-tendencies" of rats previously made physically dependent on morphine, *Psychopharmacologia 16*:375–384.

Wikler, A., Fraser, H. F., and Isbell, H., 1953, N-allylnormorphine: effects of single doses and precipitation of acute "abstinence syndromes" during addiction to morphine, methadone or heroin in man (post-addicts), *J. Pharmacol. Exp. Ther. 109*:8–20.

Wikler, A., Green, C. P., Smith, H. D., and Pescor, F. T., 1960, Use of a dilute solution (5 mcg/ml) of a benzimidazol derivative with potent morphine-like actions orally as a presumptive reinforcing agent in conditioning of drug-seeking behavior in rats, *Fed. Proc. 19*:22.

Wikler, A., Martin, W. R., Pescor, F. T., and Eades, C. G., 1963, Factors regulating oral consumption of an opioid (etonitazene) by morphine-addicted rats, *Psychopharmacologia 5*:55–76.

Wikler, A., Pescor, F. T., Miller, D., and Norrell, H., 1971, Persistent potency of a secondary (conditioned) reinforcer following withdrawal of morphine from physically dependent rats, *Psychopharmacologia 20*:103–117.

Woods, A., Makous, W., and Hutton, A., 1968, A new technique for conditioned hypoglycemia, *Psychon. Sci. 10*:389–390.

Woods, J. G., and Schuster, C. R., 1968, Reinforcement properties of morphine, cocaine and SPA as a function of unit dose, *Int. J. Addictions 3*:231–237.

CHAPTER 8

Diagnosis and Treatment of Opioid Dependence

DIAGNOSIS

Physical Dependence

The diagnosis of physical dependence on opioids can be established only by the demonstration of typical opioid-abstinence phenomena, either by isolating the patient without abstinence-suppressing medication for at least 48 hr and observing the development of pupillary dilatation, frequent yawning, lacrimation, rhinorrhea, piloerection, sweating, restlessness, vomiting, and rise in pulse rate, respiratory rate, and rectal temperature, or by administering a narcotic antagonist and observing the appearance of such opioid-abstinence signs within a few minutes. For this purpose, either nalorphine (Nalline) or naloxone (Narcan) may be used. As a narcotic antagonist, naloxone is about 10 times as potent as nalorphine, which also possesses some opioid-agonist properties. An experienced physician may administer the narcotic antagonist (1–4 mg of nalorphine or 0.1–0.4 mg of naloxone) *slowly* by intravenous injection, constantly observing the patient for early opioid-abstinence signs such as pupillary dilatation, increase in respiratory rate, lacrimation, rhinorrhea, and sweating. The appearance of these signs establishes the diagnosis of physical dependence on opioids, and further intravenous injection of the narcotic antagonist should be stopped, as it may precipitate a more severe and potentially dangerous abstinence syndrome. For less experienced physicians, the subcutaneous route is safer. The initial dose of narcotic antagonist should be 3 mg of nalorphine or 0.4 mg of naloxone, subcutaneously. If no or equivocal signs of opioid abstinence appear within 15 min, a second dose of 5 mg of nalorphine or 0.7 mg of naloxone should be given subcutaneously; if no or equivocal sign of abstinence appear within the next 15 min, a final dose of 7 mg of nalorphine or 1 mg of naloxone should be given subcutaneously. If no clear-cut signs of abstinence are produced after these three subcutaneous doses, it may be concluded that the patient is not physically dependent on opioids. Attempts to reverse an opioid-abstinence syndrome precipitated by a narcotic antagonist by administration of an opioid agonist (e.g., morphine) are likely to fail because the narcotic antagonist will block access of the opioid agonist to the opioid receptors, unless the dose of opioid agonist is relatively high; because the duration of action of a large dose of morphine outlasts the duration of the antagonistic actions of nalorphine or naloxone, severe central depression may ensue when the narcotic antagonist has been metabolized or otherwise eliminated. Since the peak time-action of nalorphine or naloxone is relatively short (30–60 min) it is preferable to "wait out" the subsidence of the abstinence syndrome precipitated by these narcotic antagonists.

The "clinical significance" of a *mild* opioid-abstinence syndrome demonstrated by either of these two methods is difficult to judge. Fraser *et al.* (1961) demonstrated that in long-detoxified former opioid addicts, statistically significant abstinence syndromes developed after experimental administration of morphine subcutaneously (starting with 32 mg/day and increasing gradually to a maximum of 207 mg/day or 240 mg/day in four divided doses each day), morphine orally (32–240 mg/day), heroin subcutaneously (13–86.8 mg/day) or codeine orally (200–1500 mg/day) *over a period of 18–20 days,* when these opioids were withdrawn abruptly. Whether or not statistically significant abstinence syndromes would have occurred if the daily doses of these opioids had been smaller, and/or if the period of daily administration of them had been shorter, is unknown. On the other hand, Wikler *et al.* (1953) reported precipitation of mild but clear-cut abstinence signs by administration of nalorphine (15 mg) in similar subjects who had received, experimentally, a total of nine subcutaneous injections of morphine 15 mg or equivalent doses of methadone or heroin *over a period of only 3 days;* as administration of these opioids continued and the daily dose increased, the amount of nalorphine required to precipitate abstinence decreased. Using naloxone, Nutt and Jasinski (1974) precipitated mild abstinence syndromes in long-detoxified former opioid addicts following a *single* dose of methadone or morphine. An analogy may be drawn between an opioid user in whom mild abstinence phenomena have been precipitated by narcotic antagonists but who showed no abstinence signs on abrupt withdrawal of the drug and a person with abnormally high blood glucose concentrations postprandially or in response to ingested glucose but who has a normal fasting blood glucose concentration and no glycosuria (chemical diabetes). Strictly speaking, such an opioid user is physically dependent, but the clinician may deem it advisable not to admit the opioid user to a methadone-maintenance program and thereby increase the degree of physical dependence. Similarly, the clinician may refrain from prescribing insulin or oral hypoglycemic agents for the "chemical diabetic," preferring to treat him by weight reduction, exercise, and dietary regulation alone.

In patients who are not physically dependent on opioids, nalorphine (but not naloxone) may produce opioid-agonistic effects, including pupillary constriction and respiratory depression; psychotomimetic effects, such as hallucinations, may also occur in some individuals after ordinary physical-dependence–testing doses (e.g., a total of 15 mg of nalorphine subcutaneously).

Opioid Use

Chronic or intermittent self-administration of opioid drugs (usually illicit) in the past may be suspected if blue or black pigmented streaks or pinhead-sized needle marks are noted in the skin, particularly in the antecubital regions, arms, volar surfaces of the forearms, dorsum of hands and feet, and (especially in women) needle marks on the abdomen and thighs. Round, shallow, punched-out healed ulcers may be seen in any of these areas of persons who have self-administered meperidine (Demerol) subcutaneously or in whom subcutaneous extravasations have occurred on attempted intravenous self-administration. Current opioid use may be suspected if the subject is "on the nod," if the pupils are markedly constricted, and if respirations are slow or periodic. Current or very recent use of morphine, heroin, methadone, or some other opioids may be confirmed by detection of the drug or its metabolic products (e.g., morphine from heroin) in the urine by various techniques, including thin-layer chromatography, the immunoassays (free radical assay technique, Abuscreen radioimmunoassay, homogeneous enzyme immunoassay technique, latex agglutination inhibition), and gas chromatography. These techniques and the principles underlying them have been reviewed by Gorodetzky (1977a). The durations of time after intravenous administration of doses of 2.5, 5, and 10 mg/70 kg of heroin or 6 and 12 mg/70 kg of morphine (heroin and morphine doses considered equieuphorigenic in nontolerant individuals) in long-detoxified former opioid addicts over which morphine could be detected in 50% or more of urine samples by the methods mentioned were investigated by Gorodetzky and his collaborators (Gorodetzky, 1977a, pp. 388–389; 1977b). Such durations varied with the dose of the opioid administered and the particular technique used: thus, after heroin, 2.5 mg/70 kg, 0–8 to 32–40 hr; 5 mg/70 kg, 8 to 48–56 hr; and 10 mg/70 kg, 16–56 hr (80 hr by gas chromatography using trimethylsilyl derivatization preceded by acid hydrolysis of the urine); after morphine; 6 mg/70 kg, 8–72 hr, and 12 mg/70 kg, 8–16 to 80 hr. In general, the shortest durations over which morphine could be detected in 50% or more of urine samples were found with thin-layer chromatography without prior acid hydrolysis, and the longest durations were found with radioimmunoassay and gas chromatography. In patients who were dependent on heroin (150–450 mg/day parenterally), Way *et al.* (1966) found that 100% of urines were positive (for morphine) in the first 24 hr after withdrawal, 90% in the second 24 hr, and 75% in the third withdrawal day, using thin-layer chromatography with prior acid hydrolysis of the urine. From the data available, it would be reasonable to expect a high probability of detecting morphine in the urine of a chronic heroin user, taking as little as 2.5–5.0 mg of heroin three times daily, even with the least sensitive technique (thin-layer chromatography without prior acid hydrolysis of the urine).

TREATMENT

Opioid Poisoning

The cardinal signs of opioid poisoning include stupor or coma, miosis, and slowed or periodic respirations. However, in very severe opioid poisoning with hypoxia, the pupils may be dilated and nonreactive to light, the corneal and tendon reflexes absent, and rectal temperature markedly subnormal. Generalized convulsions may also occur in patients poisoned by meperidine or *d*-propoxyphene. These syndromes may be mimicked wholly or in part by certain neurological conditions (bilateral subdural hematoma, particularly with herniation of the brain stem; subarachnoid or intracerebral hemorrhage; thrombosis of the basilar artery; idiopathic status epilepticus; severe carbon monoxide poisoning) and severe hypoglycemia. Coma due to diabetic acidosis or poisoning with barbiturate or other sedative drugs is usually characterized by shallow, rapid respirations.

The first duty of the physician in the treatment of a patient in coma is to ensure respiratory and circulatory function adequate for immediate survival. Tracheopharyngeal secretions should be aspirated, and an oropharyngeal airway or a cuffed endotracheal tube should be inserted; in some cases, tracheostomy may prove necessary (the assistance of an anethesiologist would be very helpful). If cyanosis, or a respiratory rate of less than 12/min, is present, artifical respiration by positive pressure should be instituted by any means at hand (mechanical resuscitator, anesthesia breathing bag, or mouth-to-mouth insufflation). The rate and depth of artificially maintained respiration are best regulated by frequent measurements of arterial pCO_2 and oxyhemoglobin saturation. If facilities for these measurements are not available, reliance may be put on judgments of the degree of cyanosis based on the appearance of the lips, fingernail beds, and mucous membranes. To facilitate circulatory support, as well as to correct dehydration, an intravenous infusion of 5% dextrose in water should be started immediately, by cutdown, if necessary. Hypotension (e.g., 60 mm Hg systolic or less) may be combated by *slow* intravenous injection of methoxamine hydrochloride, 3–5 mg followed by intramuscular injection of 10–15 mg; to maintain adequate levels of systolic blood pressure, intramuscular injection of methoxamine (10–15 mg) may be repeated at intervals of not less than 15 min.

If a reliable history suggestive of opioid poisoning is available and physical examination (including ophthalmoscopic examination of the optic discs and retinae) tends to rule out other diagnoses, attempts may be made to arouse the patient and restore spontaneous, adequate respiration by mild sensory stimulation (however, the patient should not be walked, as this may induce vomiting with aspiration in the absence of an endotracheal tube). During this time, blood and urine samples should be obtained for further differential diagnosis if necessary (see below). If the patient does not respond quickly to mild sensory stimulation, treatment with a narcotic antagonist should be started. Naloxone is preferable to nalorphine because, as already noted, the latter exerts opioid-agonist actions as well as opioid-antagonist actions, and the agonist actions may enhance central depression should the presumed signs of opioid poisoning actually be due to other causes. The initial dose of naloxone should be 0.01 mg/kg (0.7 mg/70 kg) by *slow* intravenous injection. The cardinal signs of successful opioid antagonism are *increase in respiratory rate* (and minute volume) and *pupillary dilatation;* effects of naloxone on opioid-produced coma are less striking. *Caution:* In physically dependent persons who have self-administered or have otherwise received an overdose of an opioid, relatively small doses of a narcotic antagonist may produce not only increase in respiratory rate and pupillary dilatation but also lacrimation, rhinorrhea, piloerection, profuse sweating, restlessness, vomiting, and other signs of a precipitated opioid-abstinence syndrome. If no increase in respiratory rate and pupillary dilatation are observed after the first dose of naloxone, it may be repeated once or twice at intervals of 5 min, but if no response is again observed, the diagnosis of opioid poisoning should be questioned, the differential diagnosis should be pursued (see below), and naloxone should be discontinued. If an adequate response to naloxone was obtained, the patient should be watched carefully for 24 hr or more, as the antagonistic actions of naloxone last only 2–3 hr, while the agonist actions of large doses of heroin last much longer, and those of methadone as much as 24–48 hr. If the respiratory rate falls to unacceptable levels after the initial opioid-antagonistic actions of naloxone have subsided, naloxone may be given again by the intramuscular route as often as necessary in doses 50% larger than that found to be adequate intravenously (Dole *et al.*, 1971).

Should no opioid-antagonist response to naloxone be observed, the blood and urine samples obtained should be sent to the laboratory for immediate analyses. The blood should be typed and determinations should be made for hemoglobin, hematocrit, erythrocyte and leukocyte counts (with differential), glucose, electrolytes, albumin, globulin, and levels of bromides, barbiturates, and other sedative drugs, including minor tranquilizers, and if indicated, blood cultures should be done. The urine should be analyzed for glucose, acetone, albumin, casts, and cells, and it should be subjected to a drug screen for as many pharmacological agents as the laboratory is equipped to detect. Other diagnostic procedures (X rays of the skull, electroencephalograms, examinations of the cerebrospinal fluid where not contraindicated, etc.) may have to be carried out as well. Treatment of the patient in coma not due solely to opioid poisoning is beyond the scope of this book.

Opioid Dependence

In general, two main approaches are used in the treatment of opioid-dependent patients: one involves "detoxification," followed by efforts of reeducation, rehabilitation, and prevention of relapse; the other involves transfer of dependence to orally administered methadone or *L*-alpha-acetyl-methadol (LAAM) under supervision, with attempts at social rehabilitation and, in some cases, eventual withdrawal from the opioids.

Detoxification

In patients with low degrees of physical dependence, withdrawal may be accomplished by administering the particular opioid of addiction (except heroin and other Schedule I opioids) orally (d-propoxyphene, methadone) or intramuscularly in daily amounts in divided doses just sufficient to suppress all abstinence phenomena and then progressively reducing the daily dose each day over a period of 5–10 days to zero. In patients who have a high degree of physical dependence, or whose opioid of addiction was heroin or other Schedule I opioid drug, either morphine (subcutaneously or intramuscularly) or methadone (orally) may be substituted for the opioid of addiction in daily amounts and at intervals just sufficient to suppress all abstinence phenomena for 3–5 days; then the daily dose of morphine or methadone is progressively reduced over a period of 7–10 days to zero. Care should be taken not to overdose the patient, as consciously or unconsciously, opioid addicts tend to exaggerate the amount of drug they have been taking. When morphine is used as the drug of substitution, experience has shown that it is rarely necessary to administer more than 30 mg subcutaneously every 6 hr in order to suppress all abstinence phenomena, regardless of the daily amount of opioid to which the patient, by history, has been accustomed. When methadone is used as the drug of substitution, the daily dose theoretically needed for suppression of all abstinence phenomena may be calculated on the basis of 1 mg of methadone (orally) for 3–4 mg of morphine, or 1 mg of heroin, or 0.5 mg of hydromorphone, or 20 mg of meperidine; in practice, 10–20 mg of methadone (orally) two or three times a day has been found sufficient. For the use of methadone in detoxification, FDA regulations (FDA, 1972) require that the hospital pharmacy be approved for this purpose by the FDA and state authorities, and that the procedures for methadone substitution and withdrawal be completed within 21 days. Administration of methadone for more than 21 days constitutes "methadone maintenance," for which special authority and facilities are required.

The clinical course of morphine substitution and progressive withdrawal is apt to be trying for the physicians, nurses, and patients, the latter complaining of discomfort as the daily dose of morphine is reduced. On the last day of morphine administration, codeine (30 mg) may be combined with one or more doses or morphine, and codeine alone may be continued for an additional day or two. Subsequently, one or two "pick-up" doses of morphine (6–10 mg) may be given if there are persistent complaints of muscular aching, anorexia, nausea, and/or vomiting. Intravenous infusions of 5% glucose in saline should be given to combat dehydration due to excessive sweating, vomiting, or diarrhea. Warm flow baths are useful for restlessness and aspirin for muscular aching. Hypnotics may be prescribed at bedtime to promote sleep. Compared with morphine, methadone is more effective by mouth (probably because of more complete absorption) and has a longer duration of action. Methadone does produce physical dependence, but the abstinence syndrome is delayed 2–3 days after abrupt withdrawal of the drug and is characterized by a lesser "point score" than after abrupt withdrawal of morphine, though complaints of bony and muscular aching and insomnia may be more prolonged (Isbell et al., 1948b). Methadone substitution and withdrawal are generally preferred to morphine substitution and withdrawal because the former is much less "stormy."

At least in the United States, relapse to habitual self-administration of opioid drugs is very common after detoxification, despite efforts at conventional methods of rehabilitation (individual or group psychotherapy, vocational training, education, job counseling). Thus, more than 90% of 1881 (of a total of 1912) opioid addicts who had been detoxified and institutionalized for variable periods of time at the federal hospital in Lexington, Kentucky, between 1952 and 1955 relapsed to heroin addiction within two years, and of these, more than 90% relapsed within six months after discharge from the hospital (Hunt & Odoroff, 1962). On longer follow-up, the relapse rate appears to decrease. Thus, Duvall et al. (1963) found that by the fifth year after discharge from the Lexington hospital, only 46% of 453 addicts (included in the 1881 reported on by Hunt & Odoroff, 1962) had become readdicted. A similar relapse rate (46%) after 12 years was found by Vaillant (1966), but this dropped to 35% after 20 years (Vaillant, 1973) following discharge from the Lexington hospital. Progressive decrease in the relapse rate of residents in rural areas of Kentucky who had been detoxified in the Lexington hospital was also reported by O'Donnell in a long-term (2–18 years) follow-up study. The reasons for such progressive decline in relapse rate over many years are obscure. Winick (1962) noted a sudden decline in the number of "active addicts" between the ages of 35 and 40 years in the file of active addicts of the former Bureau of Narcotics; he suggested that in some cases, "maturation" may lead to permanent abstention from opioids with or without previous treatment and despite repeated previous relapses. In a test of this maturation hypothesis, Ball and Snarr (1969) interviewed 108 males residing in Puerto Rico 15.8–19.5 years after the onset of opioid use. Of these, 23 had abstained from opioids during the 3-year period prior to interview ("cured"), while the rest were in prison or using opioids continuously or intermittently ("not cured"). All had, at one time or another, been patients at the Lexington hospital. Ball and Snarr concluded that the maturation hypothesis may be valid for roughly one-third of opioid addicts. The mean age of onset of opioid use in the cured group was 23 years, while in the noncured group it was about 19 years. Possibly, the age of onset of opioid use may be an important factor in the maturing-out process, as Zahn and Ball (1972) found that onset of opioid use at 16 or 17 years of age was associated with the worst prognosis for eventual cure, while onset at 32 years was most likely to result in eventual cure.

The effectiveness of other (or additional) methods of rehabilitation of detoxified opioid addicts in prevention relapse is difficult to assess. Therapeutic communities, in which addicts are detoxified (usually by abrupt withdrawal of the drug) and in which they reside permanently or after some months in "halfway houses" before reentering general society, claim great success, but their data, if made public at all, have been extremely difficult to evaluate (Glasscote *et al.*, 1972). Behavior therapy of one sort or another is currently being applied, but the results are not clear (Ulmer, 1977; Beatty, 1978).

Detoxification Followed by Narcotic-Antagonist Maintenance

Of special interest are current clinical investigations, restricted to investigators whose investigational new drug applications have been approved by the FDA, on the safety and efficacy of narcotic antagonists in preventing relapse of detoxified opioid addicts. The rationale for this treatment was stated by Martin *et al.* (1966) in their pioneering report on the use of cyclazocine:

> On the basis of our studies, 4 mg per day of cyclazocine will provide protection against the euphorogenic actions of large doses of narcotics, prevent the development of physical dependence, and will thereby control the pharmacological actions which are held responsible for narcotic addiction. . . . There may be other benefits. Wikler (1965) stated that two of the important reasons for relapse of the abstinent narcotic addict are conditioned abstinence which may be evoked by stimuli that have been associated with the addict's hustling activity to acquire drugs, and reinforcement of drug-seeking behavior through repeated reductions of abstinence by drug. It is possible that in subjects who attempt to readdict themselves while receiving a narcotic antagonist such as cyclazocine, there may be extinction of physical dependence and drug-seeking behavior. (pp. 463–464)

Emphasizing the importance of *active* extinction of classically conditioned abstinence and of operantly conditioned opioid-seeking behavior in minimizing the probability of relapse *after administration of the narcotic antagonist has been discontinued*, Wikler (1974, 1976) proposed that prior to temporary outpatient maintenance (up to one year, if possible) on daily opioid-blocking doses of a narcotic antagonist, the detoxified opioid addict be exposed as an inpatient to facsimiles of his drug-ridden environment and its conditioned reinforcers (other addicts, needles, syringes, bags of heroin) and be encouraged to self-inject heroin, at first under the unblocked condition and then repeatedly under narcotic-antagonist blockade, until signs of conditioned abstinence have disappeared and he desists from further self-injections (extinction). After discharge to the outpatient department and maintenance on daily blocking doses of the narcotic antagonist, it may be presumed that in the presence of his real drug-ridden environment, partial "recovery from extinction" and illicit opioid self-administration are likely to occur, but because of the blockade afforded by the narcotic antagonist, extinction should be reestablished quickly.

Since the original paper of Martin *et al.* (1966), some preliminary evaluations of narcotic-antagonist treatment have appeared, first on cyclazocine and more recently on naltrexone. These evaluations are discussed in some detail below. Only two groups of investigators (O'Brien, personal communication; O'Brien & Greenstein, 1976; Altman *et al.*, 1976; Meyer *et al.*, 1976a,b) have attempted to carry out inpatient extinction. O'Brien's group (O'Brien & Greenstein, 1976) found increase in "craving" and decrease in skin temperature (conditioned abstinence) during the "cooking-up" and other preinjection rituals; after self-injection of hydromorphone or saline under naltrexone blockade, the initial effects, if any, were in the direction of mild agonist opioidlike actions, but on repetition of self-injection, the effects became neutral and finally annoying (a judgment presumably associated with conditioned abstinence); at this point, the patients refused to self-inject further, thus leaving the presumptive conditioned abstinence syndrome unextinguished. Meyer's group (1976a,b), including Altman *et al.* (1976), found that when detoxified heroin addicts were permitted to work an operant device for purchase of intravenous injections of heroin in the unblocked condition, they did so avidly and reported marked increase in craving. Under naloxone or naltrexone blockade, their work avidity for heroin decreased markedly: of six patients, two did not purchase heroin at all, while the remaining four purchased and used heroin six, five, two, and eight times over the 10-day period of this phase of the study (Meyer *et al.*, 1976a); subsequently, three patients who, as individuals, were blocked on naltrexone in the presence of numerous peers getting high on heroin in the unblocked condition tended to maintain heroin self-administration for longer periods of time (Meyer *et al.*, 1976b). According to Meyer *et al.* (1976b), craving scores remained elevated under narcotic antagonist blockade as long as heroin self-administration continued. When the subjects realized that heroin was "unavailable" (i.e., that they were blocked by naltrexone), their craving scores fell dramatically and they stopped injections of heroin. Meyer *et al.* (1976b) felt that their data did not permit assessment of whether or not classically conditioned abstinence phenomena had been extinguished during naltrexone blockade and repeated self-injections of heroin, but they concluded that the data suggested that active extinction did not take place in the presence of naltrexone. Meyer and his associates (Altman et al., 1976) attributed the loss of interest in heroin under narcotic-antagonist blockade to "expectancy," "set," or "instructional control" and called attention to Wikler's (1974) report of the power of "cognitive labeling" in man to abolish signs and symptoms of conditioned nalorphine-precipitated opioid abstinence, observed in 1952 (Meyer et al., 1976b). Such a phenomenon may also explain the observation of Freedman et al. (1968) that cyclazocine appeared to obtund interest in opioids (but not in marijuana, amphetamines, barbiturates, or alcohol), and of Kleber et al. (1974) that patients on cyclazocine rarely challenged the opioid blockade by self-administration of illicit heroin. Emphasizing the importance of the cognitive labeling process in the successful treatment of the narcotic user with naltrexone, Meyer et al. (1976b) stated:

> During conditions when the stimulus properties of the environment (interoceptive and exteroceptive) suggest the availability of heroin, patients experience a dysphoric response that may not only be marked by classically conditioned abstinence, but also by anxiety and tension associated with an approach–avoidance conflict associated with the euphoric high generated by previous opioid administrations, as well as previous encounters with the aversive consequences of drug use. In this circumstance, tension escalates and relief can be obtained by the administration of an opioid. The dysphoria is labeled "craving" and is associated with a feeling of inevitability. Conditioned abstinence phenomena may only be one part of the symptom picture, but we suspect that the ambivalence in the conflict may be more central to the relapsing phenomenon as it manifests in human beings. Naltrexone consumption is a conscious act by the patient to enter a drug-free seeting for a period of 24–48 hours. It is marked by tension reduction because in the circumstances the stimuli associated with heroin availability (including classically conditioned abstinence) are not present.... Our data suggest that contingent reinforcement of naltrexone consumption may offer some short-term advantages relative to the initiation of naltrexone consumption by the patient in the community. Motivation to continue naltrexone consumption, however, appears to be a function if the availability of alternative reinforcers (e.g., job; meaningful, affectional relationships, etc.). We would urge that programs utilizing naltrexone consider these needs in developing their treatment programs.... Moreover our data on patients who have been on naltrexone for six months suggest that, even the patient on long-term antagonist treatment must eventually confront the time when he is naltrexone free and opioids are again available. (pp. 132–133)

In this view, extinction of conditioned abstinence and opioid-seeking behavior under naltrexone blockade is impossible because of cognitive labeling by the patient, and therefore, a high probability of relapse is to be expected after the patient ceases to take the narcotic antagonist. Wikler (1976) has suggested experimental designs other than those used in most of the studies by Meyer and his group to achieve extinction under hospital conditions, but to date, these have not been employed, at least extensively. Nevertheless, follow-up studies recently reported (see below) indicate that the percentage of patients who remain opioid-free *after outpatient cyclazocine or naltrexone maintenance has been discontinued* is directly related to the duration of prior outpatient narcotic antagonist maintenance.

Earlier reports dealt with the results of cyclazocine maintenance. Freedman *et al.* (1968) reported on 58 detoxified opioid addicts who volunteered for cyclazocine maintenance. Of these, 27 remained in regular treatment with cyclazocine for at least two months, while 31 were dropped. Induction on cyclazocine began with 0.2 mg/day; the dosage was increased slowly over a total period of 20 days to a maintenance level of 4 mg/day. During the induction period, half of the patients reported increased libido, constipation, elation, anxiety, dizziness, headaches, restlessness, and/or insomnia, which, presumably, were agonistic affects of cyclazocine to which tolerance eventually developed (without diminution of the opioid-antagonistic effects). On eventual withdrawal of cyclazocine, features of the typical cyclazocine-abstinence syndrome ("electric-shock" sensations in the head and neck, paranoid ideation, suspiciousness, depression, increased irritability, and headaches) appeared transitorily. After withdrawal of cyclazocine was completed, 21 of the 27 patients were found to be opioid-free (Fink, 1973). Similarly, Kissin *et al.* (1973) reported on a cyclazocine treatment program that had been in operation only 17 months. They found that 34 out of 77 (40%) of the patients then currently active in the cyclazocine outpatient program had achieved a totally drug-free state and were no longer on cyclazocine nor involved in either heroin or other secondary drug abuse. Most of these patients had been abstinent for about six months. The absence of antisocial behavior in this population was notable.

Retention rates on cyclazocine maintenance after detoxification has improved from about 20% when no other treatment was offered to about 50% when, initially, the patient was offered a choice of methadone maintenance, detoxification and a drug-free program, or detoxification and cyclazocine maintenance (Resnick *et al.*, 1971; Fink, 1973). The relative efficacy of "self-selection" for narcotic-antagonist treatment appears to be related to a lesser personal need for opioids and the presence of a stable heterosexual relationship (Resnick *et al.*, 1970). Nevertheless, the dropout rate from cyclazocine treatment remains inordinately high, presumably because of the disturbing (albeit) transitory agonistic actions of cyclazocine and of the cyclazocine withdrawal syndrome. With the advent of the orally efficacious narcotic antagonist naltrexone, which is practically devoid of clinically significant agonistic actions (Martin et al., 1973b; Thomas et al., 1976), it was thought that retention rates would increase dramatically. However, Thomas et al. (1976) have pointed out that cyclazocine has advantages in that it requires longer hospitalization for induction, thus permitting the establishment of a therapeutic relationship between the patient and the staff; in the outpatient clinic, skipping a dose or two of cyclazocine results in an abstinence syndrome that reminds the patient to return to the clinic and resume his cyclazocine medication. Naltrexone induction is much easier, requiring only a day or two in the hospital after detoxification, and skipping naltrexone doses as an outpatient has no ill consequences (except disappearance of the opioid blockade). Hence, most patients discontinue taking naltrexone after one or a few doses. The high dropout rate from naltrexone-maintenance treatment is illustrated by the report of Hollister et al. (1978) on the results of a *double-blind* random assignment of naltrexone or placebo in syrup similar in appearance and taste to a total of 735 detoxified opioid addicts in five clinics. Of these, 543 dropped out of the study before study–medication (naltrexone or placebo) was begun, 170 terminated study–medication before nine months, 13 completed nine months on study–medication, and 9 were still in active treatment at the data cutoff point. Six months after the end of each patient's study–medication (naltrexone or placebo), the duration of which was highly variable, "global" follow-up evaluations were made on 54 naltrexone-treated and 64 placebo-treated patients who could be found; there was no significant difference in opioid or other drug abuse or alcoholism, but 49 naltrexone patients reported a significant decrease in their subjective craving, compared with 51 placebo-treated patients ($p = 0.024$). Interestingly, in 60 naltrexone-treated and 64 placebo-treated patients submitting five or more urine samples, 26% were positive for morphine in the naltrexone-treated group, and 38% were positive in the placebo-treated group, but following the first positive urine sample, 10% of naltrexone-treated and 33% of placebo-treated patients were positive ($p = 0.002$); presumably these urine samples were obtained while the patients were still on study–medication. Cumulative retention curves for the entire study show slightly high retention rates for the naltrexone-treated group compared with placebo, particularly at 3–4 months. The main purposes of this study were to evaluate the safety and feasibility of chronic naltrexone maintenance and, if possible, to obtain some impression of its efficacy. Very few adverse effects were encountered, and these appeared to be due mainly to precipitated abstinence in patients on naltrexone who were covertly using opioids, or to prior infections. The authors concluded that naltrexone is safe and probably relatively efficacious.

The high dropout rate in this study may be attributed, in part, to the absence or insufficiency of positive reinforcement to continue to take naltrexone, inherent in the double-blind, placebo-controlled design. As Dr. Lee Schwartz, quoted by Resnick and Schuyten-Resnick (1976), stated, "It takes more than a pill to cure an ill." Emphasizing the role of the therapist in a narcotic-antagonist treatment program, these investigators stated further:

> Gradually, the patient can learn to look to the therapist—rather than to the opiate—for gratification of dependency needs, relief of anxieties and solutions to the problems and dilemmas of his life. It is through this therapeutic relationship that a patient can get *positive reinforcement* for making choices that will contribute to his achieving a more stable, socially acceptable lifestyle, while deconditioning (or at least *non*reinforcement) of his drug-seeking behavior is taking place.

The authors explained conditioning theory to their patients, so the latter could look for symptoms of conditioned abstinence within themselves and could also be alerted to the possibility of readdiction even after a long period of successful antagonist treatment.

> Stopping antagonist and resuming opiate use is, by itself, an insufficient criterion for labeling the treatment a failure. Would you say digitalis is not clinically efficacious if a patient with congestive heart failure stops taking it? In our studies we have found that the length of time patients take naltrexone increases with each successive readmission. . . . The model we use should be similar to the one we use in treating chronic medical illnesses. A patient must be told that whenever medication is discontinued, he can and should ask to be put back on the antagonist whenever he feels tempted or has begun to use opiate drugs again. Imagine the positive affect it has on patients and their families when they can view addiction as no worse than other recurrent medical problems for which treatment *is* available. The emotional impact on the patient is usually profound, since he has previously experienced negative attitudes and rejection—if only by being labeled a "failure"—whenever he has become readdicted. When the treatment staff is non-judgmental about his opiate use, it just "blows their minds." We've seen this happen over and over again—"You mean, Doc, if I goof up, I really *can* come back to the program???" (pp. 85–86)

Resnick *et al.* (1976) reported on the results of naltrexone treatment in 81 patients who took naltrexone one week or longer (110 applicants for naltrexone treatment were excluded because they were unable to complete detoxification, or took naltrexone for less than one week, or were transfers from cyclazocine, or were medically and/or psychiatrically ineligible) during the period, May 1, 1974–February 28, 1975. After one year, 27 of the 81 patients (33%) were judged opioid-free (by personal contacts, urine tests, naloxone tests), while 54 (67%) were opioid-dependent. Time on naltrexone significantly differentiated the opioid-free (mean, 12.1 weeks) from the opioid-dependent (mean, 6.8 weeks) patients at 1 year. During the period February 1975–June 1977, Resnick and Washton (1978) presented the results of a follow-up study on 267 patients who had been on naltrexone treatment for varying periods of time before voluntarily discontinuing it, and who had been off naltrexone for at least 6 months by the time of follow-up (June 1977). Of 59 patients who had taken naltrexone for 3–24 months (mean, 26.8 weeks), 18 (31%) were opioid-free 32 (54%) were readdicted, and the status of 9 was unknown. Of 143 patients who had taken naltrexone for 1 week to 3 months (mean, 4.8 months), 3 (2%) were opioid-free, 109 (76%) were readdicted, and the status of 31 (22%) was unknown; similar distributions were found in the remaining 65 patients who had taken naltrexone for 1 week or less. The results of this study and of the preceding one (Resnick *et al.*, 1976) concur in suggesting that the clinical efficacy of naltrexone is a function of treatment duration. This impression is in agreement with the findings of Greenstein *et al.* (1976), who reported on the results of chemical detection methods on 44 urine samples obtained from 41 individual patients at 1 month and 6 months (no significant differences) after termination of naltrexone treatment. Of 9 urines from patients who had taken naltrexone for more than 8 weeks, 78% were opioid-free; of 19 urines (naltrexone for less than 1 week), 19% were opioid-free. Resnick and Washton (1978) found that differentiating patients on naltrexone from those unable to complete detoxification was significantly lesser involvement with heroin (judged in terms of dollar amounts spent) in the 6-month period immediately preceding admission to the program. Also, they cite Parwatikar (1976), who reported that those who were found to be drug-free 6–9 months after discharge from naltrexone treatment tended to be better educated, had higher-status occupations and higher rates of employment, and displayed less criminal behavior than patients who became readdicted; Hurzeler *et al.* (1976), who found that the patient's "stability of living pattern" was the only variable that discriminated between the more successful and less successful patients treated with naltrexone; and Meyer *et al.* (1976b), who stated that patients living with a spouse, parents, or relatives did better in naltrexone treatment than those living with friends, living alone, or having no stable living arrangement. Very recently, Lewis *et al.* (1978) reported on the results of naltrexone treatment of 22 opioid addicts over a period of 29 months. The mean duration of naltrexone treatment was 6.2 weeks, and 12 patients (55%) continued in treatment for an average of 5.6 weeks after cessation of naltrexone. Follow-up after an average of 45.3 weeks after cessation of naltrexone indicated that 11 (58%) were known to be abstinent from opioids, and 9 (47%) were employed, compared with 3 (16%) who were employed at the onset of treatment. These investigators feel that ingestion of naltrexone provides a degree of external control, reducing the preoccupation with heroin and releasing energy for the pursuit of other goals.

For patients who voluntarily seek such external control in order to remain abstinent from opioids, "depot" preparations of naltrexone or other suitable narcotic antagonist that releases the narcotic antagonist continuously for long periods (e.g., a month) would eliminate the recurring conflict over whether to take the next dose of orally administered narcotic antagonist or to skip it and thus make opioids again available. For use in man, such depot preparations or drug-delivery systems must be nontoxic, painless, biodegradable, and capable of being removed by the physician or surgeon if, for any reason, termination of the narcotic blockade is deemed necessary. Currently, several drug-delivery systems are under investigation with *in vitro* and *in vivo* methods, the latter including the mouse tail-flick for evaluation of the narcotic-antagonist blockade of morphine analgesia, and monkeys trained to self-inject morphine intravenously for evaluation of narcotic-antagonist–produced extinction (Willette, 1976). Meyer *et al.* (1976b) stated, "It is our impression that depot preparations will be seen by patients as a "sentence" to a drug-free setting and that extinction will no more take place under conditions of depot administration than under conditions which we have observed." However, as the data of Greenstein *et al.* (1976) and of Resnick and Washton (1978) indicate, the percentage of patients remaining opioid-free after naltrexone has been discontinued increases substantially if naltrexone has been taken for 2 or 3 months or longer. It is true, as O'Brien and Greenstein (1976) have remarked, that up to now no one has shown that the remission rate for patients on naltrexone exceeds spontaneous remissions in similar untreated patients, but the opioid-free rates after naltrexone maintenance reported by Greenstein *et al.* (1976), Resnick and Washton (1978), and Lewis *et al.* (1978) greatly exceed those formerly found after *involuntary* detoxification without narcotic-antagonist maintenance (Hunt & Odoroff, 1962) and are therefore encouraging.

Methadone Maintenance (with or without Eventual Detoxification)

Postulating that the high relapse rate of detoxified heroin addicts is due to a persistent metabolic defect experienced as "drug hunger," Dole and Nyswander (1965, 1968) found that when administered by the oral route, methadone does not produce euphoria and that despite the development of a high degree of tolerance, addicts do not seek to increase the daily dose; that is, drug hunger continues to be suppressed (by daily "stabilization" doses of methadone). Because of cross-tolerance between methadone and heroin, Dole and Nyswander (1965) postulated that should the methadone-tolerant addict self-inject heroin intravenously, he would not experience the expected euphoria, and such attempts to obtain an opioid high would soon be abandoned (extinction of heroin self-administration behavior). Freed from the drug-hunger drive to hustle, from heroin, and from the criminalism involved therein, the methadone-tolerant addict can, with some assistance, find a place to live, obtain employment or go back to school, and otherwise rehabilitate himself into society. Methadone maintenance is, perhaps, the most widely used single treatment modality for opioid dependence in the United States. Martin (1977) stated that in 1973, when the estimated number of addicts in the United States was about 360,000, approximately 80,000 were on methadone maintenance (22%). In New York City, where the addict population was approximately 150,000, 30,000 were in methadone-maintenance programs (20%).

Psychological test performance in methadone-tolerant patients appear to be within normal limits. Appel and Gordon (1976) administered the Digit Symbol Substitution Test (DSST) of the Wechsler Adult Intelligence Scale (WAIS) to working and nonworking methadone patients who had been maintained on 80–120 mg/day of methadone for a year or more and two comparison groups: former heroin addicts who had been drug-free for a year or longer and persons with no history of narcotic dependence. The individual's score on the DSST is the number of symbols correctly substituted in 90 sec; a score significantly lower than normal is considered an indicator of impaired attention and/or cognitive ability. There were no significant differences between the scores of the working methadone-maintained patients and either of the two drug-free comparison groups, but the scores of the nonworking methadone-maintained patients were lower than those of any of the three other groups; however, when the DSST scores of the nonworking methadone-maintained patients were converted to T or scaled scores, they were in the normal range according to the WAIS. Appel and Gordon(1976) tentatively ascribed the lower DSST scores of the nonworking methadone-maintained patients to "overly high levels of arousal" in some of them. They also stated that in previous research they had found that methadone patients performed adequately on psychomotor and intellectual tasks. Performance on memory tests is not impaired in patients maintained on either methadone or LAAM (Grevert *et al.*, 1977).

Physical complaints and disabilities ascribable to methadone are quite common during the first six months of methadone maintenance. These include (Kreek, 1978): primary narcotic effects (drowsiness, nodding, high); constipation; excessive sweating; insomnia (often with nightmares while sleeping); interference with sexual function; menstrual irregularities; transient difficulty in urination, edema of lower extremities joint pains and swelling, and skin rash; upper gastrointestinal symptoms (pain, nausea, vomiting); bradycardia; and hypotension. In patients maintained on methadone for more than six months, the most common complaints and disabilities are, according to Kreek (1978): increased sweating, constipation, libido and orgasm abnormalities, insomnia and abnormalities of appetite. Other problems (nausea, drowsiness, nervousness–tenseness, headaches, body aches and pain, chills) may have been due to incomplete tolerance or insufficient doses of methadone. Extensive biochemical, endocrinological, and physiological studies on methadone-maintained patients have been reported by Kreek (1973, 1978). No significant abnormalities were found that could be attributed to methadone, uncomplicated by prior infections or alcoholism, except possibly for the following: hypomotility of the small bowel (Kreek, 1973); lowering of the plasma levels of FSH and LH during the first 6–12 months (only) of methadone maintenance; impaired ability of the hypothalamus to release ACTH in response to metyrapone blockade of cortison production during the first 2 months (only) of methadone maintenance; a distorted diurnal variation of plasma prolactin levels (mean prolactin levels were normal); increased levels of both thyroxine (T4) and triiodothyronine (T3) in some methadone-maintenance patients (ascribed to the increased levels of thyroxine-binding globulin in these patients); increased levels of serum albumin in some methadone-maintained patients; and persistent reduction in sensitivity of the central nervous system receptors to hypoxia, even after tolerance to the respiratory-depressant actions of methadone and the accompanying increase in pCO_2 and decrease in pO_2 had developed (Kreek, 1978).

In addition, Mendelson *et al.* (1975) reported that heroin addicts or patients maintained on high-dosage methadone (80–150 mg/day) had depressed plasma testosterone levels; patients on lower-dosage methadone maintenance (10–60 mg/day) had testosterone levels that were not significantly different from those of normal adult male controls. Martin *et al.* (1973a) found that in postaddicts experimentally stabilized on oral doses of methadone (100 mg/day), electroencephalograms showed increased delta bursts and rapid eye movement (REM) sleep and more vocalization during REM periods, as well as decreased respiratory rate, pulse rate, pupillary diameter, and blood pressure, and increased body temperature. About one-third of babies born to mothers maintained on methadone are underweight at birth and are considered premature (Wilmarth & Goldstein, 1974). Davis *et al.* (1973) reported that about 80% of babies born to mothers maintained on 60 mg/day or more of methadone exhibit methadone-withdrawal phenomena, such as irritability, hypertoxicity, tremors, excessive sucking needs, and excessive crying.

Kaim (1976) has summarized the criticisms that have been made of methadone, that is: (1) the substitution of one addiction for another; (2) the side effects from the agonist properties of methadone; (3) the logistic problems in providing a daily treatment; (4) the dangerous diversion of methadone to the illicit market; and (5) the negative image of methadone as a method of social control of minority groups. In regard to the substitution of one addiction for another, it should be noted that especially after chronic administration of methadone in the high daily doses used in methadone maintenance, withdrawal of the drug is followed by a prolonged, distressing abstinence syndrome. Thus, Martin *et al.* (1973a) found that after abrupt withdrawal of methadone from experimental subjects who had received methadone orally for 15 weeks, attaining a dose of 100 mg/day by the 7th week, a protracted abstinence syndrome ensued lasting 6–8 weeks generally, and up to 24 weeks in some respects. If the metabolic defect and drug hunger postulated by Dole and Nyswander (1965) are consequences of long-term heroin addiction, then they should be aggravated by prolonged maintenance on another opioid, namely, methadone, which likewise produces physical dependence with protracted abstinence. Senay *et al.* (1977) carried out methadone withdrawal in a double-blind manner according to two schedules, namely, "rapid withdrawal" (dose of methadone reduced by 10% per week over 10 weeks, followed by dextromethorphan placebo for 20 weeks) and "gradual withdrawal" (dose of methadone reduced by 3% per week over 30 weeks). In the rapid-withdrawal group, 8 (24%) completed the withdrawal, while 25 (76%) dropped out; in the "gradual withdrawal" group, 16 (53%) completed withdrawal and 14 (47%) dropped out. In contrast, completions occurred in 76% of a group of 33 patients who were maintained on their starting dose of methadone nonblind, and in 94% of a group of 31 patients who were likewise maintained on methadone under double-blind conditions for 30 weeks. Senay *et al.* (1977) commented that the data indicate that the withdrawal process should be carried out with a dose decrement of approximately 3% per week; larger dose decrements are associated with increased dropout rates, illicit narcotic use, and subjective distress. They also noted that in the rapid-withdrawal group, mean symptom scores were higher in the 20-week postwithdrawal period than during the preceding 10-week withdrawal phase, supporting the notion of a clinically significant protracted abstinence syndrome as suggested by Martin *et al.* (1973a).

In connection with the problem of "the dangerous diversion of methadone to the illicit market" (Kaim, 1976), it should be recalled that like heroin or morphine, methadone *intravenously* does produce an intense high or euphoria (Isbell *et al.*, 1948). Puzzling is the reason why it took so long for methadone to become an illicit opioid of addiction on the street, but a black market for methadone came into existence after the establishment of methadone-maintenance clinics, and in some cities, the number of deaths from methadone "overdoses" exceeded those attributable to heroin (Bourne, 1973). Thus, Dupont and Greene (1974) found that from July 1971 through December 1972 in the District of Columbia, the number of deaths from heroin declined progressively from about eight per month to a total of only two in the last six months of 1972. In contrast, deaths from methadone peaked in January and February 1972 at about seven per month and declined to about three per month by the end of 1972. Deaths from intravenously self-administered methadone or heroin are characterized by pulmonary edema (Kjeldgaard *et al.*, 1971).

When a patient is admitted to a methadone-maintenance program, the initial dose of methadone is 10 or 20 mg/day given orally in divided doses. As tolerance develops, the dose is gradually increased to a stabilization level, after which the patient is maintained at this level by a single daily oral dose of methadone. Induction of methadone maintenance and stabilization may take as long as six weeks and, preferably, should be carried out in a hospital. After stabilization has been achieved, the patient may be discharged to the outpatient clinic where methadone (orally) is dispensed (for limitations on dosage and take-home supplies, see below and FDA regulations governing methadone, 1972). Also, the outpatient clinic should provide assistance in finding a job and a place to live and in making arrangements for education or vocational training. In addition, the patient should be required to submit a urine specimen at random intervals for detection of morphine (heroin), other opioids, and quinine (a common adulterant of illicit heroin), as well as barbiturates, amphetamines, and cocaine. Effective June 17, 1973, the FDA requires that admission to methadone-maintenance programs be voluntary (with written consent, and in those under 18 years of age, with written consent from their parents or legal guardians also); the patient must be over 16 years of age; documentary evidence must be furnished that all patients admitted to methadone-maintenance programs have been dependent on opioids for at least two years (and in patients 16–18 years of age, have had at least two unsuccessful attempts at detoxification). At time of admission, evidence of current physical dependence must be documented (except in the cases of addicts within one week after discharge from prison or other institutions where they have spent one month or longer). Besides personal and medical histories and a physical examination, it is recommended that all new admissions have a complete blood count, liver function tests, and a serologic test for syphilis. In methadone maintenance, all methadone must be dispensed in liquid form for oral administration. The initial dose of methadone should be that sufficient to suppress opioid-withdrawal signs. Subsequently, the daily dose of methadone may be increased as tolerance develops to a maximum of 100 mg/day; higher doses, up to 120 mg/day must be justified in the medical record, and for doses over 120 mg/day (or over 100 mg/day for take-home methadone), approval must be obtained from the FDA and state authorities. During the first three months, methadone must be administered under close observation daily or at least six days a week; after three months of satisfactory cooperation, three times weekly (with no more than a two-day take-home supply); after two years of satisfactory progress two times weekly (with no more than a three-day supply). These rules may be relaxed in cases of acute illness, family crises, or necessary travel (for further details, see Methadone Treatment Manual, U.S. Department of Justice, 1973).

According to Dole and Nyswander (1968), the stabilization dose of methadone should be between 80 and 120 mg/day. However, Wilmarth and Goldstein (1974) noted that blind studies have failed to reveal important differences in the use of heroin (or other program criteria) at daily doses as widely different as 40 or 160 mg (a daily dose of 30 mg of methadone appeared to be less effective). They feel that daily oral doses of 50–80 mg/day are generally sufficient, providing there is no evidence of an unusually low plasma level. Comparing outcome results in three different methadone-maintenance programs, Wilmarth and Goldstein (1974) found that retention rates (over a period of about four years) varied from 53% to 77%. In a New York City methadone-maintenance program, there was an annual dropout rate of 13% each year. In all three programs, heroin use decreased profoundly and there was no increase in use of barbiturates, alcohol, or amphetamines. Also, employment rates increased and arrest rates decreased. Wilmarth and Goldstein (1974) emphasized the roles of rehabilitative efforts and of outreaching, nonpunitive, and nonjudgmental attitudes on the part of the staff in achieving these results. Whether or not patients on methadone maintenance can eventually be detoxified and remain opioid-free is another question. Writing in 1973, Dole stated that there was no evidence in the medical literature to support the assumption that detoxification could be achieved in most cases without compromising the patient's rehabilitation. Reviewing the long-term outcome of patients treated with methadone maintenance, Dole and Joseph (1978) found that of 1413 patients included in the files of the Community Treatment Foundation (New York), 567 remained in continuous methadone treatment, while 846 had been discharged one or more times when followed up (19.57–25.70 months after first discharge from treatment). Of the 846 patients, 167 (20%) were discharged in "good standing," and of these 58 (34%) were "apparently well"; that is, they denied any illicit opioid use during the rating period whether or not data from urinalysis were available to confirm the claim and regardless of any relapse prior to the rating period; also, there were no serious nonopioid problems such as disabling alcoholism, heavy use of nonopioid drugs, criminal activity leading to arrest, and death. The "apparently well" status was negligible in the other categories of discharge (dropouts, administrative, unknown). Of the total of 846 patients who had been discharged, only a small proportion did "apparently well," and Dole and Joseph noted that even this estimate of success may be too high since claims of abstention from opioids were accepted without urine testing. They also noted that of those doing "apparently well," 55% had been in methadone-maintenance programs for more than three years, 88% had no behavioral problems while in the clinic, and 78% had a steady or occasional job. A relationship between duration of methadone maintenance and opioid-free outcome 5–89 months after detoxification was found by Stimmel et al. (1978), that is, less than three years, 40%. These investigators found that of 1220 patients in the Mount Sinai Methadone Maintenance and Aftercare Treatment Program (New York), 429 were detoxified; on follow-up (at an average of 31.1 months from discharge), 98 in all categories of discharge (22.9%) were found to be "narcotic-free"; of these, 50 had "completed treatment," 26 had undergone "voluntary detoxification," 18 had "violated the rules," and 4 were in jail. Among the 50 who had completed treatment, 56% were "narcotic-free," while among the 48 in the other categories of discharge, the status "narcotic-free" was found in 4.5–22.4%. Similar results were reported by Cushman (1978) in a follow-up of 225 patients at an average of 2.4 years since time of discharge from St. Luke's Methadone Clinic (New York), from a total of 513 patients, 288 of whom remained in methadone-maintenance treatment. Of the 225 discharged patients, 49 (21.8%) in all categories of discharge were "apparently narcotic-free"; of these, 41 had been "therapeutically discharged" (46% of 89 in this discharge category), while 2 had been "administratively discharged" (3% of 66), and 6 had "absconded" (14% of 42), Cushman commented that about 10% of patients in methadone-maintenance treatment will detoxify "in time" and "appear to function in society without the use of nonprescribed opioids." He also noted that posttreatment mortality rates were strikingly high: in the "therapeutically detoxified," 3.3%; in the combined "administratively discharged–absconded," 2.8%, compared with 1.5% in patients still under treatment.

Levomethadyl Maintenance

A modification of methadone maintenance, using LAAM (1-alph-acetylmethadol; levomethadyl; methadyl acetate) is now under restricted investigation. In 1952, Fraser and Isbell reported that when given *orally*, LAAM produced morphinelike effects that appeared within 1 hr and persisted for 48 hr (when given subcutaneously or intravenously, there was a delay of 4–6 hr, after which morphinelike effects appeared that persisted for 24–72 hr). In a dose of 1 mg of LAAM orally for 6–8 mg of morphine, LAAM completely suppressed the morphine-abstinence syndrome in physically dependent subjects, even when LAAM was given once every three days; on abrupt withdrawal of LAAM, a mild, slowly developing abstinence syndrome appeared, resembling that seen following withdrawal of methadone from methadone-dependent subjects. Fraser and Isbell (1952) noted that because of its long duration of action, LAAM is likely to produce cumulative toxic effects if doses of LAAM are not widely spaced in time.

Use of LAAM instead of methadone for maintenance of opioid addicts would reduce the number of clinic visits per week and eliminate take-home medication with the attendant dangers of accidental ingestion by children in the addict's household and of diversion into illicit drug traffic on the street. Jaffe and Senay (1971) divided 10 patients stabilized on methadone into two groups: a control group of 5 patients who continued on methadone (average dose 68 mg/day) ingested daily at the clinic except for take-home doses for Sundays or for Saturdays and Sundays; an experimental group of 5 patients who ingested methadone (average dose 50 mg/day) daily at the clinic for 5 days, ingested a dose of 50 mg of LAAM on Saturdays, and received dextromethorphan hydrobromide placebo to take home on Sunday, or who ingested methadone (same dose/day) daily at the clinic for 4 days, a dose of 60 mg of LAAM on Fridays., with dextromethorphan hydrobromide placebo to take home for Saturdays and Sundays (later, the dose of LAAM was increased to 65 mg). A checklist of symptoms revealed no differences between groups, and a physician blind to the experiment was unable to discriminate patients on methadone from patients on LAAM. Zaks *et al.* (1972) compared 20 heroin addicts who, after detoxification, were randomly assigned to maintenance on methadone (final maintenance level, 100 mg/day), which was ingested in the clinic every day for the first month, then twice weekly, with take-home supplies of the drug for the nonclinic days, or on LAAM ingested in the clinic on Mondays, Wednesdays, and Fridays (no take-home medications). The maintenance dose levels of LAAM were of two kinds: "low," 30–50 mg, and "high," 80 mg. Over a period of 4–6 months of maintenance in the outpatient clinic, the methadone and the high-dose LAAM patients reported no withdrawal symptoms, no response to cross-tolerance test doses of 50 mg of heroin intravenously, and about equal frequency of morphine-positive urines (2.0–2.8%), indicating illicit use of heroin; however, some of the high-dose LAAM patients reported increased "irritability," "jerky movements" of arms and/or legs, and constipation. In contrast, the low-dose LAAM patients reported withdrawal symptoms beginning 40–48 hr after the last previous dose of LAAM, the majority showed some response to cross-tolerance test doses of 50 mg of heroin intravenously, and in a far greater proportion than in methadone or high-dose LAAM patients, urines were positive for morphine (18.9%); as in high-dose LAAM patients, some of those on low-dose LAAM complained of increased "irritability," "jerky movements," and constipation. Zaks *et al.* (1972) concluded that 80 mg of LAAM ingested three times weekly suppressed narcotic hunger as effectively as 100 mg of methadone ingested daily. Similarly, in a double-blind study, Jaffe *et al.* (1972) found no differences in acceptability to patients, reduction of illicit drug use, increase in legitimate employment, reduction of criminal activity, frequency of clinic visits, and medical safety between patients maintained on methadone (30–80 mg/day ingested daily or three times a week, with take-home methadone for the other days) or LAAM (on Mondays, Wednesdays, and Fridays, with take-home supplies of dextromethorphan hydrobromide placebo, 30 mg, for the other days) over a period of 15 weeks of maintenance. However, 2 of the 19 patients on LAAM complained of "jerking" and "twitching" of their arms or legs when at rest. In an "open" study comparing patients maintained solely on methadone or methadone Mondays through Thursdays plus LAAM on Fridays (no take-home medications), or solely on LAAM ingested every other day or Mondays, Wednesdays, and Fridays (LAAM: methadone dose ratios, 1.2 to last 48 hr; 1.5 to last 72 hr). Wilson *et al.* (1976) likewise found no difference in social adjustment, occupational participation, clinic attendance, or drug abuse patterns; however, they observed a variety of disturbing effects of LAAM in some of the patients, namely, a mild amphetaminelike effect most marked in the early phases of treatment, which was manifested by increased motor activity, irritability, tenseness, and restlessness. Wilson *et al.* concluded that LAAM may exaggerate a loss of impulse control in hysterical and explosive personality patterns, and they noted that increased aggresive behavior was observed in participants with such personalities throughout their study. They also observed an "allergic" reaction to LAAM in one patient and early opioid-abstinence signs on the third day after the last previous dose of LAAM in another. In five of six patients who were hospitalized for laboratory tests at the beginning and at the end of the study, serum glutamic oxalacetic transaminase (SGOT) levels were elevated, and also in five of six patients, the hematocrit percentage was slightly decreased at the end of the study. Wilson *et al.* regarded as major unanswered questions about LAAM the frequency of allergic reactions, the significance of alterations in blood count and liver function tests, and the relation of LAAM to increased aggressive behavior. In a large-scale nonblind study of 308 patients maintained on methadone (average dose, 59.78 mg/day) ingested in the clinic with take-home days and 328 patients crossed over from methadone to LAAM (average dose, 59.35 mg) ingested in the clinic on Mondays, Wednesdays, and Fridays, Ling *et al.* (1978) found that 11 patients on LAAM terminated from the study because of allergic reactions, amphetaminelike effects, "spaced-out" feelings, irritability, sexual problems, severe constipation, leg and foot edema, and/or severe headache. Nevertheless, these investigators concluded that LAAM is as safe as methadone and, when given three times a week, is an acceptable and effective maintenance drug for many heroin addicts. In a comparison of methadone and LAAM by addicts who had been maintained on both drugs for at least three months each, Trueblood *et al.* (1978) found that the majority of the patients reported that LAAM provided a better blockade, that actual use of heroin was less on LAAM, and that LAAM was more effective than methadone in reducing craving. Most patients perceived no difference between LAAM and methadone in respect of adverse effects on sleep, appetite, and sexual performance. Trueblood *et al.* concluded that LAAM will be an acceptable maintenance drug.

From this brief review, it appears that except for a minority of heroin addicts who react adversely to LAAM, this drug may help solve two of the problems mentioned by Kaim (1976) that have arisen with methadone maintenance, namely, the logistical problems in providing a daily treatment and the dangerous diversion of methadone to the illicit market. However, there is no evidence that the persistent, adverse agonistic effects of LAAM, its perpetuation of physical dependence and presumably of the "metabolic defect" that underlies drug hunger, and the negative image of social control of addicts through pharmacological reinforcement will be any less for LAAM than for methadone.

REFERENCES

Altman, J. L., Meyer, R. E., Mirin, S. M., McNamee, H. B., and McDougle, M., 1976, Opiate antagonists and the modification of heroin self-administration behavior in man: An experimental study, *Int. J. Addictions 11:*485–500.

Appel, P. W., and Gordon, N. B., 1976, Digit-symbol performance in methadone-treated ex-heroin addicts, *Amer. J. Psychiat. 133:*1337–1340.

Ball, J. C., and Snarr, R. W., 1969, A test of the maturation hypothesis with respect to opiate addiction, *UN Bull. Narcotics 21:*9–13.

Beatty, D., 1978, Contingency contracting with heroin addicts, *Int. J. Addictions 13:*509–527.

Bourne, P. G., 1973, Methadone diversion, in *Proceedings of the Fifth National Conference on Methadone Treatment*, pp. 839–841. National Association for the Prevention of Addiction to Narcotics, New York.

Cushman, P., 1978, Methadone maintenance: Long-term follow-up of detoxified patients, in *Recent Developments in Chemotherapy of Narcotic Addiction, Annals of the New York Academy of Sciences*, Vol. 113 (B. Kissin, J. H. Lowinson, and R. B. Millman, Eds.), pp. 165–172. The New York Academy of Sciences, New York.

Davis, M. M., Brown, B. S., and Glendenning, S. T., 1973, Neonatal effects of heroin addiction and methadone-treated pregnancies. Preliminary report of 70 live births, in *Proceedings of the Fifth National Conference on Methadone Treatment*, pp. 1153–1162. National Association for the Prevention of Addiction to Narcotics, New York.

Dole, V. P., 1973, Detoxification of methadone patients and public policy, *J. Amer. Med. Ass. 226:*780–781.

Dole, V. P., and Joseph, H., 1978, Long-term outcome of patients treated with methadone maintenance, in *Recent Developments in Chemotherapy of Narcotic Addiction, Annals of the New York Academy of Sciences*, Vol. 311 (B. Kissin, J. H. Lowinson, and R. B. Millman, Eds), pp. 181–189. The New York Academy of Sciences, New York.

Dole, V. P., and Nyswander, M., 1965, A medical treatment for diacetylmorphine (heroin) addiction, *J. Amer. Med. Ass. 193:*646–650.

Dole, V. P., and Nyswander, M., 1968, Methadone maintenance and its implications for theories of narcotic addiction, in *The Addictive States: Research Publications of the Association for Nervous and Mental Disease*, Vol. 46 (A. Wikler, Ed.), pp. 359–366. Williams & Wilkins, Baltimore, Maryland.

Dole, V. P., Foldes, F. F., Trigg, H., Robinson, J. W., and Blatman, S., 1971, Methadone poisoning—Diagnosis and treatment, *New York State J. Med. 71:*541–543.

Dupont, R. L., and Greene, M. H., 1974, Beginning to dissect a heroin addiction epidemic, in *Addiction* (P. G. Bourne, Ed.), pp. 101–112. Academic Press, New York.

Duvall, H. J., Locke, B. Z., and Brill, L., 1963, Follow-up study of narcotic drug addicts five years after hospitalization, *Pub. Health Rep. 78:*185–196.

FDA regulations governing methadone, in *Federal Register*, Vol. 37, Section 130.44, *Conditions for the Use of Methadone*, Dec. 15, 1972.

Fink, M., 1973, Questions in cyclazocine therapy of opiate dependence, in *Opiate Addiction: Origins and Treatment* (S. Fisher and A. M. Freedman, Eds.), pp. 203–209. V. H. Winston and Sons, Washington, D.C.

Fraser, H. F., and Isbell, H., 1952, Actions and addiction liabilities of alpha-acetylmethadols in man, *J. Pharmacol. Exp. Ther.* 105:458–465.

Fraser, H. F., Van Horn, G. D., Martin, W. R., Wolbach, A. B., and Isbell, H., 1961, Methods for evaluating addiction liability. (A) "Attitude" of addicts toward opiate-like drugs, (B) A short-term "direct" addiction test, *J. Pharmacol. Exp. Ther.* 133:371–387.

Freedman, A. M., Fink, M., Sharoff, R., and Zaks, A., 1968, Clinical studies of cyclazocine in the treatment of narcotic addiction, *Amer. J. Psychiat.* 124:1499–1504.

Glasscote, R. M., Sussex, J. N., Jaffe, J. H., Ball, J., and Brill, L., 1972, *The Treatment of Drug Abuse: Programs, Problems, Prospects,* American Psychiatric Association, Washington, D.C.

Gorodetzky, C. W., 1977a, Detection of drugs of abuse in biological fluids, in *Drug Addiction. I. Morphine, Sedative/Hypnotic and Alcohol Dependence* (W. R. Martin, Ed.), pp. 319–409. Springer-Verlag, New York.

Gorodetzky, C. W., 1977b, Time course of morphine (M) detection in human urine after i.v. heroin (H) by latex agglutination inhibition (LAI), *The Pharmacologist* 19:142.

Greenstein, R., O'Brien, C. P., Mintz, J., Woody, G., and Hanna, H., 1976, Clinical experience with naltrexone in a behavioral research study: An interim report, in *Narcotic Antagonists: Naltrexone. Progress Report* (D. Julius and P. Renault, Eds.), pp. 141–149. NIDA Research Monogr. 9, DHEW Publ. No. (ADM) 76–387, National Technical Information Service, Springfield, Virginia 22161.

Grevert, P., Masover, B., and Goldstein, A., 1977, Failure of methadone and levomethadyl acetate (levo-alpha-aceylmethadol, LAAM) maintenance to affect memory, *Arch. Gen. Psychiat.* 34:849–853.

Hollister, L. E., Bearman, J. E., Duster, T. S., Freedman, D. X., Gallant, D. M., Harris, L. S., Jarvik, M. E., Jasinski, D. R., and Klett, C. J., 1978, Clinical evaluation of naltrexone treatment of opiate-dependent individuals. *Arch. Gen. Psychiat.* 35:335–340.

Hunt, G. H., and Odoroff, M. E., 1962, Follow-up study of narcotic drug addicts after hospitalization, *Pub. Health Rep.* 77:41–54.

Hurzeler, M., Gewirtz, D., and Kleber, H., 1976, Varying clinical contexts for administering naltrexone, in *Narcotic Antagonists: Naltrexone. Progress Report* (D. Julius and P. Renault, Eds.), pp. 48–66. NIDA Research Monogr. 9, DHEW Publ. No. (ADM) 76–387, National Technical Information Service, Springfield, Virginia 22161.

Isbell, H., Eisenman, A. J., Wikler, A., and Frank, K., 1948a, The effects of single doses of 6-dimethylamino-4,4-diphenyl-3-heptanone (amidone, methadon or "10820") on human subjects, *J. Pharmacol. Exp. Ther.* 92:83–89.

Isbell, H., Wikler, A., Eisenman, A., Daingerfield, M., and Frank, K., 1948b, Liability of addiction to 6-dimethylamino-4,4-diphenyl-3-heptanone (methadon, "amidone" or "10820") in man, *Arch. Intern. Med.* 82:362–396.

Jaffe, J. H., and Senay, E. C., 1971, Methadone and *l*-methadyl acetate: Use in management of narcotic addicts, *J. Amer. Med. Ass.* 216:1303–1305.

Jaffe, J. H., Senay, E. C., Schuster, C. R., Renault, P. R., Smith, B., and DiMenza, S., 1972, Methadyl acetate *vs.* methadone: A double-blind study in heroin users. *J. Amer. Med. Ass.* 222:437–442.

Kaim, S. C., 1976, Evolution of the National Academy of Sciences study of naltrexone, in *Narcotic Antagonists: Naltrexone. Progress Report* (D. Julius and P. Renault, Eds.), pp. 37–44. NIDA Research Monogr. 9, DHEW Publ. No. (ADM) 76–387, National Technical Information Service, Springfield, Virginia 22161.

Kissin, B., Ottomanelli, G., Sang, E., and Halloran, G., 1973, Cyclazocine treatment for heroin addicts, in *Proceedings of the Fifth National Conference on Methadone Treatment*, pp. 658–666. National Association for the Prevention of Addiction to Narcotics, New York.

Kjelgaard, J. M., Halm, G. W., and Heckenlively, J. R., 1971, Methadone-induced pulmonary edema, *J. Amer. Med. Ass.* 218:882–883.

Kleber, H. D., Kinsella, J. K., Riordan, C., Greaves, C., and Sweeney, D., 1974, The use of cyclazocine in treating narcotic addicts in a low-intervention setting, *Arch. Gen. Psychiat.* 30:37–42.

Kreek, M. J., 1973, Medical safety and side effects of methadone in tolerant individuals, *J. Amer. Med. Ass.* 223:665–668.

Kreek, M. J., 1978, Medical complications in methadone patients, in *Recent Developments in Chemotherapy of Narcotic Addiction, Annals of the New York Academy of Sciences*, Vol. 311 (B. Kissin, J. H. Lowinson, and R. B. Millman, Eds.), pp. 110–132. The New York Academy of Sciences, New York.

Lewis, D. C., Mayer, J., Hersch, R. G., and Black, R., 1978, Narcotic antagonist treatment: Clinical experience with naltrexone, *Int. J. Addictions* 13:961–973.

Ling, W., Klett, C. J., and Gillis, R. D., 1978, A cooperative clinical study of methadyl acetate. I. Three-times-a-week regimen, *Arch. Gen. Psychiat.* 35:345–353.

Martin, W. R., 1977, Chemotherapy of narcotic addiction, in *Drug Addiction. I. Morphine, Sedative/Hypnotic and Alcohol Dependence* (W. R. Martin, Ed.), pp. 279–318. Springer-Verlag, New York.

Martin, W. R., Gorodetzky, C. W., and McClane, T. K., 1966, An experimental study in the treatment of narcotic addicts with cyclazocine, *Clin. Pharmacol. Ther.* 7:455–465.

Martin, W. R., Jasinski, D. R., Haertzen, C. A., Kay, D. C., Jones, B. E., Mansky, P. A., and Carpenter, R. W., 1973a, Methadone—A re-evaluation, *Arch. Gen. Psychiat.* 28:286–295.

Martin, W. R., Jasinski, D. R., and Mansky, P. A., 1973b, Naltrexone, an antagonist for the treatment of heroin dependence: Effects in man, *Arch. Gen. Psychiat.* 28:782–791.

Mendelson, J. H., Mendelson, J. E., and Patch, V. D., 1975, Plasma testosterone levels in heroin addiction and during methadone maintenance, *J. Pharmacol. Exp. Ther.* 192:211–217.

Methadone Treatment Manual. Prescriptive Package, 1973, U.S. Department of Justice, Washington, D.C.

Meyer, R. E., Mirin, S. M. Altman, J. L., and McNamee, H. B., 1976a, A behavioral paradigm for the evaluation of narcotic antagonists, *Arch. Gen. Psychiat.* 33:371–377.

Meyer, R., Randall, M. Barington, C., Mirin, S., and Greenberg, I., 1976b, Limitations of an extinction approach to narcotic antagonist treatment, in *Narcotic Antagonists: Naltrexone. Progress Report* (D. Julius and P. Renault, Eds.), pp. 123–135. NIDA Research Monogr. 9, DHEW Publ. No. (ADM) 76–387, National Technical Information Service, Springfield, Virginia 22161.

Nutt, J. G., and Jasinski, D. R., 1974, Methadone–naloxone mixtures for use in methadone maintenance programs. I. An evaluation in man of their pharmacological feasibility. II. Demonstration of acute physical dependence, *Clin. Pharmacol. Ther.* 15:156–166.

O'Brien, C. O., and Greenstein, R., 1976, Naltrexone in a behavioral treatment program, in *Narcotic Antagonists: Naltrexone. Progress Report* (D. Julius and P. Renault, Eds.), pp. 136–140. NIDA Research Monogr. 9, DHEW Publ. No. (ADM) 76–387, National Technical Information Service, Springfield, Virginia 22161.

O'Brien, C. P., Personal communication (letter), Spetember 5, 1978.

Parwatikar, S., Crawford, J., Nekulpa, J. V., and DeGracia, C., 1976, Factors influencing success in an antagonistic treatment program, in *Narcotic Antagonists: Naltrexone. Progress Report* (D. Julius and P. Renault, Eds.), pp. 77–81. NIDA Research Monogr. 9, DHEW Publ. No. (ADM) 76–387, National Technical Information Service, Springfield, Virginia 22161.

Resnick, R. B., and Schuyten-Resnick, E., 1976, A point of view concerning treatment approaches with narcotic antagonists, in *Narcotic Antagonists: Naltrexone. Progress Report* (D. Julius and P. Renault, Eds.), pp. 84–87. NIDA Reseach Monogr. 9, DHEW Publ. No. (ADM) 76–387, National Technical Information Service, Springfield, Virginia 22161.

Resnick, R. B., and Washton, A. M., 1978, Clinical outcome with naltrexone, in *Recent Developments in Chemotherapy of Narcotic Addiction, Annals of the New York Academy of Sciences*, Vol. 311 (B. Kissin, J. H. Lowinson, and R. B. Millman, Eds.), pp. 241–246. The New York Academy of Sciences, New York.

Resnick, R. B., Fink, M., and Freedman, A. M., 1970, A cyclazocine typology in opiate dependence, *Amer. J. Psychiat.* 126:1256–1260.

Resnick, R. B., Fink, M., and Freedman, A. M., 1971, Cyclazocine treatment of opiate dependence: A progress report, *Compr. Psychiat.* 12:491–502.

Resnick, R. B., Aronoff, M., Lonborg, G., Kestenbaum, R., Kauders, F., Washton, A., and Hough, G., 1976, Clinical efficacy of naltrexone: A one year follow up, in *Narcotic Antagonists: Naltrexone. Progress Report* (D. Julius and P. Renault, Eds.), pp. 114–117. NIDA Research Monogr. No. (ADM) 76–387, National Technical Information Service, Springfield, Virginia 22161.

Senay, E. C., Dorus, W., Goldberg, F., and Thornton, W., 1977, Withdrawal from methadone maintenance, *Arch. Gen. Psychiat.* 34:361–367.

Stimmel, B., Goldberg, J., Cohen, M., and Rotkopf, E., 1978, Detoxification from methadone maintenance: Risk factors associated with relapse to narcotic use, in *Recent Developments of Chemotherapy of Narcotic Addiction, Annals of the New York Academy of Sciences*, Vol. 311 (B. Kissin, J. H. Lowinson, and R. B. Millman, Eds.), pp. 173–180. The New York Academy of Sciences, New York.

Thomas, M., Kauders, F., Harris, M., Cooperstein, J., Hough, G., and Resnick, R., 1976, Clinical experiences with naltrexone in 370 detoxified addicts, in *Narcotic Antagonists: Naltrexone. Progress Report* (D. Julius and P. Renault, Eds.), pp. 88–91. NIDA Research Monogr. 9, DHEW Publ. No. (ADM) 76–387, National Technical Information Service, Springfield, Virginia 22161.

Trueblood, B., Judso, B. A., and Goldstein, A., 1978, Acceptability of methadyl acetate (LAAM) as compared with methadone in a treatment program for heroin addicts, *Drug and Alcohol Dependence* 3:125–132.

Ulmer, R. A., 1977, Behavior therapy: A promising drug abuse treatment and research approach of choice, *Int. J. Addictions* 12:777–784.

Vaillant, G. E., 1966, A twelve year follow-up of New York narcotic addicts. I. The relation of treatment to outcome, *Amer. J. Psychiat.* 122:727–736.

Vaillant, G. E., 1973, A twenty year follow-up of New York narcotic addicts, *Arch. Gen. Psychiat.* 29:237–241.

Way, E. L., Mo, B. P. N., and Quock, C. P. (in collaboration with: Yap, P. M., Ou, G., Chan, S. C., and Cheng, J.), 1966, Evaluation of the nalorphine pupil diagnostic test for narcotic usage in long-term heroin and opium addicts, *Clin. Pharmacol. Ther.* 7:300–311.

Wikler, A., 1965, Conditioning factors in opiate addiction and relapse, in *Narcotics* (D. I. Willner and G. G. Kassebaum, Eds.), pp. 85–100. McGraw-Hill, New York.

Wikler, A., 1974, Requirements for extinction of relapse-facilitating variables and for rehabilitation in a narcotic-antagonist treatment program, in *Narcotic Antagonists: Advances in Biochemical Psychopharmacology*, Vol. 8 (M. C. Braude, L. S. Harris, E. L. May, J. P. Smith, and J. E. Villareal, Eds.), pp. 399–414. Raven Press, New York.

Wikler, A., 1976, The theoretical basis of narcotic addiction treatment with narcotic antagonists, in *Narcotic Antagonists: Naltrexone. Progress Report* (D. Julius and P. Renault, Eds.), pp. 119–122. NIDA Research Monogr. 9, DHEW Publ. No. (ADM) 76–387, National Technical Information Service, Springfield, Virginia 22161.

Wikler, A., Fraser, H. F., and Isbell, H., 1953, *N*-allylnormorphine: Effects of single doses and precipitation of acute "abstinence syndromes" during addiction to morphine, methadone or heroin in man (postaddicts), *J. Pharmacol. Exp. Ther.* 109:8–20.

Willette, R. E., 1976, The development of sustained action preparations of narcotic antagonists, in *Narcotic Antagonists: Naltrexone. Progress Report* (D. Julius and P. Renault, Eds.), pp. 31–44. NIDA Research Monogr. 9, DHEW Publ. No. (ADM) 76–387, National Technical Information Service, Springfield, Virginia 22161.

Wilmarth, S. S. and Goldstein, A., 1974, *Therapeutic Effectiveness of Methadone Maintenance Programs in the Management of Drug Dependence of Morphine-Type in the U.S.A.*, World Health Organization, Geneva.

Wilson, B. K., Spannagel, V., and Thomson, C. P., 1976, The use of *l*-alpha-acetylmethadol in treatment of heroin addiction: An open study, *Int. J. Addictions* 11:1091–1100.

Winick, C., 1962, Maturing out of narcotic addiction, *U.N. Bull. Narcotics* 14:1–7.

Zahn, M. A., and Ball, J. C., 1972, Factors related to cure of opiate addiction among Puerto Rican addicts, *Int. J. Addictions* 7:237–245.

Zaks, A., Fink, M., and Freedman, A. M., 1972, Levomethadyl in maintenance treatment of opiate dependence, *J. Amer. Med. Ass.* 220:811–813.

Index

Analgesics, opioid, 37–51
  agents, 37–51, 95–132, 141–162
    codeine, 37–38, 50
    diacetylmorphine (heroin), 37, 48
    etorphine (Immobilon), 38
    fentanyl (Sublimaze), 132
    hydromorphone (Dilaudid), 37–38
    levorphanol (Levo-Dromoran), 37
    meperidine (Demerol), 37, 49–50
    methadone (Dolophine), 37–38,
      48–49
    morphine. see Morphine actions;
      Tolerance and physical depen-
      dence, opioid
    oxycodone (Percodan), 37–38
    oxymorphone (Numorphan), 37–38
    pentazocine (Talwin), 38, 51
    phenazocine (Prinadol), 37–38
    d-propoxyphene (Darvon), 37–38,
      50–51
  receptor interactions, 70–75
    agonists (at μ and/or κ and/or σ
      and/or δ receptors), 70–75
    benzomorphans, 72–73
    β-endorphin, 73
    cyclazocine, 70–72, 75
    ^{3}H-dihydromorphine, 74–75
    etorphine, 73
    ketocyclazocine, 71
    leucine-enkephalin, 73–74
    methionine-enkephalin, 73–74
    morphine, 71–73

Analgesics, opioid (cont.)
  receptor interactions (cont.)
    agonists (cont.)
      N-allylnormetazocine (N-allyl-
        norphenazocine, SKF 10,047), 71
      normorphine, 73–74
      pentazocine, 72
    partial agonists (at μ and/or κ and/or
      σ receptors), 70–72
      buprenorphine, 72
      diprenorphine, 72
      nalorphine, 70, 72
      oxilorphan, 72
      propiram, 72
Antagonists, opioid, 51–61
  agents, 53–61
    cyclazocine, 57–59
      attenuation of physical depen-
        dence on morphine, 59
      effects of single and repeated
        doses, 57–59
      opioid-antagonistic actions, 58–59
      tolerance and physical depen-
        dence, 58
    nalorphine (N-allylnormorphine),
      53–57
      attenuation of physical depen-
        dence on opioids, 56–57
      effects of single doses in the drug-
        free state, 53–54
      opioid-antagonistic actions in the
        non-tolerant state, 55

Antagonists, opioid (*cont.*)
  agents (*cont.*)
    nalorphine (*cont.*)
      opioid-antagonistic actions in the
        tolerant state, 55–56
      tolerance and physical depen-
        dence, 54–55
    naloxone (Narcan), 59–60
      opioid-antagonistic actions, 59–60
    naltrexone, 60–61
      attenuation of physical depen-
        dence on morphine, 61
      opioid-antagonistic actions, 60–61
      physical dependence, absence of,
        61
    competitive antagonism at μ receptor,
      71–72
      buprenorphine, 72
      cyclazocine, 71–72
      diprenorphine, 72
      nalorphine, 72
      naloxone, 72
      naltrexone, 72
      oxilorphan, 72
      pentazocine, 72
      propiram, 72
    history of, 51–53

Brain stem, 114–131
  and morphine analgesia, 114–123
    anterior thalamic nuclei, 123
    decerebrate preparations, 120–121
    floor of fourth ventricle, 115–116
    mesencephalic reticular formation,
      123
    monoamine systems, 116–120
    nucleus gigantocellularis, 114, 119–
      120
    nucleus paragigantocellularis, 114,
      119–120
    nucleus raphé magnus, 114, 116,
      117–119
    periaqueductal gray matter (PAG),
      114, 121–123
    periventricular gray matter (PVG),
      115, 121–123
  and effects of electrical stimulation,
    123–131
    flight-fear reactions, 123–124

Brain stem (*cont.*)
  and effects of electrical stimulation (*cont.*)
    stimulation-produced analgesia
      (SPA), 124–131
      contrasts between SPA and
        morphine, 130–131
      cross-tolerance to morphine
        analgesia, 127
      due to activation of nucleus
        paragigantocellularis, 119–120
      due to activation of nucleus raphé
        dorsalis, 129
      due to activation of nucleus raphé
        magnus, 129
      due to activation of periaqueductal
        gray matter (PAG), 121–123, 127,
        129–131
      due to activation of periventricular
        gray matter (PVG), 127
      due to activation of PVG-PAG re-
        gion, 127
      monoamines in SPA and morphine
        analgesia, similarities, 127–128
      similarities between SPA and
        morphine analgesia, 127–128

Cerebral cortex, 131–132
  orbitofrontal, 131
    opioid receptor binding in frontal
      pole, 131
    pain relief by prefrontal lobotomy,
      131
    pain relief by rostral cingulum-
      otomy, 131
  sensorimotor, 131–132
    effects of morphine on, 132
Conditioning processes, 28–30, 159–162,
  167–215
  clasical conditioning, 29–30, 160–162,
    168, 178–213
    of atropine salivation and mydriasis,
      179
    of insulin hyperglycemia, 179
    of insulin hypoglycemia, 179
    of morphine salivation, 178–179
    of morphine sleep, 178–179
    of saccharine hypoglycemia, 179
    of the opioid agonist-abstinence cy-
      cle, 178–198

Conditioning processes (*cont.*)
  classical conditioning (*cont.*)
    of the opioid antagonist-precipitated
      abstinence syndrome, 207–211
    in monkeys, with nalorphine,
      208–210
    in man, with nalorphine, 207–208
    in man (methadone maintenance
      patients), with naloxone, 210–
      211
  conditioned abstinence, 30, 171, 180–
    182, 186–198, 207–215
    a disease, *sui generis*, 30, 213. *See also*
      Preface
    cognitive relabeling, 208, 214, 229
    extinction of, 211–214, 227–229
    implications for relapse and treat-
      ment, 213–215
    in postaddicts, 171, 180–182
    in street-addicts, under naltrexone
      blockade, 211–213
  conditioned reinforcers and relapse, 29,
    171–178, 180–182, 200–207
    in dogs, 172
    in man, 29, 171–172, 180–182
    in monkeys, 175–176
    in rats, 174–178, 200–207
  conditioning theory of relapse, 180–181
  interoceptive conditioning, 177, 200–
    207
    extinction of, 177, 214–215
  operant conditioning, 28–29, 168–169,
    172–178
    in chimpanzees, 172–173
    in dogs, 172
    in man, 28–29, 168–169, 172
    in monkeys, 172, 175–176
    in rats, 172–178
    relation to classical conditioning, 178

Diagnosis. *See* Opioid dependence, diagnosis

Endorphins. *See* Enkephalins and endorphins
Enkephalins and endorphins, 76–90
  agents, 73–89
    adrenocorticotrophin (ACTH, pre-
      cursor of β-lipotropin and

Enkephalins and endorphins (*cont.*)
  agents (*cont.*)
      β-endorphin), 77–79, 84–85,
        88–89
    α-endorphin, 78–79, 86
    β-endorphin, 73–74, 78–79, 84–89
    γ-endorphin, 78, 86–87
    δ-endorphin, 73–74
    enkephalins, 73–74, 77, 85–86
    leucine-enkephalin, 73–74, 77
    β-lipotropin (precursor of
      β-endorphin), 75
    methionine-enkephalin, 73–74, 77, 86
    morphine-like factors, 76–77
  in analgesia, 79–84
    acupuncture, 81–83
    animals, 79–83
      cats, 82
      mice, 81–83
      rats, 79–80, 83
    man, 82–84
      absence of role in ischemic pain, 83
      absence of role in hypnotic
        analgesia, 83–84
  in mental disorders, 86–90
    catatonia in rats, 86–88
      produced by β-endorphin, revers-
        ible by naloxone, 86–87
      produced by β-endorphin, com-
        pared with haloperidol, 87–88
    effects of DTγE on schizophrenic pa-
      tients, 89–90
    effects of β-endorphin on depressed
      and schizophrenic patients, 89
    effects of hemodialysis on schizo-
      phrenic patients, 90
    effects of naloxone on schizophrenic
      hallucinations, 88–89
    effects of naloxone in depressions, 89
    β_H-Leu^5-endorphin in dialysates of
      schizophrenic patients, 90
  in physical dependence, 84–86
    dual action of morphine on ACTH
      and β-endorphin receptors,
      84–85
    increase in intraneural cyclic AMP by
      chronic morphine, 86
    inhibition of enkephalin release by
      chronic morphine, 85

Enkephalins and endorphins (*cont.*)
   in physical dependence (*cont.*)
      naloxone-precipitated abstinence
         after β-endorphin intracereb-
         rally, 84
Etiology of opioid dependence, 25–34
   definitions and dynamics, 25–30
      a disease, *sui generis*, 30, 213. *See also*
         Preface
      conditioning processes in, 28–30,
         159–162, 167–215
         classical conditioning, 29–30, 160–
         162, 168, 178–213
         operant conditioning, 28–29, 168–
         169, 172–178
      reinforcement, 26, 171–172
         and arousal, 26
         direct and indirect sources of, 26
         history of schedules of, 28–29
      dependence, psychic and physical,
         25–26
      euphoria, dysphoria, 27–28, 104–106
      tolerance, 26, 45–48, 141–162
      WHO (World Health Organization)
         definitions, 25
   mode of spread, 23–33
   personality studies, 30–31
      increased needs, 31
      psychopathy, 30–31
   prognosis, 33–34
      maturation hypothesis, 33
      Vietnam War veterans, 33–34
Etonitazene, effects on normal and
   morphine-dependent rats, 184–
   187
Euphoria and dysphoria, 27–28, 104–106
   after barbiturates, 105–106
   after morphine, 27–28, 104–105

Hypothalamus and pituitary gland, 40–42

Locus ceruleus, 86, 116
   tolerance to inhibitory effects of opioids
      on, 86
      no cross-tolerance to inhibitory effect
         of clonidine on, 86

Morphine actions, 38–45, 95–132
   analgesic, 95–132

Morphine actions (*cont.*)
   analgesic, conditioned emotional re-
      sponse, 100–102
   analgesic, pain and alarm thresholds,
      96–97
   analgesic, pain-anticipatory anxiety,
      97–100, 102–103
   analgesic, sites of. *See* Brain stem;
      Cerebral cortex; Spinal cord
   other, 38–45, 102–104
      electroencephalographic, 39, 43–44
      emetic, 44
      endocrine, 40–42
      performance under varying incen-
         tives, 103–104
      pupillary, 42–43
      respiratory and vasomotor, 43–44
      spinal reflexes, 44–45, 107–114
      temperature regulation, 41–42
Morphine tolerance and physical dependence. *See* Tolerance and physical dependence, opioids

Non-opioid drug dependence syndromes, 5*l*20
   alcohol, 9–11
   amphetamines, 11–12
   cannabis (marihuana, hashish, Δ⁹-
      THC), 16–18
   cocaine, 12–14
   hallucinogens, 14–16
   sedatives, 5–9
   tobacco, 18–20

Opioid dependence, 1–4, 25–61; 76–80,
   141–162, 167–215, 219–244
   complications, 4
      crime, 4
      deaths, 4
      marital instability, 4
      medical problems, 4
      psychiatric problems, 4
      unemployment, 4
   diagnosis, 219–222
      of opioid use, by clinical criteria,
         221
      of opioid use, by urinary drug-
         detection methods, 221–222

Opioid dependence (*cont.*)
  diagnosis (*cont.*)
    of physical dependence, by abrupt
      opioid withdrawal, 219
    of physical dependence, by use of
      narcotic antagonists, 219–221
  etiology. *See* Etiology of opioid depen-
    dence
  prevalence, 1–4
  relation to use of marihuana and other
    drugs, 2–3
  treatment. *See* Treatment of opioid de-
    pendence

Pain
  effects of barbiturates on, 105
  effects of morphine on. *See* Morphine,
    actions, analgesic
  nature of, 95–107
  neurophysiological models of, 106–107
Physical dependence. *See* Tolerance and
    physical dependence, opioids
Pituitary gland and hypothalamus, 40–42

Receptors, 69–76
  molecular pharmacology, 69–70
    definitions and measurements, 69–70
      affinity, 70
      agonists, 69
      antagonists, 70
      competitive dualism, 70
      intrinsic activity, 70
      partial agonists, 70
      receptor dualism, 70
  opioid, drugs acting on, 59–61, 70–75
    benzomorphans, 72–73
    β-endorphin, 73
    buprenorphine, 72
    cyclazocine, 70–72, 75
    ³H-dihydromorphine, 74–75
    diprenorphine, 72, 75
    etorphine, 73
    ketocyclazocine, 71
    leucine-enkephalin, 73–74
    ³H-leucine-enkephalin binding,
      73–74
    methionine-enkephalin, 73–74
    morphine, 71–73

Receptors (*cont.*)
  opioid, drugs acting on (*cont.*)
    N-allylnormetazocine (N-allyl-
      norphenazocine, SKF 10,047), 71
    nalorphine, 70, 72
    naloxone, 59–60
    ³H-naloxone binding, 74–75
    naltrexone, 60–61
    normorphine, 73–74
    oxilorphan, 72
    propiram, 72
    stereospecific binding to, 74–76
    distribution in nervous system and
      intestine, 74–75
    effect of sodium ion on, 75
  types of, 70–74
    in chronic spinal dog, 71–72
    in guinea pig ileum and mouse vas
      deferens, 72–74
    δ-receptors, 73–74
    κ-receptors, 73
    μ-receptors, 73–74
Reinforcement, 19, 26, 171–172
  and arousal, 19, 26
  appetitive, aversive, 171–172
  positive, negative, 171–172
  sources of, direct and indirect, 26
Relapse, 33–34, 168–210
  conditioning theory of, 180–182
  in postaddicts, 33–34, 226–227
  in rats (etonitazene drinking), 188–207
  role of conditioned reinforcers, 29,
    171–178, 180–182, 200–207
  in dogs, 172
  in man, 29, 171–172, 180–182
  in monkeys, 175–176
  in rats, 174–178, 200–207

Self regulated readdiction to morphine in
    man, 168–171
Spinal cord, 107–132
  analgesic test responses, 107–108, 114
  effects of decortication, spinal tran-
    section and morphine on, 107–
    108
  effects of lumbar intrathecal opioids
    on, 114, 121
  skin-twitch, 107
  tail-flick, 107

Spinal cord (*cont.*)
    reflexes, effects of opioids on, 107–114
        in spinal cats, 108–113
        in spinal cats, inhibitory processes,
            110–111
            role of acetylcholine, 111
        in spinal cats, monosynaptic arcs,
            109–110
        in spinal cats, polysynaptic arcs,
            108–109
            post-δ and C fiber arcs, 111
        in spinal cats, supraspinal inhibitory
            and facilitatory mechanisms,
            107–109, 113
        in spinal cats, unit responding in
            dorsal gray laminae, 111–113
        in spinal dogs, 107–108
        in spinal man, 108
        in spinal man (paraplegic patients),
            108
    transmission of pain, 113

Tolerance and physical dependence,
        opioids, 45–51, 141–162, 183–
        184. *See also* Non-opioid drug
        dependence syndromes; Opioid
        dependence, diagnosis, treat-
        ment
    phenomena, 28–30, 45–48, 141–142,
        159–162, 167–215, 219–220
    abstinence syndromes, early and
        protracted, 46–48
    abstinence syndromes, effects of pre-
        frontal lobotomy on, 48
    abstinence syndromes, precipitated
        by narcotic antagonists, 47,
        219–220
    conditioning processes. *See* Condi-
        tioning processes
    in chronic decorticated dogs, 168
    in chronic spinal dogs, 141–142, 167
    in chronic spinal man, 142
    in man, 45–48, 141
    in rats, 183–184
    residual tolerance, 45
    reversal of abstinence hypothermia
        by conditioned stimuli, 184
    blockade by naloxone, 184
    theories of, 141–162
    cellular counteradaptation, 143

Tolerance and physical dependence (*cont.*)
    theories of (*cont.*)
        disuse supersensitivity, 145–147
        disuse supersensitivity, to
            catecholamines, 146
        disuse supersensitivity, to pen-
            tylenetetrazol, 146
        disuse supersensitivity, to pilocar-
            pine, 146–147
        dual action, 143–145
            stimulant actions of opioids, 143–
            145
        enzyme expansion, 157–158
            protein synthesis in, 157–158
            protein synthesis, inhibition by ac-
                tinomycin, 158
            protein synthesis, inhibition by
                8-azaguanine, 158
            protein synthesis, inhibition by
                cycloheximide, 158
        homeostatic counteradaptation, 142
        immune mechanisms, 158–159
            morphine dose-intervals and tol-
                erance, 158
        learning factors, 159–162
            associative (Pavlovian), 160–162
            nonassociative, 159
        new receptors, 150–157
            silent and pharmacological recep-
                tors, 151
            tolerance without physical depen-
                dence, 151–152
            increase in number of silent re-
                ceptors, 152
            decrease in number of phar-
                macological receptors, 152
            tolerance with physical depen-
                dence, 152–157
            increase in number of phar-
                macological receptors, 152–153,
                156–157
            decrease in number of phar-
                macological receptors, 153–156
        pharmacological redundancy, 147–
            150
            evidence for, in chronic spinal
                dogs, 149
            evidence for, in man, 148
            evidence for, in rats, 149–150
            neural model of, 147–148

Tolerance and physical dependence (*cont.*)
  theories of (*cont.*)
    pharmacological redundancy (*cont.*)
      effects of chronic morphine and
        morphine-withdrawal, 147–148
      persistence of morphine effect on
        respiratory center during tol-
        erance, 148
  transmitters involved in, 152–157
    acetylcholine, 152–153
    catecholamines, 153–155
      synthesis of ^{14}C-catecholamines,
        154
      turnover of ^{3}H-dopamine, 155
      turnover of ^{3}H-dopamine, con-
        ditionability of, 155
    serotonin, 155–157
      turnover of, 156
      blockade by morphine, 155–156
Treatment of opioid dependence, 222–244
  detoxification, 224–227
    methadone substitution and with-
      drawal, 225
    rapid withdrawal, 225–226
    relapse after, 226–227
    therapeutic communities, 227
  levomethadyl (LAAM) maintenance,
    241–244
    comparisons with methadone main-
      tenance, 241–243
    human pharmacology of, 241–243

Treatment of opioid dependence (*cont.*)
  methadone maintenance, 234–241
    criticisms of, 237–238
    FDA regulations governing, 238–239
    induction of, 238
    maintenance dosage in, 239
    medical complications of, 236–237
    rationale, 234–235
    results of, 239–241
      eventual methadone detoxifica-
        tion, 240–241
      tolerance to methadone, 235–236
  narcotic antagonist maintenance after
    detoxification, 227–234
    depot preparations, 234
    rationale, 227–228
      cognitive labeling, 208, 214, 229
      extinction of conditioned absti-
        nence, 211–214, 227–229
    with cyclazocine, 227, 230–231
    with naltrexone, 228–230, 231–234
      drop-out rate in, 231–234
      results of, 231–234
  of opioid poisoning, 222–224
    differential diagnosis, 222–224
    general supportive measures, 222–
      223
    with naloxone, 223–224
      signs of opioid-antagonism, 223
      signs of precipitated opioid-
        abstinence, 223